Preventive Cardiology

A Guide for Clinical Practice

Edited by

Killian Robinson, MD

The Cleveland Clinic Foundation
Departments of Cardiology and Internal Medicine
Cleveland, Ohio

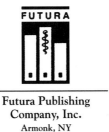

Futura Publishing
Company, Inc.
Armonk, NY

Library of Congress Cataloging-in-Publication Data

Preventive cardiology: a guide for clinical practice/edited
  by Killian C. Robinson.
      p. cm.
    Includes bibliographical references and index.
    ISBN 0-87993-692-4
    1. Cardiovascular system—Diseases—Prevention. I. Robinson,
Killian C.
    [DNLM; 1. Heart Diseases—prevention & control. 2. Vascular Dis-
eases—prevention & control. WG 210 P944 1998]
    RC669.P665 1998
    616.1'05—dc21
    DNLM/DLC
    for Library of Congress   98-6277
                                                                  CIP

Published by
Futura Publishing Company, Inc.
135 Bedford Road
Armonk, New York 10504

LC #: 98-6277
ISBN #: 0-87993-692-4

Every effort has been made to ensure that the information in this book is
as up to date and accurate as possible at the time of publication. However,
due to the constant developments in medicine, neither the author, nor the
editor, nor the publisher can accept any legal or any other responsibility
for any errors or omissions that may occur.

Printed in the United States of America on acid-free paper.

To Jackie Yew Ming, Síofra, Ríoghnach,

Liam, and Kate.

And Séamus.

Introduction

Although this book is directed toward all those interested in preventive medicine, it is particularly oriented toward those who wish to further their knowledge and understanding of how these principles are applied in general cardiac practice. For many reasons, there has been a rapid growth in interest in this field in general, and in preventive cardiology in particular, over the last several years. Apart from the obvious necessity to avoid the massive social and financial costs associated with cardiovascular diseases, recent intervention studies have shown that the progress of these disorders may be arrested and potentially reversed. Furthermore, other important investigations have shown that primary prevention of cardiovascular disease is feasible with the use of simple interventions. This book presents some of the more recent advances in the management of risk factors from a clinical perspective.

The background for hypertension is presented first, which summarizes the prevalence of this condition as well as its potential hazards in the general population and in the elderly. The importance of left ventricular hypertrophy and heart rate are also discussed. This is followed by a comprehensive discussion of the pharmacological management of arterial hypertension including recommendations for primary prevention of elevated blood pressure and clinical evaluation of the hypertensive patient. Management of hypertension in the elderly and individualization of therapy are discussed as well as the advantages and disadvantages of the different pharmacological preparations.

Physiological and metabolic effects of physical activity are discussed as well as the relationship between physical activity, interrelationships with other risk factors, and coronary artery disease. The role of diabetes and insulin resistance in development of coronary disease is discussed as well as the effect of diabetes on outcomes following cardiac interventions. Congestive heart failure and conduction disorders and the management of other risk factors in diabetics are discussed.

Diet and dietary interventions for secondary prevention, including the use of antioxidants, are outlined. The management of hyperlipidemia focuses on a number of special issues including isolated low high-density lipoprotein cholesterol, severe hypertriglyceridemia, and dyslipidemia in patients who have undergone cardiac and renal transplantation. Clinical utility of apolipoprotein and lipoprotein (a) measurement are placed in context and the role of combination drug therapy is highlighted. This is followed by a discussion of homocysteine, which is receiving greater attention as a risk factor. The biochemistry and metabolism of homocysteine are then reviewed. This review includes the role of the essential vitamins folic acid and vitamins B_6 and B_{12} and the molecular biology of relevent enzymes. The causes of high circulating levels of homocysteine, interelationships with, and possible mechanisms of, vascular disease and the treatment of high homocysteine are then covered in detail.

This section is followed by a detailed discussion of preventive cardiology in specialized population groups, including children and adolescents, women, and minorities. The pathology of atherosclerosis in high-risk children and adolescents is outlined and is followed by an individualized approach to lipid and risk factor management. Dietary and pharmacological interventions are discussed and evaluation and follow-up of these patients is also covered.

Women are discussed in detail in a separate chapter that deals with the role of estrogen in cardiovascular disease. Hypercholesterolemia, lipoprotein (a), diabetes mellitus, obesity, and hypertension are discussed in relation to gender, as are smoking and lifestyle. Nonclassical risk factors such as psychosocial issues and menopause are also discussed. Primary and secondary preventive measures in women are also reviewed, including lipid-lowering drugs, antioxidant therapy, hormone replacement therapy, and smoking cessation. Cultural, socioeconomic, and genetic aspects of preventive cardiology in minorities follow, emphasising coronary heart disease in African-Americans and other ethnic minorities. Risk factor interventions in these groups and aspects of access to medical care are also discussed.

Gene therapy of vascular disease is reviewed with emphasis on familial hypercholesterolemia as a model for this form of treatment. New targets are discussed, including high-density lipoprotein cholesterol, antithrombotic strategies, and valvular prosthetic devices. Current approaches for this form of treatment are reviewed.

The subject of smoking cessation is covered in detail with the emphasis on methods and management of smoking cessation. There are overviews of both behavioral and pharmacological techniques as well as alternatives such as hypnosis and multimodal treatment. The role of the physician in the process of smoking cessation is highlighted.

Antiplatelet and anticoagulant therapy in the prevention of ischemic heart disease are covered in detail and this includes a review of antiplatelet drugs. The uses of aspirin in primary and secondary prevention of coronary artery disease and in other cardiovascular disorders are followed by a discussion of dipyridamole, ticlopidine, and sulfinpyrazone, as well as inhibitors of thromboxane formation and/or binding and platelet glycoprotein II_b/III_a inhibitors. Heparin and the role of warfarin in primary and secondary prevention and combination antiplatelet and anticoagulant therapy are then covered.

Finally, establishment of a clinical prevention program is discussed. This includes guidelines for organizational design and operation of a preventive cardiology clinic, core concepts, an outline of algorithm-driven clinical practice, and cost effectiveness as well as programmatic issues such as patient flow and resource requirements.

The intention has been to give a clinically orientated summary of the importance and management of the major risk factors likely to be encountered by primary care physicians, internists, cardiologists, nurse practitioners, and others who are involved in the care of patients with vascular diseases. Hopefully, the approaches and interventions outlined in this volume will make the treatment of patients with coronary artery disease more successful.

Killian Robinson, MD

Contributors

Mary E. Bower, PhD   Co-Director, Department of Psychiatry and Psychology, Cleveland Clinic Smoking Cessation Program, Section of Psychology, Cleveland Clinic Foundation, Cleveland, Ohio

Garland Y. DeNelsky, PhD   Director, Department of Psychiatry and Psychology, Cleveland Clinic Smoking Cessation Program, Head, Section of Psychology, Cleveland Clinic Foundation, Cleveland, Ohio

Patricia J. Elmer, PhD   Division of Epidemiology, University of Minnesota, Minneapolis, Minnesota

Laurent J. Feldman, MD   Departments of Medicine (Cardiology) and Biomedical Research, St. Elizabeth's Medical Center, Tufts University School of Medicine, Boston, Massachusetts

JoAnne Micale Foody, MD   Department of Cardiology, Section of Cardiovascular Prevention and Rehabilitation, The Cleveland Clinic Foundation, Cleveland, Ohio

Antonio M. Gotto, Jr, MD, PhD   Distinguished Service Professor and Chairman, Department of Medicine, Baylor College of Medicine, Chief, Internal Medicine Service, The Methodist Hospital, Houston, Texas

Anjan Gupta, MD   Departments of Cardiology and Internal Medicine, The Cleveland Clinic Foundation, Cleveland, Ohio

Robert Hunter, MA   Department of Cardiology, The Cleveland Clinic Foundation, Cleveland, Ohio

Jeffrey M. Isner, MD   Departments of Medicine (Cardiology) and Biomedical Research, St. Elizabeth's Medical Center, Tufts University School of Medicine, Boston, Massachusetts

Donald W. Jacobsen, PhD   Department of Cell Biology, Lerner Research Institute, Cleveland Clinic Foundation, CCF Professor of Chemistry, Department of Chemistry, Cleveland State University, Cleveland, Ohio

Peter H. Jones, MD Associate Professor, Department of Medicine, Section of Atherosclerosis and Lipid Research, Baylor College of Medicine, Director, Lipid Metabolism and Atherosclerosis Clinic, The Methodist Hospital, Houston, Texas

William B. Kannel, MD, MPH, FACC Department of Medicine, Section of Preventive Medicine and Epidemiology, Evans Memorial Research Foundation, Boston University School of Medicine/Framingham Heart Study, Boston, Massachusetts

Peter O. Kwiterovich, Jr, MD Professor, Departments of Pediatrics and Medicine, Chief, Lipid-Research Atherosclerosis Division, Director, Lipid Clinic, Johns Hopkins University School of Medicine, Baltimore, Maryland 21287–3654

David J. Moliterno, MD Department of Cardiology, The Cleveland Clinic Foundation, Cleveland, Ohio

Fredric J. Pashkow, MD Director, Cardiac Health Improvement and Rehabilitation Program, The Cleveland Clinic Foundation, Cleveland, Ohio

Thomas A. Pearson, MD, PhD Mary Imogene Bassett Research Institute, Columbia University College of Physicians and Surgeons, New York, New York

Killian Robinson, MD Departments of Cardiology and Internal Medicine, The Cleveland Clinic Foundation, Cleveland, Ohio

Dennis L. Sprecher, MD Section Head, Department of Preventive Cardiology, The Cleveland Clinic Foundation, Cleveland, Ohio

Steven R. Steinhubl, MD Department of Cardiology, The Cleveland Clinic Foundation, Cleveland, Ohio

Corinne Varin-LeBreton, MD Service de Cardiologie, Centre Hospitalier Universitaire, Rennes, France

Donald G. Vidt, MD Senior Physician, Cleveland Clinic Foundation, Department of Nephrology and Hypertension, Cleveland, Professor of Internal Medicine Ohio State University, Columbus, Ohio

Peter W. F. Wilson, MD Clinical Associate Professor, Department of Medicine, Boston University Medical School and Tufts University Medical School, Framingham, Massachusetts

Contents

Chapter 1

Hypertension
Epidemiological Appraisal

William B. Kannel, MD, MPH, FACC

Introduction

The high prevalence and potent contribution of hypertension to the occurrence of cardiovascular disease (CVD) assign it a high priority for intervention to prevent cardiovascular events. Most hypertension is classified as "benign essential hypertension" despite its importance as a cardiovascular risk factor. Ignorance about its cause makes it difficult to prevent, although a wide range of factors has been shown to influence blood pressure (BP). Nevertheless, we were successful in reducing cardiovascular morbidity and mortality by detecting and controlling hypertension with antihypertensive therapy. Treatment is likely to be even more effective when it is tailored to the patient's risk profile using the array of pharmaceuticals available with different modes of action and side-effect profiles.

Prevalence and Incidence

Hypertension is a highly prevalent condition worldwide. As commonly defined it is the most prevalent vascular disease. The prevalence

Dr. Kannel was supported by National Institutes of Health grants N01-HV-92922 and N01-HV-52971 and the Visiting Scientist Program.

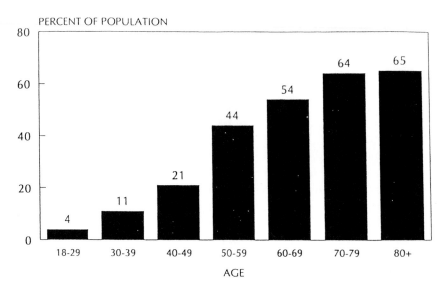

Figure 1. *Percent prevalence of hypertension by age, United States, 1988–1991. SBP 140+ mm Hg or 90+ DBP or on medication.*

of hypertension increases sharply with age (Figure 1). By middle age (50–59 years) 44% have BPs of 140/90 mm Hg or greater and two-thirds of persons over age 70 have such hypertension. The prevalence is substantially higher in blacks than in whites.[1] For hypertension as currently defined (140/90 mm Hg or greater BP or being on hypertensive medication), 65% of hypertensive persons in the United States were aware of it in 1988–1991; 48% were on treatment and 21% were controlled on treatment. These percentages were substantially lower in 1976–1980 (Figure 2).[2]

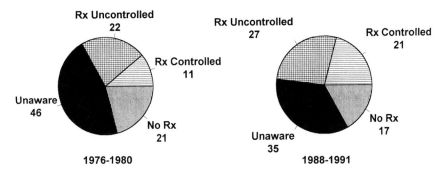

Figure 2. *Percent hypertension awareness, treatment, and control, United States, 1976–1980 and 1988–1991. SBP 140+ mm Hg or 90+ DBP or on medication. Rx = on medication.*

In most populations BP rises with age. In the Framingham Study cohort there was an average 20 mm Hg systolic BP (SBP) and 10 mm Hg diastolic BP (DBP) rise as subjects aged from 30 to 60 years. SBPs in women continue to rise until age 80 and in men until age 70 and thereafter decline. DBPs peak earlier and then decline after age 55–60. This disproportionate rise in SBP in advanced age results in a high prevalence of isolated SBP, making it the most common variety of hypertension in the elderly. Some 65% of hypertension in the elderly is isolated systolic hypertension. Whereas isolated systolic hypertension increases with age, isolated diastolic hypertension decreases in prevalence as people get older.

The incidence of new onset of hypertension also increases with age. Over three decades of follow-up of the Framingham Study cohort, two-thirds developed elevated BPs. These tended to occur in those with high normal BPs, those who were obese, and those with impaired glucose tolerance.[3,4] The high incidence and prevalence of hypertension poses an urgent need for primary prevention targeted at persons who have BPs in the upper end of the normal BP distribution from which the bulk of future hypertension arises.[3,4]

Cardiovascular Hazards

Hypertension is one of the most powerful contributors to the leading causes of death. Every 10-mm Hg increment in SBP increases age-

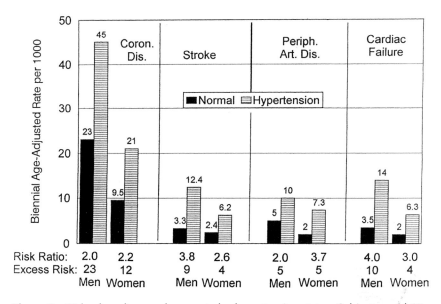

Figure 3. *Risk of cardiovascular events by hypertensive status. Subjects aged 35–64; Framingham Study; 36-year follow-up.*

adjusted the risk of cardiovascular events, 20% at age 35–64 and 13% at age 65–94. The corresponding increments in risk for DBP are 13% and 19%.

Hypertension is a major promoter of CVD, inflicting a two- to four-fold increase in risk of cardiovascular events compared to normotensive persons of the same age (Figure 3). It is a powerful risk factor for all of the major CVDs in middle-aged and elderly persons of both sexes. Atherosclerotic CVD and coronary heart disease (CHD) in particular are now the most common sequelae of hypertension. Its relative impact is greatest for stroke and cardiac failure, but coronary disease is by far the most common and most lethal of all the cardiovascular sequelae of hypertension. The risk of developing coronary disease in hypertensive persons is equal to the sum of the risks for all the other major cardiovascular sequelae (Figure 3). Women appear less vulnerable in terms of absolute risk, but risk ratios are just as large as those for men. Although the risk ratio for hypertension diminishes somewhat with advancing age, the absolute risk of cardiovascular events in the elderly is about double that of persons under age 65.

Components of Blood Pressure

There has long been a conviction that the cardiovascular sequelae of hypertension derive chiefly from the diastolic component of the BP.[5,6] It is difficult to find evidence to support this contention, which was expressed in Cecil's first edition of the *Textbook of Medicine* and maintained again in the sixth edition in 1943, despite actuarial data linking mortality to SBP.[5,6] Prospective epidemiological studies consistently showed that the SBP is a better predictor of cardiovascular events than DBP.[6,7]

Rutan et al,[6] in a review of the evidence from epidemiological studies and trials, concluded that there is no support for the clinical concept that elevated DBP rather than SBP is the chief risk factor for CVD.

Nevertheless, DBP is tenaciously considered the hallmark of essential hypertension, and entry criteria for trials, goals of therapy, and success of intervention were generally based on DBP. This is unjustified judging from 36 years of follow-up in the Framingham Study during which occurrence of cardiovascular events was evaluated in relation to SBP and DBP. For every cardiovascular sequela of hypertension, risk was more closely related to SBP than to DBP. Comparing the predictive power of SBP, DBP, mean arterial pressure, and pulse pressure on an equal footing for the different range of values, SBP emerges as the best predictor of cardiovascular morbidity and mortality (Table 1). An examination of the impact of a standard deviation increase in each component of BP or incidence of CVD indicates a consistently greater impact of SBP than DBP at all ages in both sexes. No other component of BP appears to consistently impact greater than SBP.

Table 1
Impact of Blood Pressure Components on Risk of Cardiovascular Disease by Age and Sex

	Men		Women	
	35–64 y	65–94 y	35–64 y	65–94 y
Systolic	0.302***	0.259***	0.288***	0.089†
Diastolic	0.341***	0.410***	0.361***	0.207***
Mean arterial	0.345***	0.364***	0.350***	0.167***
Pulse pressure	0.256***	0.354***	0.309***	0.200***

Thirty-year follow-up to Framingham Study. Values represent standardized logistic regression coefficients in mm Hg.

*** $P < 0.001$.

† Not significant.

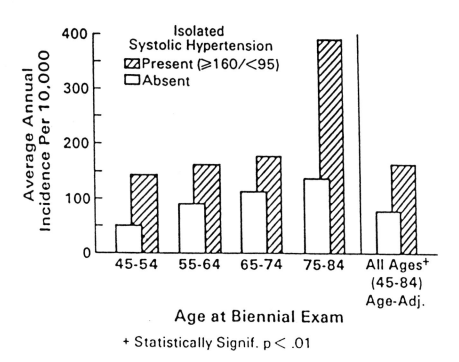

Figure 4. *Risk of MI with isolated systolic hypertension; 24-year follow-up, Framingham Study; men aged 45–84.*

Although taken alone DBP is a reasonable predictor of cardiovascular events, its impact wanes with advancing age and may be misleading in the elderly. In contrast, the SBP continues to be highly predictive in advanced age. In persons with systolic hypertension in the Framingham Study, the accompanying DBP was weakly related to risk of CVD, whereas in persons with diastolic hypertension, the risk was strikingly related to accompanying SBP.[8] Among subjects whose DBP never exceeded 95 mm Hg, cardiovascular risk increased sharply in relation to SBP at all ages, including the elderly.[8]

Isolated systolic hypertension in the Framingham Cohort was associated with a two- to threefold excess occurrence of cardiovascular morbidity and mortality in general and myocardial infarction (MI) in particular (Figure 4). Because of the foregoing and the fact that SBP is more accurately measured and provides a wider range of values for evaluation of risk, greater emphasis on SBP is warranted in estimating the hazard of hypertension and in evaluating the efficacy of antihypertensive therapy.

The Elderly

Hypertension is a particularly powerful predisposing factor for the major cardiovascular problems that afflict the elderly. It doubles the risk of cardiovascular events in both sexes over age 65.[9] The relative risk imposed exceeds that induced by cholesterol, smoking, and diabetes. The decrease in risk ratio for hypertension with advancing age is offset by a doubling of CVD incidence, resulting in greater excess risk and attributable risk (Table 2 and Figure 3). This makes antihypertensive treatment in the elderly more cost-effective than in the middle aged.

Table 2

Relation of Hypertension to Cardiovascular Outcomes in Patients Aged 65–94 from the Framingham Study

Cardiovascular Sequelae	Biennial Aged-Adjusted Rate/1000		Risk Ratios		Excess Risk/ 1000*	
	Men	Women	Men	Women	Men	Women
Coronary disease	72.6	44.2	1.6	1.9	27.7	20.5
Stroke	36.0	38.8	1.9	2.3	17.3	18.0
Peripheral arterial disease	16.5	9.6	1.6	2.0	6.0	4.8
Cardiac failure	33.0	23.5	1.9	1.9	15.8	11.4
Cardiovascular disease	124.9	80.6	1.8	1.8	56.0	35.2

* All differences were significant, $P < 0.0001$ except $P < 0.03$ in peripheral arterial disease.
Reproduced with permission from Reference 8.

The prevalence of hypertension in the elderly is high with about 50% afflicted. Because of the disproportionate increase in SBP with age, the prevalence of isolated systolic hypertension rises so that this is the chief variety of hypertension in the elderly. This isolated systolic hypertension in the elderly is associated with a distinct excess risk of all the cardiovascular sequelae, including coronary disease, stroke, cardiac failure, and peripheral arterial disease.[8,9]

Hypertension in the elderly, as in the middle aged, tends to cluster with other risk factors, so that there is a higher prevalence of hypercholesterolemia, diabetes, obesity, triglyceride, and left ventricular hypertrophy (LVH), all of which enhance the risk. Also, some 25% already have some evidence of CVD such as coronary disease, stroke, cardiac failure, or peripheral arterial disease.[9] These associated cardiovascular conditions and risk factors that commonly accompany hypertension in the elderly determine the urgency for treatment and the choice for therapy, particularly in the elderly.

Left Ventricular Hypertrophy

LVH showed to be causally related to hypertension, the risk of its occurrence increasing with the height of the BP.[10] Development of LVH in the hypertensive patient is evidence that target organ damage occurred.[11,12] The most convenient office procedure for detecting LVH is recording of the electrocardiogram (ECG), and persons found to have ECG-LVH showed to be at increased risk of clinical manifestations of CHD, cardiac failure, and strokes.[11]

Echocardiographic investigation provides more sensitive data on LVH that quantify the relation. These quantified data on LVH indicate that cardiovascular morbidity and mortality increase with left ventricular (LV) mass.[12] Echocardiographic studies indicate that antihypertensive therapy can regress LVH in hypertensive patients.[13] However, it is not clear whether regression of LVH in either the echocardiogram or ECG reduces the hazard of CVD.

Subjects in the Framingham Study with higher baseline voltage and more severe repolarization abnormalities characteristic of ECG-LVH had higher SBP and DBP.[10] Furthermore, in the Framingham Study, serial changes in voltage under observation were associated with corresponding changes in BP.[10] Serial changes in BP were, however, only marginally related to serial repolarization ECG changes and more so in men than women.[10]

In the Framingham Study cohort, the incidence of CVD was shown to increase over a threefold range in relation to voltage on ECG (Figure 5). Also, compared with a normal repolarization pattern, severe repolar-

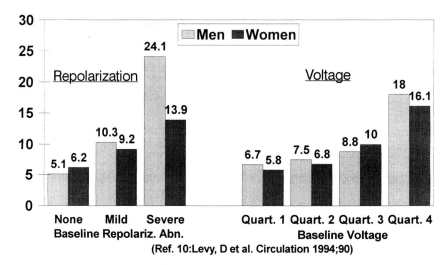

Figure 5. *Biennial age-adjusted rate of CVD incidence per 1000 by ECG features of LVH; Framingham Study.*

ization abnormality increased risk of cardiovascular events almost 6-fold in men and 2.5-fold in women. Subjects who had a serial decline in voltage under observation had only 50% the risk of cardiovascular events of those who had no change (Table 3). Those who increased their voltage increased their risk (2-fold in men and 1.6-fold in women). Improvement in repolarization was associated with a similar reduction in cardiovascular risk only in men (almost 50%), whereas worsening of repolarization increased risk twofold in both sexes.

Hypertrophy increases the myocardial oxygen requirement, imposing a hazard of ischemia when there is coronary atherosclerosis and decreased coronary reserve. This is especially the case when repolarization abnormality is present.[14] When LVH occurs there is also an increased risk of arrhythmia and sudden death.[15]

Persons who improve their voltage and repolarization abnormality tend to have a concomitant decline in BP,[10] linking BP to the evolution of LVH, as was demonstrated in trials of antihypertensive therapy. However, serial changes in ECG and echocardiograms are not highly correlated.[11,12] Both anatomic (as by roentgenogram) and ECG evidence of LVH contribute independently to occurrence of CVD, and those who have both have greater risk than those with either alone.[7,11]

Hypertensive persons who develop LVH greatly escalate their risk of CVD. Despite its limitations, the ECG is valuable in detecting LVH in office practice and is an essential test in monitoring of hypertensive patients for organ damage and response to therapy.

Table 3

Risk for Cardiovascular Disease Events as a Function of Serial
Electrocardiogram Changes

	Odds Ratio (95% Confidence Interval)	
	Men	Women
Voltage change*		
Serial voltage decrease	0.46 (0.26–0.84)	0.56 (0.30–1.04)
No changes	1.00	1.00
Serial voltage increase	1.86 (1.14–3.03)	1.61 (0.91–2.84)
Repolarization changes†		
Improved	0.45 (0.20–1.01)	1.19 (0.56–2.49)
No change	1.00	1.00
Worsened	1.89 (1.05–3.40)	2.02 (1.07–3.81)

Follow-up interval was from examination $n + 1$ to examination $n + 2$.

* Odds ratios for serial voltage changes (between examination n and examination $n + 1$) reflect adjustment for age and baseline voltage quartile at examination n.

† Odds ratios for serial repolarization changes (between examination n and examination $n + 1$) reflect adjustment for age and baseline repolarization at examination n.

Reproduced with permission from Reference 13.

Heart Rate

As hypertension exacts its toll on the heart, it must speed up its rate in order to compensate for a decreased stroke output. Also, persons with a more rapid heart rate (HR) tend to have and develop more hypertension than persons with slower HRs. An increased HR is an independent contributor to CVD and CHD mortality in persons with hypertension. This effect is greater for fatal than nonfatal cardiovascular events in both sexes.[16]

Each 10 beat-per-minute increment in HR in hypertensive persons, adjusted for age and BP, was found to be associated with a 20% increase in all-cause and a 14% increase in cardiovascular mortality in both sexes. CHD mortality increased 16% in men and 12% in women.[16] Data suggest a direct effect of HR on cardiovascular sequelae of hypertension that may be mediated through the autonomic nervous system so that treatment of hypertension with medications that slow the HR may be particularly beneficial.

Cardiac Failure

Cardiac failure is a disabling and lethal end stage to CVD, and sudden death is a common mode of exitus.[17] Once the heart used up

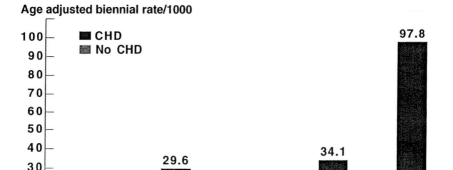

Age adjusted biennial rate/1000

Risk variables: age, cardiac enlargement by X-ray, ECG-LV hypertrophy, glucose intolerance, heart rate, systolic BP

Figure 6. *Risk of cardiac failure by quintile of multivariate risk and CHD status; Framingham Study; 32-year follow-up; men aged 35–94.*

all its reserve and compensatory mechanisms, the survival rate is little better than that for cancer. Median survival is only 1.7 years in men and 3.2 years in women once overt cardiac failure ensues.[17] Declines in death rates from CVD were not accompanied by a reduced incidence of cardiac failure or improved survival.[18] Candidates for cardiac failure with CHD or hypertension, the chief causes, can be readily detected from a cardiovascular risk profile made up of ingredients easily ascertained in outpatient office practice (Figure 6). Persons in the upper quintile of multivariate risk are high-yield candidates for echocardiographic and other costly procedures to detect LV dysfunction. A substantial reduction in the incidence and mortality from congestive heart failure (CHF) can be achieved only by detection and correction of presymptomatic LV dysfunction, which is often induced by hypertension. Among the various correctable risk factors for CVD that promote cardiac failure, hypertension is dominant.[18]

Renin

Much effort went into seeking out factors that increase risk of CHD in hypertensive patients. One such proposed risk factor is a high renin-sodium profile.[19] A high renin activity for the level of sodium excretion was proposed as a predictor of MI in persons with hypertension in retrospective and prospective studies. However, several studies failed to confirm these claims.[19]

The renin hypothesis is plausible because renin secretion is influenced by sodium intake, BP, sympathetic activity, and sodium balance. An activated renin-angiotensin system can cause vasoconstriction and have direct metabolic effects on the heart and blood vessels, including stimulation of smooth muscle cell migration and growth and intimal hyperplasia after vascular surgery.[19] Also, local tissue angiotensin may be important in hypertensive CVD. Inhibition of angiotensin-converting enzymes (ACEs) was shown to reduce myocardial ischemia, decrease atherosclerosis, and retard stenosis after injury.[19]

Multivariate Risk

Hypertension in middle-aged and elderly persons seldom occurs in isolation. It tends to cluster with other metabolically linked risk factors.[7] The biological determinant of this clustering is uncertain, but insulin resistance promoted by abdominal obesity seems a likely candidate (Figure 7). The risk of cardiovascular events in general and of coronary disease in particular is quite variable, depending on the associated burden of risk factors that accompanies the hypertension (Figure 8). High risk of cardiovascular sequelae is concentrated in those hypertensive persons who have dyslipidemia, glucose intolerance, or LVH. About 50% of the cardiovascular events in hypertension occur in those in the upper quintile of multivariate risk.

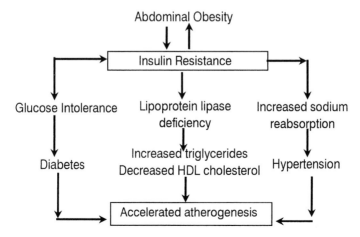

Figure 7. *Atherogenic pathways of insulin resistance to accelerated atherosclerosis.*

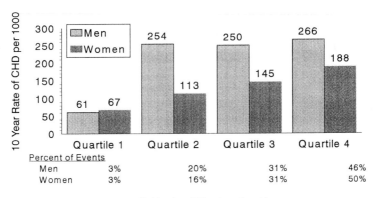

Multivariate RF's: Age, Smoking,

Figure 8. *Rate of CHD by quartile of multivariate risk; Framingham Study; hypertensives aged 49–81.*

Preventive Implications

New onset of hypertension continues unabated, despite improved detection and massive treatment of the general population. The chief hazards are atherosclerosis and CHD now that severe hypertension is seldom left uncontrolled. Systolic as well as diastolic hypertension must now be recognized as a cardiovascular hazard at all ages in both sexes. It is important to recognize that hypertension usually occurs in conjunction with blood lipid abnormalities, impaired glucose tolerance, obesity, hyperuricemia, and LVH. The hypertensive risk of CHD is concentrated in those with one or more of the following: a high total/high-density lipoprotein-cholesterol ratio, impaired glucose tolerance, high fibrinogen, ECG abnormalities, or cigarette smoking. Measurement of these cardiovascular risk factors is required to properly evaluate the need for antihypertensive treatment and to select the best treatment. Optimal treatment must improve not only the BP but also the composite risk profile.

In more advanced situations, long-standing hypertension is commonly associated with angina, MI, cardiac failure, renal insufficiency, peripheral vascular disease, retinopathy, stroke, or LVH. Choice of drug therapy for hypertension accompanied by these conditions will vary and should be individualized to maximize benefit against the associated conditions as well as the hypertension. Silent or unrecognized MIs must be sought out since they occur in marked excess in hypertensive persons.[20]

ECG-LVH is an ominous harbinger of dangerous cardiovascular events and must not be taken as an incidental accompaniment of hypertension, despite lack of symptoms. Awaiting evidence of organ damage before treating is unwarranted since the first such evidence is often a MI, stroke, or sudden death.

Controlled trials tested the efficacy of treating mild hypertension and showed treatment to prevent strokes and cardiac failure. Evidence for benefit in preventing CHD is less consistent. This was attributed to metabolic penalties of diuretics and β-blockers used and failure to tailor therapy to take into account the accompanying lipid profile, LVH, or diabetes.

Treatment of hypertension to prevent CHD would appear to require control of blood lipids and cigarette smoking. Diuretics and some β-blockers may make management of the lipids more difficult. Agents such as α-1−blockers, ACE inhibitors, and calcium antagonists, which either do not affect or improve lipids, would appear preferable if coexistent dyslipidemia is present.

For impaired cardiac function, ACE inhibitors and diuretics should be preferred. For associated ischemia, β-blockers and calcium antagonists are preferable and, for associated peripheral vascular disease, β-blockers are best avoided. Thus therapy for hypertension must take into consideration associated risk factors, concomitant disease, age, race, and side-effect profile. Treatment must also give more attention to step-down therapy and hygienic control of mild hypertension with weight control and less salt, alcohol, and fat in the diet, potassium and magnesium supplementation, and comprehensive risk reduction. Hypertension is, after all, only one ingredient of the cardiovascular risk profile.

References

1. National Heart, Lung, and Blood Institute. National High Pressure Education Program. Working group report on hypertension in the elderly. *Hypertension* 1994;23:275–285.
2. National Heart, Lung, and Blood Institute. *The Fifth Report of the Joint Committee on Detection, Evaluation and Treatment of High Blood Pressure*. Bethesda Md: 1993. NIH publication 93–1088.
3. Kannel WB, Garrison RJ, Dannenberg AL. Secular blood pressure trends in normotensive persons: the Framingham Study. *Am Heart J* 1993;124:1154–1158.
4. Leitschuh M, Cupples LA, Kannel WB, et al. High normal blood pressure progression to hypertension in the Framingham Study. *Hypertension* 1991;17:22–27.
5. Gubner RS. Systolic hypertension: a pathogenetic entity. *Am J Cardiol* 1962;9:773–776.
6. Rutan GH, McDonald RH, Kuller LH. A historical perspective of elevated systolic vs diastolic blood pressure from an epidemiolgical and clinical trial viewpoint. *J Clin Epidemiol* 1989;42:663–673.
7. Kannel WB. Epidemiology of essential hypertension: the Framingham experience. *Proc R Coll Phys Edinb* 1991;21:273–287.
8. Kannel WB. Hypertension in the elderly: epidemiologic appraisal from the Framingham Study. *Cardiol Elderly* 1993;1:359–363.
9. Levy D, Anderson KM, Savage DD, et al. Echocardiographically detected left ventricular hypertrophy: prevalence and risk factors: the Framingham Heart Study. *Ann Intern Med* 1988;108:7–13.

10. Levy D, Salomon M, D'Agostino RB, et al. Prognostic implications of baseline electrocadiographic features and their serial changes in subjects with left ventricular hypertrophy. *Circulation* 1994;90:1780–1793.
11. Kannel WB, Dannenberg AL, Levy D. Population implications of electrocardiographic left ventricular hypertrophy. *Am J Cardiol* 1987;60:851–931.
12. Levy D, Garrison RJ, Savage DD, et al. Prognostic implications of echocardiographically determined left ventricular mass in the Framingham Heart Study. *N Engl J Med* 1990;322:1561–1566.
13. Dahloff B, Pennert K, Hansson L. Reversal of left ventricular hypertrophy in hypertensive patient: a meta-analysis of 109 treatment studies. *Am J Hypertens* 1992;5:95–110.
14. Pringle SD, Macfarlane PW, McKillop JH, et al. Pathophysiologic assessment of left ventricular hypertrophy and strain in asymptomatic patients with essential hypertension. *J Am Coll Cardiol* 1989;13:1377–1381.
15. Levy D, Anderson KM, Savage DD, et al. Risk of ventricular arrhythmias in left ventricular hypertrophy. The Framingham Heart Study. *Am J Cardiol* 1987;60:560–585.
16. Gillman MW, Kannel WB, Belanger AJ, et al. Influence of heart rate on mortality among persons with hypertension: the Framingham Study. *Am Heart J* 1993;125:1148–1154.
17. Ho K, Anderson KM, Kannel WB, et al. Survival after onset of congestive heart failure in Framingham Heart Study subjects. *Circulation* 1993;888:107–115.
18. Kannel WB, Ho K, Thom T. Changing epidemiologic features of cardiac failure. *Br Heart J* 1994;72(suppl):3–9.
19. Dzau VJ. Renin and myocardial infarction in hypertension. *N Engl J Med* 1991;324:1128–1130.
20. Kannel WB, Dannenberg A, Abbott R. Unrecognized myocardial infarction and hypertension: The Framingham Study. *Am Heart J* 1985;109:581–585.

Chapter 2

Pharmacologic Management of Arterial Hypertension

Donald G. Vidt, MD

Introduction

The Report of the Fifth Joint National Committee on Detection, Evaluation and Treatment of High Blood Pressure (JNC-V)[1] provided a new working system for classifying adult blood pressure (BP). As noted in Table 1, stages of hypertension replace the traditional terms, "mild hypertension" and "moderate hypertension," which failed to convey the impact of these levels of high BP on cardiovascular disease (CVD) risks. High BP stage 1, previously termed "mild," is the most common form of high BP in the adult population, and, as such, is responsible for a large proportion of the excess morbidity, disability, and mortality attributable to hypertension.

I modified this classification to combine stage 3 and 4 for further simplification. Any patient with BP ≥180/110 mm Hg deserves further evaluation or referral with considerable expediency. Patients with BP in this range certainly require aggressive pharmacologic therapy.

When systolic BP (SBP) and diastolic BP (DBP) fall into different stages, the higher stage should be selected to classify the individual's BP status. For instance, 160/92 mm Hg should be classified as stage 2, and 180/106 should be classified as stage 3. Isolated systolic hypertension (ISH) is defined as an SBP ≥140 mm Hg and DBP <90 mm Hg and staged

From Robinson K, (ed): *Preventive Cardiology*. Armonk, NY: Futura Publishing Company, Inc. © 1998.

Table 1
Classification of Blood Pressure for Adults Age 18
and Older (Modified)

	Systolic (mm Hg)*	Diastolic (mm Hg)*
Optimal	<120	<80
Normal[†]	<130	<85
High normal	130–139	85–89
	Hypertension[‡]	
Stage 1	140–159	90–99
Stage 2	160–179	100–109
Stage 3	≥180	≥110

In addition to classifying stages of hypertension based on average blood pressure levels, the clinician should specify presence or absence of target organ disease and additional risk factors. For example, a patient with diabetes and a blood pressure of 142/94 mm Hg plus left ventricular hypertrophy should be classified as "stage 1 hypertension with target organ disease (left ventricular hypertrophy) and with another major risk factor (diabetes)." This specificity is important for risk classification and management.

* Patients not taking antihypertensive drugs and not acutely ill.

[†] Optimal blood pressure with respect to cardiovascular risk is SBP <120 mm Hg and DBP <80 mm Hg. However, usually low readings should be evaluated for clinical significance.

[‡] Based on the average of two or more readings taken at each of two or more visits following an initial screening.

Adapted with permission from Reference 1.

appropriately (eg, 170/85 mm Hg is defined as stage 2 ISH). The new classification system recognizes that all stages of hypertension are associated with increased cardiovascular morbidity and mortality. The higher the BP, the greater the risk. The new system also focuses on the presence or absence of additional risk factors, encouraging identification of lipid disorders, cigarette smoking, diabetes mellitus (DM), physical inactivity, and obesity. Detection and treatment of these added risk factors are critical to the successful management of the patient with hypertension.

Clinical manifestations of target organ damage are also specified in the new classification system. The risks of vascular complications at any level of high BP are increased severalfold for persons with target organ disease (Table 2). The identification of other cardiovascular risk factors and target organ damage is important for a more precise risk stratification of the hypertensive patient and will facilitate the clinician's decision to treat or not to treat and determine the aggressiveness of therapy warranted. In some situations, this classification may also help in the selection of antihypertensive therapy.

Table 2
Manifestations of Target Organ Disease

Organ System	Manifestations
Cardiac	Clinical, electrocardiographic, or radiological evidence of coronary artery disease
	Left ventricular hypertrophy or "strain" by electrocardiography or left ventricular hypertrophy by echocardiography
	Left ventricular dysfunction or cardiac failure
Cerebrovascular	Transient ischemic attack or stroke
Peripheral vascular	Absence of one or more major pulses in the extremities (except for dorsalis pedis) with or without intermittent claudication; aneurysm
Renal	Serum creatinine ≥ 130 μmol/L (1.5 mg/dL)
	Proteinuria (1+ or greater)
	Microalbuminuria
Retinopathy	Hemorrhages or exudates, with or without papilledema

Reproduced with permission from Reference 1.

Current Status of Therapy

Considerable emphasis was placed on the sustained declines in coronary and stroke mortality observed in the United States from 1972 to 1990. During the last two decades the mortality rate for the number one cause of death, coronary heart disease (CHD), decreased approximately 50% and that from stroke fell by 57%. Since high BP is recognized as one of the major risk factors for CHD, and the most important risk factor for cerebrovascular disease, it seems reasonable to assume that progress in the detection, treatment, and control of hypertension contributed substantially to these declining mortality rates.

However, there is emerging evidence that hypertension is undertreated in the United States at present. The Third National Health and Nutritional Examination Survey (NHANES III, 1988–1991) estimated that, of 43 million hypertensive persons (BP ≥ 140 and/or ≥ 90 mm Hg) in the United States, 31% were unaware of their disease.[2] Only 53% of the total hypertensive population and 69% of persons aware of their hypertension were receiving antihypertension medication at the time of this survey. Of greater concern was that only 24% of the entire hypertensive population and 45% of those on treatment actually had BP controlled to <140/90 mm Hg. At the time of NHANES, the average BP for all treated hypertensive patients was 135/83 mm Hg, whereas the average BP in normotensive adults surveyed was 117/71 mm Hg. Only 14% of Mexican-Americans with hypertension had their BP controlled to below <140/90 mm Hg, compared with 24% of non-Hispanic whites and 25% of non-Hispanic black Americans (Figure 1).

The prevalence of high BP increases with age, is greater for blacks than for whites, and in both races is greater in less-educated than better-educated people. It is especially prevalent and devastating in lower socioeconomic groups. In young adulthood and early middle age, high BP is more prevalent in men than in women, but, thereafter, the reverse is true. Blacks and whites in the southeastern United States have a greater prevalence of high BP and higher stroke death rates than do blacks and whites in other areas of the country.[2] Nonfatal and fatal CVDs (eg, CHD and stroke), renal disease, and all-cause mortality increased progressively with higher levels of both SBP and DBP.

Epidemiological data suggest that the optimal BP with respect to cardiovascular risk is <120/80 mm Hg.[3,4] Long-term follow-up on 347 978 men screened for the Multiple Risk Factor Intervention Trial (MRFIT) indicated that 32% of the men who died of CHD within 11.6 years had SBPs of <140 mm Hg at the time of screening. Another 43% of excess deaths had SBPs between 140 and 160 mm Hg. In a study of 123 borderline hypertensive subjects from Tecumseh, Michigan, Julius et al[5] reported that clinic BPs averaged 131/94 mm Hg, whereas home BPs averaged 126/80 mm Hg; the average age of subjects was 31.4 years. In 822 normotensive subjects of comparable age, clinic BPs averaged 112/75 mm Hg and home BPs averaged 114/72 mm Hg. On the average, the borderline hypertensive

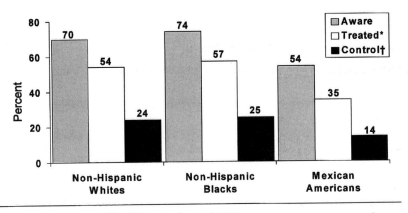

* Treated: treated with antihypertensive medication.
† Control: proportion of hypertensives whose SBP <140 and DBP <90 mmHg

Data source: NHANES III. Adapted from Burt et al.[2]

Figure 1. *The percent of people with high BP who have their BP under control, by race and ethnicity: United States 1988–1991. Data from NHANES III, phase 1. Adapted with permission from Reference 2.*

subjects had a lower stroke index and a higher peripheral resistance than normotensive subjects and already had evidence of diastolic dysfunction by echocardiography. Borderline hypertensive subjects also had a higher incidence of other cardiovascular risk factors, including higher cholesterol, lower high-density lipoprotein cholesterol (HDL-C), higher triglycerides, higher plasma insulin, and higher insulin/glucose ratios than did the normotensive subjects.

Of disturbing note are reports from several sources regarding the occurrence of target organ disease, which is closely associated with hypertension control. Hypertension is considered a major risk factor for stroke, congestive heart failure (CHF), and end-stage renal disease. Despite hypertension control efforts, hospitalization rates for heart failure in the United States between 1971 and 1993 continued to increase, particularly for persons over age 65. New cases of end-stage renal disease due to hypertension increased steadily and are second only to DM as a cause of end-stage renal disease.[6] Of great concern is a recent report from the National Stroke Association indicating that, between 1992 and 1993, the number of deaths from stroke in the United States increased for the first time in 35 years and, in particular, increased disproportionately among black men and women. Because hypertension is a major risk factor for stroke, CHF, and progressive renal disease, aggressive efforts to control high BP to more optimal levels seem appropriate. A recent working group report from the National High Blood Pressure Education Program recommended that BP be reduced to <130/85 mm Hg in an effort to reduce the rate of end-stage renal disease as a complication of hypertension.[6]

The Treatment of Mild Hypertension Study demonstrated a 33% reduction in cardiovascular events after 4.4 years in participants receiving active antihypertensive drug therapy plus lifestyle modifications, compared to those who were on lifestyle modifications and placebo.[7] Final BPs averaged 124/79 mm Hg for the drug treatment group and 132/82 mm Hg in the placebo group. This study provides further credence to the concept of "the lower the BP, the better," even for patients with mild or what we now term stage 1 or 2 hypertension.

A recent report from the Framingham Heart Study[8] shows the relative frequencies of untreated hypertension in men and women according to age. Isolated diastolic hypertension (SBP <160 mm Hg, DBP ≥90 mm Hg) is undertreated in persons younger than 60 years. Although borderline ISH (SBP 140–159 mm Hg; DBP <90 mm Hg) is grossly undertreated in patients 60 years of age and older and the Systolic Hypertension in the Elderly Program (SHEP)[9] provided impressive evidence of the benefits of treating ISH, Framingham data show that it is frequently not treated, especially in persons 70 years of age and older. ISH accounts for 60% of cases of hypertension and results from a disproportionate rise in SBP because of diminished arterial compliance. Framingham data also demon-

Table 3
Risk Factors in the Hypertensive Patient

Untreatable	Treatable
Age	Obesity
Race	Hyperlipidemia
Family history	Physical inactivity
Diabetes mellitus	Tobacco use
	Ethanol excess

strated that the risk of cardiovascular sequelae rises as the pulse pressure increases. ISH is associated with a two- to threefold increase in the risk of cardiovascular events, cardiovascular mortality, and overall mortality.[10]

Finally, the importance of a comprehensive risk factor analysis in each hypertensive patient must be emphasized. Careful assessment of the individual patient's risk profile will facilitate the decision as to when drug treatment should be initiated and how aggressively that treatment should be pursued (Table 3). The presence of untreatable risk factors or of target organ disease should prompt initiation of pharmacologic treatment at lower BP levels and treatment to a lower goal level than if there were no other risk factors or target organ disease present. Other treatable risk factors must also be effectively managed if optimal control and prevention of CVD events are to be achieved. Observational studies and clinical trials clearly showed the additive influences of multiple risk factors on cardio-

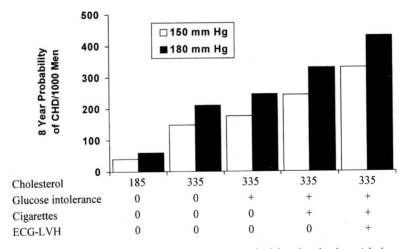

Figure 2. *Risk of CVD according to SBP at specified levels of other risk factors. Adapted with permission from Reference 11.*

vascular events, together with the benefits of controlling not only BP but other risk factors as well (Figure 2).[11] As of 1997, all physicians must be responsible for multiple risk factor control in managing their hypertension patients. Only by aggressive management of all treatable risk factors can maximal reduction in total cardiovascular risk be obtained.

Primary Prevention of High Blood Pressure

Primary prevention of hypertension can be accomplished by application of intervention techniques to the general population in an effort to achieve a downward shift in the distribution of BP. Special focus can be narrowed to persons who are most likely to develop hypertension (eg, those with high-normal BP, a family history of hypertension, and with one or more of the several lifestyle factors that appear to be important contributors to age-related increases in BP).[12] These lifestyle factors include a high sodium intake, excessive consumption of calories with subsequent obesity, physical inactivity, excessive alcohol consumption, and low intake of potassium. These changes form the basis for interventions that showed promise in preventing high BP.

Evidence is less convincing for other lifestyle interventions such as stress management; supplementation of the diet with calcium, magnesium, fish oils, or fiber; or alterations in macronutrient consumption. However, in many instances, available data are insufficient to make a final judgment on the potential role of these factors in the primary prevention of hypertension.

Evaluation of the Hypertensive Patient

Except when hypertension is severe and life threatening, evaluation should precede the initiation of treatment. The initial evaluation should be thorough, cost-effective, and informative regarding the following questions:

1. Does the patient have primary or secondary (and possibly reversible) hypertension?
2. Is target organ disease present?
3. Are cardiovascular risk factors present in addition to high BP?

For most patients, repeated determinations of BP should be obtained before proceeding with evaluation. Repeated measurements are especially important for patients with borderline or labile hypertension. Patients with average SBP of 140 mm Hg or greater and/or DBP of 90 mm Hg or higher should be evaluated.

The most important component of the pretreatment evaluation is a complete history and physical examination. For patients previously found to have hypertension, the duration of the disease should be established. Response to any prescribed antihypertensive therapy and adverse effects of treatment should be noted. The history of prescription and over-the-counter medications should be obtained, since many drugs interact with antihypertensive agents, raising BP or reducing the efficacy of antihypertensive drugs. Other risk factors such as smoking, hyperlipidemia, DM, and obesity must be documented. Emotional stress, socioeconomic status, or specific food practices possibly affecting BP control or compliance should be noted. In particular, an estimate of daily sodium intake and alcohol use should be established. The use of oral contraceptives in younger women and excessive alcohol intake in both men and women represent the two most common causes of potentially reversible hypertension. An inquiry regarding the use of recreational drugs (eg, marijuana and cocaine) should be made in all age groups. Any family history of hypertension, premature CVD or mortality, DM, renal disease, or pheochromocytoma should be documented.

Symptoms of target organ involvement may be revealed by obtaining a history of transient ischemic attack, stroke, myocardial infarction, angina pectoris, atherosclerotic heart disease, or lower-extremity arteriosclerosis obliterans. A change in the diurnal pattern of urine flow may be an early clue to concentrating defects secondary to hypertension-induced renal disease or other forms of renal parenchymal disease.

The physical examination should help verify the degree of target organ involvement and may also provide additional clues to secondary causes of hypertension. Careful measurement of BP, height, and weight and a thorough fundoscopic evaluation for evidence of arteriolar narrowing, arteriovenous compression, hemorrhages, exudates, or papilloedema should be made. Auscultation and palpation of the neck should be performed for evidence of carotid bruits, distended neck veins, or an enlarged thyroid gland. Examination of the heart should establish its size, rate, and rhythm as well as the presence or absence of murmurs. Auscultation of the lungs for rhonchi, rales, or wheezes will establish the presence or absence of congestive heart failure or, possibly, chronic pulmonary disease. Examination of the abdomen should include both auscultation and palpation for evidence of bruits, enlarged kidneys, other abdominal masses, or dilation of the abdominal aorta. Examination of the extremities may disclose diminished or absent peripheral pulses, bruits, or edema, and careful neurological assessment will establish the presence of fixed neurological deficits.

The history and physical examination should be complemented by a few carefully selected laboratory studies, preferably performed before initiating therapy. Measurements of hemoglobin, hematocrit, urinalysis, se-

---

Table 4

Clues to Selected Secondary Causes of Hypertension

Renovascular hypertension
    Systolic-diastolic epigastric bruit
    Accelerated or malignant hypertension
    Unilateral small kidney discovered by any investigative procedure
    Onset of hypertension under age 30 or after age 55
    Resistant hypertension
    Hypertension and unexplained impairment in renal function
    Acute impairment in renal function in response to ACE inhibitor
    Evidence of extensive ASO: carotid, coronary, peripheral
Primary hyperaldosteronism
    Hypokalemia with inappropriate kaliuresis
    Resistant hypertension
    Weakness, periodic paralysis, paresthesias, in tetany (rare)
    Aldosterone/renin ratio >10
Pheochromocytoma
    Paroxysms of hypertension and headache, tachycardia, palpitations, tremor, and
        sweating
    History of labile blood pressure
    Substandard weight or recent weight loss
    A pressor response to antihypertensive drugs or during induction of anesthesia
    Resistant hypertension
    Occasional occurrence with neurocutaneous syndromes
    Unusual lability of blood pressure or orthostatic hypotension
    Abnormal glucose tolerance
Cushing's syndrome
    Recent change in appearance and weight gain
    Extreme weakness with muscle wasting
    Typical body habitus with moon facies, skin changes, and hirsutism
    Glucose intolerance
    Neutrophilia with relative lymphocytopenia
Coarctation of the aorta
    Absent or reduced pulses in the lower extremities
    Palpable pulsations over intercostal arteries in the posterior thorax
    Bruits over intercostal arteries
    Rib notching on chest X-ray
    Absent aortic knob
Renal parenchymal disease
    Abnormal urinalysis, particularly heavy proteinuria
    Abnormal urogram, renal ultrasound, or isotopic renography
    Abnormal renal biopsy

---

rum potassium, and creatinine plus an electrocardiogram (ECG) will help to determine the severity of vascular disease or the presence of target organ involvement and may provide clues to secondary hypertension. The addition of a lipid profile and measurements of serum calcium, fasting blood sugar, and serum uric acid will help identify other cardiovascular risk factors. Many of these studies are easily obtainable today as part of an automated blood chemistry profile. The decision to perform additional diagnostic studies should be determined by the presence or absence of clinical clues to secondary hypertension uncovered in the course of the history, physical examination, and screening laboratory studies. Indications for pursuing specialized diagnostic procedures to rule out curable hypertension include the following:

- the onset of hypertension before age 30 or after age 55
- an abrupt onset of hypertension at any age
- DBP >110 mm Hg or SBP >180 mm Hg
- hypertension refractory to three-drug therapy
- hypertensive retinopathy, group III or IV (malignant hypertension)

Fewer than 5% of the almost 50 million hypertensive patients in the United States have a curable cause of their hypertension, such as renovascular disease, pheochromocytoma, primary aldosteronism, or coarctation of the aorta. Clinical clues to the presence of specific reversible causes of hypertension are listed in Table 4.

Initiation of Therapy

Once the diagnosis of hypertension is established, the process of patient education should be started. For subsequent therapy to be successful, patients must recognize that hypertension is a lifelong disease, usually asymptomatic (since the symptoms do not correlate with BP levels) and that therapy will, in most instances, need to be maintained for life. Effective therapy will control hypertension, and optimal control is usually compatible with an excellent long-term prognosis and quality of life. Adherence with a prescribed regimen is the key to successful therapy and depends on the patient's willingness to comply with recommended medications and to undertake selected behavioral modification when indicated.

Lifestyle modification received increasing attention in recent years, while evidence continued to mount regarding selected nonpharmacologic measures in the control of BP, particularly in patients with stage 1 hypertension. Selected lifestyle interventions can also be of adjunctive value in patients with more severe hypertension receiving pharmacologic therapy. Properly used, lifestyle modification interventions offer the ability to improve the cardiovascular risk profile. Even when not adequate in themselves to control hypertension, they may reduce the number or doses of antihypertensive medications required. Effective lifestyle modification includes appropriate reduction of calorie, salt, alcohol, and fat consumption. In addition to these measures, participation in regular exercise and avoidance of tobacco need to be considered.

Moderate dietary sodium restriction carries no risk for hypertensive patients and may benefit selected patients by modest reductions in BP. Almost one-half of all patients who reduce their daily sodium intake into the range of 2 g of sodium or 5–6 g of salt will lower their BP by about 3–5 mm Hg.[13,14] In some stage 1 hypertensive patients, this change may be sufficient to normalize BP without medication, whereas, in others, sodium restriction will enhance the efficacy of antihypertensive medications. Appropriate counseling should include educational information regarding the labeling of processed foods and an increased awareness of the sodium content of frequently purchased foods.

The role of other agents such as potassium, calcium, and magnesium in the genesis of hypertension remains controversial. A modest beneficial effect on BP was noted after potassium supplementation in hypertensive patients who were rendered hypokalemic from using diuretics.[15] Preliminary nutritional data suggested that calcium intake is lower among hypertensive individuals than normotensive individuals and that calcium supplementation may lower BP in hypertensive patients.[12,16] Calcium supplements may be considered for patients in whom rigid restriction of dairy products was undertaken for control of hyperlipidemia. Similarly, lower magnesium levels were noted in hypertensive individuals. Diuretic therapy may induce hypomagnesemia and hypokalemia, and if these are documented, supplementation may be considered in the diuretic-treated patient. The need for potassium and magnesium supplementation clearly lessened in recent years with the trend of using lower doses of diuretics in the management of hypertension. Various lifestyle issues in the management of CVD are discussed elsewhere in this text.

Initial Drug Therapy

Initial therapy for stage 1 and 2 hypertension in most patients will consist of a single drug (monotherapy) (Table 5). In selected patients, however, initiation of treatment with one of the newer fixed combinations of antihypertensive agents may be appropriate for initial therapy as well as for subsequent therapy. The role of newer fixed combinations will be addressed later in this section. Recommendations outlined in the JNC-V report that favor the selection of diuretics or β-blockers as initial therapy remain suitable at this time (Figure 3). These agents were proven to reduce morbidity and mortality from hypertension in randomized clinical trials. These two classes of drugs would appear preferred for initial drug therapy if there are no contraindications to their use in the individual patient and there are no special indications for the selection of an alternative agent. Alternative drug classes include the calcium antagonists, angiotensin-converting enzyme (ACE) inhibitors, α_1-receptor blockers, the α-β-blocker (labetalol), and the angiotensin II (AII) receptor antagonists. Re-

Table 5
Antihypertensive Medications

Type of Drug	Usual Dosage Range (total mg/d)*	Frequency (once per day unless otherwise noted)
Initial antihypertensive agents		
DIURETICS		
Thiazides and related sulfonamide diuretics		
Bendroflumethiazide (Naturetin)	2.5–5	
Benzthiazide (Exna)	12.5–50	
Chlorothiazide (Diuril)	125–500	Twice
Chlorthalidone (Hygroton)	12.5–25	
Hydrochlorothiazide (HydroDiuril, Esidrix)	12.5–50	
Hydroflumethiazide (Saluron, Diurcardin)	12.5–50	
Indapamide (Lozol)	2.5–5	
Methyclothiazide (Enduron)	2.5–5	
Metolazone (Zaroxolyn)	1.25–10	
Metolazone (Mykrox)	0.5–1	
Polythiazide (Renese)	1.0–4	
Quinethazone (Hydromox)	25–100	
Trichlormethiazide	1.0–4	
Loop diuretics		
Bumetanide (Bumex)	0.5–5	Twice
Ethacrynic acid (Edecrin)	25.0–100	Twice
Furosemide (Lasix)	20.0–320	Twice
Torsemide (Demadex)	5–10	
Potassium-sparing agents		
Amiloride (Midamor)	5–10	Once or twice
Spironolactone (Aldactone)	25–100	Twice or thrice
Triamterene (Dyrenium)	50–150	Twice
ADRENERGIC INHIBITORS		
β blockers		
Atenolol (Tenormin)	25–100[†]	
Betaxolol (Kerlone)	5–40	
Bisoprolol fumarate (Zebeta, Ziac)	5–20	
Metoprolol (Lopressor)	50–20	
Metoprolol (long-acting) (Toprol XL)	50–200	
Nadolol (Corgard)	20–240[†]	
Propranolol (Inderal)	40–240	Twice
Propranolol (long-acting) (Inderal LA)	60–240	

continues

Table 5 Continued
Antihypertensive Medications

Type of Drug	Usual Dosage Range (total mg/d)*	Frequency (once per day unless otherwise noted)
β blockers		
Timolol (Blocadren)	20–40	
β blockers with intrinsic sympathomimetic activity		
Acebutolol (Sectral)	200–1200[†]	Twice
Carteolol (Cartrol)	2–10[†]	
Penbutolol (Levatol)	20–80[†]	
Pindolol (Visken)	10–60[†]	
α-β blocker		
Labetalol (Normodyne, Trandate)	200–1200	Twice
α₁-receptor blocker		
Doxazosin (Cardura)	2.0–16	
Prazosin (Minipress)	2.0–20	Twice or thrice
Terazosin (Hytrin)	1.0–20	
ACE inhibitors		
Benazepril (Lotensin)	10.0–40[†]	Once or twice
Captopril (Capoten)	12.5–150[†]	Twice
Cilazapril	2.5–5.0	Once or twice
Enalapril (Vasotec)	2.5–40[†]	Once or twice
Fosinopril (Monopril)	10.0–40	Once or twice
Lisinopril (Prinivil, Zestril)	5.0–40[†]	
Perindopril	1.0–16[†]	Once or twice
Quinapril (Accupril)	5.0–80[†]	Once or twice
Ramipril (Altace)	1.25–20[†]	Once or twice
Spirapril	12.5–50	Once or twice
Calcium antagonists		
Diltiazem (sustained release)		Twice
(Cardizem SR)	120–360	
Diltiazem (extended release)		
(Cardizem CD)	120–360	
Diltiazem (extended release)		
(Dilacor XR)	180–480	
Diltiazem (extended release)		
(Tiazac)	180–360	
Verapamil (Verelan)	120–480	
Verapamil (long-acting) (Calan SR,		Once or twice
Isoptin SR)	120–480	
Verapamil (extended release)		
(Covera HS)	240–480	
Dyhydropyridines		
Amlodopine (Norvasc)	5–10	

continues

Table 5 Continued
Antihypertensive Medications

Type of Drug	Usual Dosage Range (total mg/d)*	Frequency (once per day unless otherwise noted)
Dyhydropyridines		
Felodipine (Plendil)	5–20	Twice
Isradipine (DynaCirc)	2.5–10	Twice
Nicardipine (sustained release)		Twice
(Cardene SR)	60–120	
Nifedipine GITS (Procardia XL)	30–90	
Nisoldipine (Sular)	10–60	
Angiotensin II antagonists		
Losartan (Cozaar)	25–100	
Valsartan (Diovan)	80–320	
Supplemental antihypertensive agents		
Centrally acting α_2 agonists		
Clonidine (Catapres)	0.1–1.2	Twice
Clonidine TTS (patch)	0.1–0.3	Once weekly
(Catapres-TTS)		
Guanabenz (Wytensin)	4–64	Twice
Guanfacine (Tenex)	1–3	
Methyldopa (Aldomet)	250–2000	Twice
Peripherally acting adrenergic neuron antagonists		
Guanadrel (Hylorel)	10–75	Twice
Guanethidine (Ismelin)	10–100	
Rauwolfia alkaloids		
Rauwolfia root	50–200	
Reserpine	0.05‡–0.2	
Direct vasodilators		
Hydralazine (Apresoline)	50–300	Twice to four times
Minoxidil (Loniten)	2.5–80	Once or twice

* The lower dose indicated is the preferred initial dose, and the higher dose is the maximum daily dose. Most agents require 2–4 weeks for complete efficacy, and more frequent dosage adjustments are not advised except for severe hypertension. The dosage range may differ slightly from the recommended dosage in the *Physician's Desk Reference* or package insert.

† Indicates drugs that are excreted by the kidney and require dosage reduction in renal impairment.

‡ 0.1 mg dose may be given every other day to achieve this dosage.

Adapted from Reference 1.

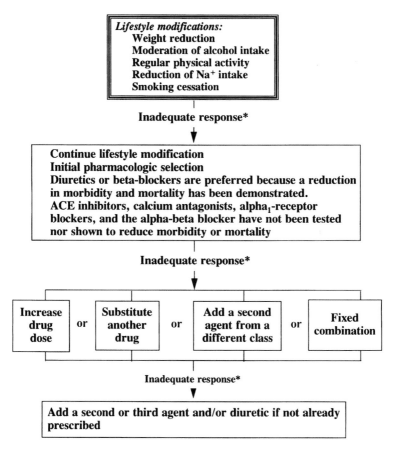

Figure 3. *Treatment algorithm.*

sults of clinical trials comparing diuretics and β-blockers with these new classes of agents are underway, but results are not yet available to influence a change in treatment recommendations.

The above appraisal of diuretics and β-blockers should not imply that all patients should be started on one of these two classes of agents. As noted, individual patients may have relative contraindications to the use of these drugs. In addition, requisite consideration of other factors, including demographic characteristics, concomitant illnesses, cost of medication, metabolic and subjective side effects, and potential drug interactions, should all influence subsequent therapeutic decisions. The stepped-care treatment algorithm included in the JNC-V report does not exclude the concept of individualizing the initial selection of an antihypertensive agent nor the selected use of a fixed combination.

Combining antihypertensive drugs with different modes of action will often allow smaller doses of drugs to be used to achieve control and minimize the potential for dose-dependent side effects. If a diuretic is not selected as the first drug, it will often be useful as a second-step agent because its addition usually enhances the effects of other agents. If addition of a second agent produces satisfactory BP control, an attempt to withdraw the first agent may be considered because monotherapy with virtually all drugs can provide BP control for upward of one-half of patients treated.

The selected use of fixed combinations is included in the modified treatment algorithm. Prior JNC reports and most clinical treatment recommmendations discouraged the use of these agents, especially for initial therapy. Many of the early fixed-drug combinations were inappropriate from the standpoint of dosages offered or the duration of action of individual drug components. Some of the earliest fixed combinations included agents with very short duration of action in the same tablet with agents of long duration of action. Newer fixed combinations (see Table 6) offer the advantage of more appropriate dosages (eg, small doses of diuretics) together with prolonged duration of action for each component to facilitate once-daily dosing. Newer combinations have also taken advantage of clinical data supporting the additive effects of the individual components when used together.

In patients with high-normal, labile, or borderline hypertension, pharmacologic therapy would not seem appropriate at this time. However, efforts at lifestyle modification would certainly be indicated, particularly in patients with other cardiovascular risk factors.

For patients with stage 1 hypertension, pharmacologic therapy is indicated, particularly if 3–6 months of lifestyle modification failed to normalize BP. For patients with stage 1 hypertension and without evident target organ damage or other major risk factors, no clear consensus exists regarding initiating drug therapy. As noted earlier, emerging information from selected clinical trials suggested that such patients may benefit from pharmacologic therapy.[7,17] For all patients with stage 2 or 3 severity hypertension, pharmacologic therapy is indicated even in the presence or absence of evident target organ damage or other major risk factors. Evidence supports the aggressive treatment of hypertension for all hypertensive patients; although the initial goal of treatment outlined in JNC-V was 140/90 mm Hg with concurrent control of other cardiovascular risk factors, the author feels that further reductions in BP should be pursued with due regard for cardiovascular function, especially in older patients. If BP of 120/80 mm Hg is indeed representative of "normal" BP in our society and with disappointing results to date in control efforts in hypertension,

Table 6
Selected Combinations Tablets

Drug	Dosage (mg)	Brand Name
β blocker/diuretic		
Atenolol/chlorthalidone	50/25	Tenoretic
	100/25	
Bisoprolol/HCTZ*	2.5/6.25	Ziac
	5/6.25	
	10/6.25	
Nadolol/bendroflumathiazide	40/5	Corzide
	80/5	
ACE[†] inhibitor/diuretic		
Lisinopril/HCTZ	10/12.5	Zestoretic
	20/12.5	Prinizide
	20/25	
Benazepril/HCTZ	5/6.25	Lotensin HCT
	10/12.5	
	20/12.5	
	20/25	
Calcium antagonist/ACE inhibitor		
Amlodipine/benazepril	2.5/10	Lotrel
	5/10	
	5/20	
Felodipine/enalapril	5/5	Lexxel
Trandolapril/verapamil	1/240	Tarka
HCL (ER)	2/180	
	2/240	
	4/240	

* HCTZ: hydrochlorothiazide.
† ACE: angiotensin-converting enzyme.

it would seem time to revise BP goals downward to 130/80 mm Hg, and even lower in patients with coexisting risk factors not amenable to treatment, or for which there is no evidence that treatment will reduce risk.[18]

For patients with stage 3 hypertension (DBP ≥110 mm Hg or SBP ≥180 mm Hg), effective treatment may require more than one agent or the possible addition of a third agent after a short interval if control is still not achieved. Initiation of therapy with a fixed-combination preparation in patients with stage 3 hypertension can be especially appropriate. Certainly, if the fixed combination does not contain a diuretic, the early addition of a diuretic as a third agent is indicated if initial control is inadequate. Achieving and maintaining target BP with the lowest possible dose of medication is a primary goal of antihypertensive therapy and will require ongoing patient follow-up, possibly involving periodic dosage readjustments. Follow-up at 3- to 4-month intervals is adequate in controlled hypertensive patients, although associated target organ damage and other cardiovascular risk factors will play a role in the frequency of visits.

Stepped-Down Therapy

After BP has been effectively controlled for 6–12 months, it may be possible to reduce antihypertensive drug dosages in a planned, progressive manner. Stepped-down therapy can be particularly successful in patients who adhered to other lifestyle modification recommendations and will often maintain controlled BP levels with reduced doses of medication or occasionally, no medication.

Supplemental Antihypertensive Agents

Other available agents such as the direct-acting vasodilators, α_2-agonists, and peripherally acting adrenergic neuron antagonists, including the rauwolfia alkaloids, are generally not well suited for initial therapy in the treatment of hypertension because they cause more side effects that may limit adherence to therapy. The direct-acting smooth muscle vasodilators (hydralazine and minoxidil) often induce reflex sympathetic stimulation of the cardiovascular system and fluid retention and are most effectively used in association with an adrenergic-blocking agent and diuretic. The α_2-agonists (clonidine, guanabenz, guanfacine, and methyldopa) induce annoying drowsiness and dry mouth in most patients. None of these agents should be withdrawn abruptly because of the risk of "rebound" hypertension, especially with moderate to higher dosages. Peripherally acting adrenergic antagonists such as guanadrel or guanethidine can cause orthostatic and exercise-induced hypotension, while the sedative and depressive effects of the rauwolfia alkaloids led to a progressive decline in use. A transdermal preparation of clonidine (TTS) can be better tolerated in small doses than the oral preparation and may be useful as monotherapy in carefully selected patients.

These supplemental agents are all effective antihypertensives and can be useful as "add-on" agents in patients with severe or refractory hypertension. They can also be useful in patients with hypertensive urgencies or emergencies.

Individualizing Antihypertensive Therapy

A knowledge of the clinical pharmacology of the different classes of antihypertensive agents together with their practical advantages, disadvantages, adverse effects, and potential drug interactions should enable the clinician to select the most appropriate initial therapy for most hypertensive patients. The following paragraphs will examine some of these issues for the classes of agents recommended for initiation of antihypertensive therapy. Additional information on the clinical pharmacology, indications, and clinical recommendations of these classes of agents is available from several sources.[19–22]

Oral Diuretics

Patients receiving thiazide or loop diuretics should receive lower doses and undergo dietary counseling to avoid metabolic changes. Diuretics are especially indicated in hypertensive patients with edema, blacks, the elderly, and obese hypertensive patients. The early tendency for sodium and water retention in patients with chronic renal insufficiency is an indication for diuretics, as is CHF. Hypertensive patients with recurrent renal calculi, particularly those who are demonstrated to hypersecrete calcium, may benefit from a nonloop diuretic.

Hyperuricemia, hypokalemia, and hypercalcemia, the most commonly observed metabolic abnormalities caused by diuretics, clearly pose less of a problem now that smaller daily doses are used. Hyperglycemia and hypercholesterolemia are occasionally observed, and sexual dysfunction may present a problem. Cholestyramine and cholestipol decrease absorption of diuretics and nonsteroidal anti-inflammatory drugs (NSAIDs) may antagonize diuretic effectiveness. As a general rule, the longer-acting thiazides are more appropriate for patients with normal renal excretory function, whereas the loop diuretics may be more useful for patients with renal insufficiency (serum creatinine >2.0 mg/dL).

Potassium-sparing combinations should be avoided in patients with renal insufficiency and may cause hyperkalemia when combined with ACE inhibitors or potassium supplements.

β-Adrenergic Blockers

For the patient who survives a myocardial infarction, a β-blocker may be especially indicated because of the cardioprotective effects of this class, particularly the agents without intrinsic sympathomimetic activity (ISA), or α-blocking properties. Young hypertensive patients, especially whites with hyperkinetic circulation, respond particularly well to β-blockers. The antianginal and antiarrhythmic effects of β-blockers make them particularly useful in hypertensive patients with coronary artery disease (CAD) or supraventricular arrhythmias. Migraine headache and senile tremor also respond well to these agents, should they represent associated problems in the hypertensive patient. Other special indications include severe hypertrophic cardiomyopathy and, possibly, severe asymmetric septal hypertrophy without flow obstruction.

β-Blockers should not be used in patients with asthma, chronic obstructive pulmonary disease (COPD), heart block more than first degree, or sick sinus syndrome. Whereas β-blockers were generally considered contraindicated in CHF with systolic dysfunction, current research suggests that they can be of benefit in low doses to patients with dilated cardiomyopathy when added to standard therapy. Dosages being tested in CHF are generally lower than those used in hypertension.

β-Blockers should be used with caution in insulin-treated diabetic patients and patients with peripheral vascular disease, in whom peripheral arterial insufficiency may be aggravated. Increased triglycerides and decreased HDL-C are observed, except with β-blockers with ISA. Fatigue, insomnia, and reduced exercise tolerance may also accompany their use.

Cimetidine may increase serum levels of β-blockers that are primarily metabolized by the liver due to enzyme inhibition, and combinations of negative inotropic calcium antagonists with β-blockers may have additive sinoatrial (SA) and atrial-ventricular depressant effects.

α-β–Blockers

The α-β–blocker labetalol has a mechanism of action similar to that of β-blockers plus α_1-blockade, which may cause postural effects. Titration should therefore be based on standing BP. This agent may be more effective in blacks than other β-blockers. Its adverse effects are similar to those of other β-active agents, but labetalol may have lesser adverse effects on blood lipids, cardiac output, and heart rate. Second-generation vasodilating β-blockers also demonstrated efficacy when used in low dosages in addition to standard therapy for patients with CHF.

α_1-Blockers

These agents block postsynaptic α_1-receptors and cause vasodilation. All may cause postural effects. Titration should be based on standing BP. Special indications include hypertension with DM or lipid abnormalities, since these agents do not adversely affect carbohydrate tolerance or lipid parameters. Hypertensive men with benign prostatic hypertrophy may experience relief of early obstructive symptoms with these agents. The major adverse effects are orthostatic hypotension, weakness, palpitations, headaches, and occasional syncope. These agents should be used cautiously in older patients because of the risk of orthostatic hypotension.

Angiotensin-Converting Enzyme Inhibitors

Special indications for ACE inhibitors include hypertension with CHF or left ventricular (LV) dysfunction following myocardial infarction

(MI). There is some evidence to indicate that favorable cardiac remodeling may occur under the influence of these agents. Younger hypertensive patients, particularly whites, appear to respond especially well to this class of drugs. Captopril and probably other ACE inhibitors proved effective in delaying the progression of chronic renal disease in patients with type I insulin-dependent DM (IDDM). Preliminary evidence suggests benefit in patients with type II diabetes with nephropathy and in other hypertensive conditions associated with renal parenchymal disease and proteinuria. No adverse effects are seen on carbohydrate tolerance or lipid metabolism. The most common adverse effect is cough; rash, angioneurotic edema, hyperkalemia, and dysgeusia were also observed. Hypotension was observed especially in patients with high plasma renin activity, such as that associated with diuretic therapy. Acute reversible renal failure may be seen with bilateral renal artery stenosis or unilateral stenosis in a solitary kidney.

In patients taking ACE inhibitors, NSAIDs (including aspirin) may decrease BP control and hyperkalemia may be more prevalent with potassium supplements, potassium-sparing agents, and NSAIDs. ACE inhibitors may increase serum lithium levels.

Calcium Antagonists

Whereas all calcium antagonists block calcium transport across cell membranes and cause smooth muscle relaxation, verapamil and diltiazem may also block slow channels in the heart and may reduce sinus rate and produce heart block. The dihydropyridine calcium antagonists are more potent vasodilators and may cause dizziness, flushing, and peripheral edema. Constipation is more commonly observed with verapamil and diltiazem. Particular indications are seen in hypertensive patients with angina pectoris or paroxysmal tachyrhythmia. Elderly patients, especially blacks, respond well, whereas associated conditions such as migraine headache and esophageal spasm may provide special indications. Secondary cardioprotection in patients who had a non–Q-wave infarction and pulmonary hypertension provide further potential indications.

Verapamil and diltiazem should be used with caution in patients with CHF, whereas dihydropyridines may aggravate angina and myocardial ischemia. Use with caution in patients with second- and third-degree heart block or sick sinus syndromes. Calcium antagonists appear lipid neutral and have little effect on carbohydrate metabolism. Cimetidine may increase the pharmacologic effects of all calcium antagonists through inhibition of hepatic metabolizing enzymes, resulting in increased serum levels. Verapamil and possibly diltiazem increase the serum levels of digoxin and carbamezapine, potentially leading to toxicity. Serum levels of cyclosporine are increased by diltiazem, nicardipine, and verapamil.

Angiotensin II Receptor Antagonists

These agents are highly selective antagonists for the angiotensin-1 (AT-1) receptor and block the vasoconstrictor and aldosterone-secreting effects of AII by inhibiting the binding of AII to the AT-1 receptor. AII antagonists appear to mimic many of the effects of ACE inhibitors through their inhibition of the renin-angiotensin aldosterone system. Theoretically, AII antagonists could provide a more complete blockade than ACE inhibitors, since they act further downstream at the tissue receptors.

Although they may be beneficial in any hypertensive patients in whom an ACE inhibitor would seem particularly appropriate, AII antagonists have two distinct advantages unlike ACE inhibitors: they do not induce cough and they cause angioneurotic edema much less frequently.

The prototype AII receptor antagonist losartan may induce headache or, less frequently, complications such as back pain, diarrhea, fatigue, or nasal congestion. Several new AII receptor antagonists are undergoing development and may be available for clinical use within the next 12 months. Medications affecting the angiotensin system, such as losartan, can cause fetal and neonatal morbidity and mortality when given to pregnant women and should therefore be avoided.

Resistant Hypertension

With the availability of so many highly effective antihypertensive agents, hypertension resistant to treatment should be unusual. The incidence of resistant hypertension is variable, ranging from 0.3% in a work site control program to as high as 13% of patients seen in a referral care center.[23,24] Hypertension can be considered resistant if BP remains >140/90 mm Hg, despite administration of maximal recommended doses of three drugs, including an oral diuretic plus two of the following classes of agents: a β-adrenergic blocker or other antiadrenergic agent, a direct vasodilator or calcium antagonist, and an ACE inhibitor or AII receptor antagonist. The most frequent causes of resistance are suboptimal treatment, drug interactions, drug intolerance, and patient nonadherence. Patient factors may include the use of over-the-counter substances, excess intake of alcohol or sodium, or use of illicit drugs.[24] Volume overload is a common occurrence in patients with resistant hypertension and should be suspected in patients treated with a regimen that does not include an oral diuretic. Physicians must also recognize the superiority of thiazide diuretics in patients with normal renal function and loop diuretics to control plasma volume in patients with renal insufficiency. Obese hypertensive patients do not respond as well as leaner patients to antihypertensive therapy, particularly to centrally acting agents or β-adrenergic blockers. Those with glucose intolerance and insulin resistance may also require higher drug doses.

If drug-related causes are ruled out and the patient is compliant, look for a secondary cause of hypertension such as renal parenchymal disease, renal artery stenosis, or primary aldosteronism. Also consider the occasional occurrence of pseudohypertension,[25] especially in an older patient, and the possibility of office hypertension.

A systematic evaluation of patients with suspected resistant hypertension should identify its cause in the majority of cases. An algorithm that may be helpful in approaching such a patient appears as Figure 4.[26] If an explanation for the resistance to therapy is not found after this orderly investigation, it may be appropriate to consider arbitrary increases in medication to levels above usual recommended doses or possibly the

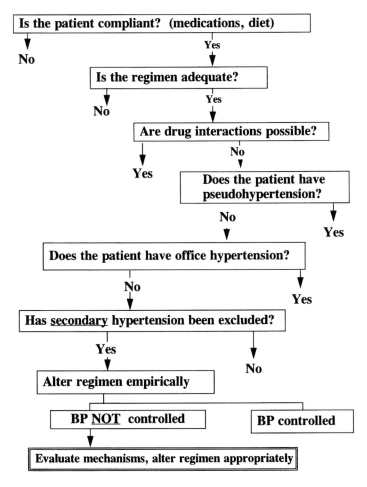

Figure 4. *Algorithm for management of resistant hypertension. Reproduced with permission from Reference 26.*

addition of a fourth or fifth agent to the regimen. In the occasional patient who remains refractory to therapy despite the above efforts, careful hemo-dynamic evaluation, including assessment of cardiac hemodynamics, blood and plasma volume, as well as concentrations of catecholamines, renin, and aldosterone, may provide clues that will enable more targeted selection of antihypertensive drug therapy.

Hypertensive Urgencies and Emergencies

Improved public health efforts over the past two decades to detect and treat arterial hypertension resulted in a sharp decrease in the prev-alence of accelerated or malignant hypertension. Most hypertensive ur-gencies and emergencies arise as a result of poorly controlled chronic hypertension. Clearly, increased awareness, widespread detection ef-forts, and more aggressive therapy for stage 1 and 2 hypertension con-tributed to this progressive decline in the incidence rate of hypertensive urgencies and emergencies. Nevertheless, a true hypertensive emer-gency still represents a clinical situation requiring immediate reduction in BP (not necessarily to normal levels) to limit or prevent target organ damage. A hypertensive emergency should be treated with a parenteral agent that enables titratable dosing to facilitate a controlled reduction in BP. The initial goal of treatment should be to reduce DBP to no more than 100–110 mm Hg or the mean arterial pressure by no more than 20% to 25% initially.[27–29] If this degree of BP reduction is well tolerated, further gradual reductions in BP can be accomplished over the next 24–48 hours.

A distinction between a true emergency and a hypertensive urgency can be helpful in determining the required expediency for therapy as well as the selection and rate of administration of appropriate drugs (Table 7). Hypertensive urgencies are associated with severely elevated BP but with-out severe symptoms or progressive target organ dysfunction. Adequate treatment of a hypertensive urgency can be achieved by lowering BP within 24–48 hours, usually with oral agents.[30,31]

In practice, most cases of hypertensive urgencies are in asymptomatic patients who are noncompliant or poorly controlled on current regimens; a few have newly diagnosed hypertension. Nonspecific symptoms are common, including headaches, dizziness, or weakness, which might be due to elevated BP. There are no data available showing any benefit in rapidly lowering the BP in asymptomatic patients with severe hyperten-sion. On the other hand, scattered reports suggest potential harm to pa-tients from precipitous reduction in BP, particularly in those with signif-icant cardiovascular risk factors.

Table 7
Hypertensive Emergencies and Urgencies

Hypertensive Emergencies

Hypertensive encephalopathy
Malignant hypertension (some cases)
Severe hypertension in association with acute cerebral, renal, or cardiac
    complications
    Intracerebral hemorrhage
    Subarachnoid hemorrhage
    Acute atherothrombotic brain infarction (with severe hypertension)
    Rapidly progressive renal failure
    Acute aortic dissection
    Acute left ventricular failure with pulmonary edema
    Acute myocardial infarction
    Unstable angina
Eclampsia
Catecholamine excess states
    Pheochromocytoma crisis
    Food or drug interactions (tyramine) with monoamine oxidase inhibitors
    Some cases of rebound hypertension following sudden withdrawal of
        antihypertensive agents (ie, clonidine, guanabenz, methyldopa)
Overdose with sympathomimetics or drugs with similar action (eg, phencyclidine,
    lysergic acid diethylamide (LSD), cocaine, phenylpropanolamine)
Head trauma
Post-coronary artery bypass hypertension
Postoperative bleeding at vascular suture lines

Hypertensive Urgencies

Accelerated and malignant hypertension
Extensive body burns*
Acute glomerulonephritis with severe hypertension*
Scleroderma crisis
Acute systemic vasculitis with severe hypertension*
Surgically related hypertension
    Severe hypertension in patients requiring immediate surgery*
    Postoperative hypertension*
    Severe hypertension after kidney transplantation
Severe epistaxis
Episodic and severe hypertension associated with chronic spinal cord injury:
    autonomic hyperreflexia syndrome*

* At times may become a true hypertensive emergency.

For the patient with a true hypertensive emergency, immediate hospitalization is warranted. The initial examination should focus on determining the degree of target organ involvement and possible clues to a secondary and possibly reversible cause of hypertension. Prompt initiation of therapy should take precedence over time-consuming diagnostic procedures. Additional diagnostic studies, if necessary, can be undertaken after BP is safely controlled.

For most patients with severe hypertension or "a hypertensive urgency," but without symptoms or evident target organ dysfunction, initiation of treatment (or resumption of prior antihypertensive therapy) is appropriate. Therapy should probably be initiated with two agents, followed by a third agent if necessary, within 24–48 hours. Drug titration to control BP can be accomplished over several days to several weeks according to general guidelines outlined earlier in this chapter for the management of stage 3 hypertension. Parenteral agents available for the treatment of hypertensive emergencies are listed in Table 8. They were divided into parenteral vasodilators and adrenergic inhibiting agents. In most instances, parenteral agents should be given for several hours to no more than 24 hours. When an initial goal BP is achieved and the patient is stable, oral medications should be considered. Any approved oral agent can be used in combination for the initial management of a hypertensive urgency. Captopril, clonidine, and labetalol may prove particularly useful by oral administration in the initial management of such an urgency, by modified loading doses, or by frequent readministration as noted in the table. These oral agents do not generally produce a precipitous reduction in BP, and their duration of action can be prolonged. In the case of captopril, there is limited evidence to suggest that it may be effective by sublingual administration.

A word of caution regarding immediate-release nifedipine: this agent was used widely during the last decade for the initial management of hypertensive urgencies and some emergencies, despite cautions expressed regarding the precipitous reduction in BP observed with its use and numerous case reports of ischemic events following its administration. In the past year these concerns were greatly heightened with additional reports attesting to increased coronary mortality,[32] association with an increased cancer risk,[33] and concerns regarding gastrointestinal bleeding in patients treated with it. Given the seriousness of the reported adverse events, the Food and Drug Administration (FDA) discouraged the use of this agent for treating hypertension, a use that does not have specific FDA approval. In view of these concerns, it is recommended that immediate-release nifedipine be deleted from hospital and emergency room formularies and specifically should not be used in the management of hypertension in either urgent or long-term care situations.[34] For optimal management of the patient with a hypertensive urgency or emergency, it is imperative that the clinician have a thorough knowledge of the pharmacologic properties and proper indications for currently available agents.

Table 8

Management of Hypertensive Emergencies and Urgencies

Agent	Dose	Onset/Duration of Action (after discontinuation)	Precautions
		Parenteral Vasodilators	
Sodium nitroprusside	0.25–10 μg/kg/min as IV infusion; maximal dose for 10 min only	Immediate/2–3 min following infusion	Nausea, vomiting, muscle twitching; with prolonged use may cause thiocyanate intoxication, methemoglobinemia; acidosis, cyanide poisoning; bags, bottles and delivery sets must be light resistant
Nitroglycerine	5–100 μg as IV infusion	2–5 min/5–10 min	Headache, tachycardia, vomiting, flushing, methemoglobinemia; requires special delivery system due to drug binding to PVC tubing
Nicardipine	5–15 mg/h IV infusion	1–5 min/15–30 min, but may exceed 12 h after prolonged infusion	Tachycardia, nausea, vomiting, headache, increased intracranial pressure; hypotension, may be promoted after prolonged infusions
Verapamil	5–10 mg IV; can follow with infusion of 3–25 mg/h	1–5 min/30–60 min	Heart block (1°, 2°, 3°), concomitant digitalis and β blockers, bradycardia
Diazoxide	50–150 mg as IV bolus, repeated, or 15–30 mg/min by IV infusion	2–5 min/3–12 h	Hypotension, tachycardia, aggravation of angina pectoris, nausea and vomiting, hyperglycemia with repeated injections
Hydralazine	10–20 mg as IV bolus or 10–40 mg IM, repeat every 4–6 h	10 min IV/>1 h (IM) 20–30 min IV/4–6 h (IM)	Tachycardia, headache, vomiting, aggravation of angina pectoris

continues

Table 8 Continued

Management of Hypertensive Emergencies and Urgencies

Agent	Dose	Onset/Duration of Action (after discontinuation)	Precautions
Enalaprilat	0.625–1.25 mg every 6 h IV	15–60 min/12–24 h	Renal failure in patients with bilateral renal artery stenosis, hypotension
Parenteral Adrenergic Inhibitors			
Labetalol	20–80 mg as IV bolus every 10 min; 2 mg/min as IV infusion	5–10 min/2–6 h	Bronchoconstriction, heart block, orthostatic hypotension
Esmolol	500 µg/kg/bolus injection IV or 25–100 µg/kg/min by infusion; may rebolus after 5 min or increase infusion rate to 300 µg/kg/min	1–5 min/18–30 min	>1° heart block, CHF, asthma
Methyldopate	250–500 mg as IV infusion every 6 h	30–60 min/4–6 h	Drowsiness
Phentolamine	5–15 mg as IV bolus	1–2 min/30–120 min	Tachycardia, orthostatic hypotension
Oral Agents			
Captopril	25 mg PO, repeat as needed SL, 25 mg	15–30 min/6–8 h SL 15–30 min/2–6 h	Hypotension, renal failure in bilateral renal artery stenosis
Clonidine	0.1–0.2 mg PO, repeat as required	30–60 min/8–16 h	Hypotension, drowsiness, dry mouth
Labetalol	200–400 mg PO, repeat every 2–3 h	30 min–2 h/2–12 h	Bronchoconstriction, heart block, orthostatic hypotension
Prazosin	1–2 mg PO; repeat each h, as needed	1–2 h/8–12 h	Syncope (1st dose), palpitations, tachycardia, orthostatic hypotension

IV, intravenous; IM, intramusculur; h, hour; PO, by mouth.

Hypertension in the Elderly

The elderly are a growing segment of the hypertensive population worldwide. It is projected that the population over age 65 in the United States will increase 40% by the year 2000 and will reach 70 million by the year 2030. Moreover, it is the oldest stratum of our society that is increasing most rapidly. Approximately 1% was over age 85 in 1985, and this figure is predicted to reach 7 million by the year 2030.

Hypertension in the elderly can be divided into systolic-diastolic hypertension (SBP 140 mm Hg or more and/or DBP 90 mm Hg or more), which is seen in younger age groups, and ISH, where SBP is 140 mm Hg or more and DBP is less than 90 mm Hg. The prevalence of hypertension among black men and women aged 64–74 years is higher (72%) than that observed among white and Mexican-American counterparts.[2] In fact, age-specific estimates of the prevalence of hypertension among non-Hispanic black men and women are higher for every age group among black women and for all ages except those over 80 years. For every age and racial group up to 59 years of age, men had a higher rate of age-specific hypertension than women. However, the reverse is true for non-Hispanic black and Mexican-American men and women 60 years of age and older and non-Hispanic men and women 70 years of age and older.

SBP and DBP elevations represent primary hypertension in the majority of cases, as is true for younger individuals for whom secondary causes of hypertension are rare. When secondary hypertension is seen in individuals over age 65, it most commonly relates to atherosclerotic renal vascular disease.

The elderly also develop ISH. Using the current definition of normotension or target BP as SBP of 140 mm Hg or more, with a DBP under 90 mm Hg, 65% of those over age 60 will have ISH. As noted earlier, SBP may represent a more important prognostic index for CVD than high DBP in the elderly.

Morbidity and mortality data clearly demonstrated the excess cardiovascular risk associated with untreated SBP and DBP elevations in the elderly, and it was established that these risks can be reduced by treatment that effectively lowers BP. Studies confirming these beneficial effects include the hypertension, detection and follow-up program (HDFP),[35] the Australian Therapeutic Trial in mild hypertension,[36] and the European Working Party on High Blood Pressure in the Elderly trial.[37] Three more recent studies on elderly hypertensives deserve mention. The Swedish Trial in Old Patients with Hypertension randomized 1627 patients aged 70–74 years to active treatment and placebo. Active treatment significantly reduced the number of primary end points and both stroke morbidity and mortality. Although the study was not designed to assess effects on total mortality, a significant reduction in deaths was noted in the active treatment group.[38] The Medical Research Council trial of treatment of hypertension in older adults reported results on 4396 patients aged 65–74 years, randomized to receive a diuretic, β-blocker, or placebo. Both treatments reduced BP below the level observed in the placebo group. The diuretics significantly reduced the risk of stroke by 31%, coronary events by 44%, and all cardiovascular events by 35%, compared with the placebo group. The β-blockers showed no significant reduction in these end points. The reduction in strokes was mainly in nonsmokers taking the diuretic.[39] The Systolic Hypertension in the Elderly program (SHEP) study demonstrated the ability of drug therapy to reduce BP among persons with ISH.[9] A total of 4936 persons age 60 and older were randomized to active treatment with a diuretic-based regimen or placebo. The primary objective of SHEP was to assess the ability of antihypertensive drug treatment to reduce the risk of nonfatal and fatal stroke in ISH. Secondary objectives included assessment of antihypertensive treatment on multiple cardiovascular morbidity and mortality end points including cardiac end points, all-cause mortality, and quality of life measures. After an average follow-up of 4 years, antihypertensive step-care drug treatment with low-dose chlorthalidone as step 1 medication reduced the incidence of total stroke by 36% and the incidence of fatal and nonfatal coronary events was reduced by 27%.

Treatment Considerations in the Elderly

The capacity of lifestyle modification to reduce morbidity and mortality in older patients with hypertension was not conclusively demonstrated. However, because of their ability to improve the cardiovascular risk profile, lifestyle modifications, properly used, may offer multiple benefits at little cost and with minimal risk to the older patient.

Dietary measures (sodium and caloric restriction) can be tried first as an alternative to drug therapy for elderly patients with stage 1 or 2 hypertension. Care must be taken to ensure through education and counseling that any new restricted diet is adequate for the older patient who may already have a marginal diet. Excessive ethanol intake presents problems for older patients similar to those in other sectors of the population. Tobacco use should be avoided since it represents a major risk factor for CVD. Physical exercise should be encouraged for the elderly to the limits of their abilities, even though it may not be achievable to those levels encouraged for younger hypertensive individuals.

The benefits of treating systolic and diastolic hypertension in the elderly are now well documented. The goal of treatment should be similar to that for younger patients, that is, to reduce DBP to <90 mm Hg and SBP to <140 mm Hg. If well tolerated, further reductions can be considered. It must be remembered that a contracted plasma volume and reduced baroreflex sensitivity may affect the responsiveness of elderly patients to therapy, particularly to those drugs that tend to induce postural changes in BP. These postural changes may further intensify the existing tendency to postural reductions in BP observed in many elderly patients with position changes.

Together with control of BP, avoidance of adverse effects should encourage the use of the lowest effective doses of any antihypertensive agents when used alone or in combination. As for younger patients, the clinician should keep in mind the potential beneficial or adverse effects on other concomitant diseases and potential adverse metabolic effects that may be associated with selected antihypertensive agents. Decreases in renal and/or hepatic function with age may increase the risk of drug accumulation since all antihypertensive agents are metabolized in the liver and/or excreted by the kidneys. Multiple other pharmacologic agents being utilized by older individuals may increase the risk of drug interactions with antihypertensive agents. Clinicians must also be aware of potential central nervous system (CNS) effects of selected agents that may cause confusion or depression in the elderly patient. A primary goal of treatment should be the maintenance of an optimal quality of life for the treated hypertensive, regardless of age.

In initiating therapy in the elderly, it is appropriate to reduce usual initial adult doses by one-half and to gradually increase daily dosages over a period of weeks. Patients should be seen frequently, every 2–4 weeks until BP is stabilized. Once control is achieved, usual follow-up at 3–4 months is advisable. Keep in mind the importance of avoiding the induction of orthostatic hypotension in older patients. In selecting initial antihypertensive therapy, JNC-V recommendations as outlined earlier in this chapter are appropriate. Older patients respond particularly well to oral diuretics. These agents together with adrenergic blockers are preferred if no contraindications exist for their use and/or there are no special indications for choosing an alternate initial agent.

Finally, how low should BP be reduced in the elderly hypertensive patients? If cardiovascular risks are increased at all levels of BP >120/80 mm Hg, what levels of BP on treatment are appropriate and safe for the elderly hypertensive patients? The goal for DBP is a bit unclear, but it would appear to be safe to reduce it to at least 85 mm Hg. In the HDFP,[35] the average DBP in the elderly group at the end of 5 years was 81 mm Hg. Although some authorities expressed concern about a "J-curve" phenomenon (in which the risk of coronary mortality might paradoxically increase if DBP is reduced below a critical level), the average DBP was 68 mm Hg at the end of the 5-year SHEP trial in the actively treated group, and there was no evidence of a J-curve in this important trial. Although there are no randomized trials to show that treatment of borderline ISH

(SBP 140–159 mm Hg, DBP <90 mm Hg) reduces cardiovascular morbidity and mortality, it is evident that these levels of BP do increase the risk of CVD and progress to more severe hypertension. The benefits of pharmacologic therapy for hypertension were demonstrated for patients in their 80s.[9,40] Fletcher and Bulpitt[18] summarized studies relating the level of BP during treatment for hypertension to the risks of stroke and CHD

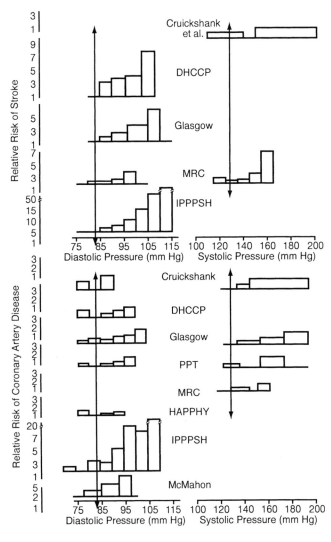

Figure 5. *Relative risks of stroke and CHD according to BP during treatment for hypertension in eight studies and meta analyses. Reproduced with permission from Reference 18.*

in an effort to identify optimal BP to be achieved by treatment (Figure 5). Based on their review of observational follow-up studies and randomized trials, primarily involving those with stage 1 to 2 hypertension, they concluded that it appeared reasonable to lower DBP to <85 mm Hg to provide maximal benefit of reducing the risks of strokes and MI compared to those risks in patients with DBP >100 mm Hg. They recommended that SBP should be lowered to <125 mm Hg since there was no indication that doing so had any adverse effects.

These treatment goals are more aggressive than those recommended in any current treatment guidelines for managing hypertension. Yet, given the disappointing treatment results outlined earlier in this chapter, it would seem appropriate and logical to consider more aggressive treatment goals on a population basis in an effort to induce further reductions in risks from hypertension. Certainly the issue of lower target levels for BP reduction will be given careful consideration by future JNC Reports and by other published hypertension treatment guidelines.

References

1. Joint National Committee on Detection. Evaluation and treatment of high blood pressure. The 5th report of the Joint National Committee on Detection, Evaluation, and Treatment of High Blood Pressure (JNCV). *Arch Intern Med* 1993;153:154–183.
2. Burt VL, Wheaton P, Roccella EJ, et al. Prevalence of hypertension in the US adult population. Results from the Third National Health and Nutrition Examination Survey, 1988–1991. *Hypertension* 1995;25:305–313.
3. MacMahon S, Peto R, Cutler J, et al. Blood pressure, stroke, and coronary heart disease. Part 1, prolonged differences in blood pressure: prospective observational studies corrected for the regression dilution bias. *Lancet* 1990; 335:765–774.
4. Stamler J, Stamler R, Neaton JD. Blood pressure, systolic and diastolic, and cardiovascular risks. US population data. *Arch Intern Med* 1993;153:598–615.
5. Julius S, Jamerson K, Mejia A, et al. The association of borderline hypertension with target organ changes and higher coronary risk. Tecumseh Blood Pressure study. *JAMA* 1990;264:354–358.
6. National High Blood Pressure Education Program Working Group. 1995 Update of the working group reports on chronic renal failure and renovascular hypertension. *Arch Intern Med* 1996;156:1938–1947.
7. Neaton JD, Grimm RH Jr, Prineas RJ, et al. Treatment of mild hypertension study. Final results. *JAMA* 1993;270:713–724.
8. Sagie A, Larson MG, Levy D. The natural history of borderline isolated systolic hypertension. *N Engl J Med* 1993;329:1912–1917.
9. SHEP Cooperative Research Group. Prevention of stroke by antihypertensive drug treatment in older persons with isolated systolic hypertension: final results of the Systolic Hypertension in the Elderly Program (SHEP). *JAMA* 1991;265:3255–3264.
10. Kannel WB. Cardiovascular risk factors in the older adult. *Hosp Pract* 1996;31:135–150.

11. Kannel WB. Hypertension. Relationship with other risk factors. *Drugs* 1986;31(suppl 1):1–11.
12. National High Blood Pressure Education Program Working Group. National High Blood Pressure Education Program Working Group report on primary prevention of hypertension. *Arch Intern Med* 1993;153:186–208.
13. Law MR, Frost CD, Wald NJ. By how much does dietary salt reduction lower blood pressure? III. Analysis of data from trials of salt reduction. *Br Med J* 1991;302:819–824.
14. Cutler JA, Follmann D, Elliott P, et al. An overview of randomized trials of sodium reduction and blood pressure. *Hypertension* 1991;17:I27–I33.
15. Kaplan NM, Carnegie A, Raskin P, et al. Potassium supplementation in hypertensive patients with diuretic-induced hypokalemia. *N Engl J Med* 1985;312:746–749.
16. Harlan WR, Hull AL, Schmouder RL, et al. Blood pressure and nutrition in adults. The National Health and Nutrition Examination Survey. *Am J Epidemiol* 1984;120:17–28.
17. Materson BJ, Reda DJ, Cushman WC, et al. Department of Veterans Affairs Cooperative Study Group on Antihypertensive Agents: single-drug therapy for hypertension in men: a comparison of six antihypertensive agents with placebo [see Correction appears in *N Engl J Med* 1994;330:1689]. *N Engl J Med* 1993;328:914–921.
18. Fletcher AE, Bulpitt CJ. How far should blood pressure be lowered? *N Engl J Med* 1992;326:251–254.
19. Swales JD, ed. *Textbook of Hypertension.* Oxford, UK: Blackwell Scientific; 1994.
20. Izzo JL, Black HR, eds. *Hypertension Primer.* Dallas, TX: American Heart Association; 1993.
21. *Drug Evaluations.* Chicago, IL: American Medical Association; 1996.
22. United States Pharmacopeia—Drug Information. *Drug Information for the Health Care Professional.* 16th ed, vol I. Rockville, MD: United States Pharmacological Convention; 1996.
23. Alderman MH, Budner N, Cohen H, et al. Prevalence of drug resistant hypertension. *Hypertension* 1988;11:II71–II75.
24. Yakovlevitch M, Black HR. Resistant hypertension in a tertiary care clinic. *Arch Intern Med* 1991;151:1786–1792.
25. Zuschke CA, Pettyjohn FS. Pseudohypertension. *South Med J* 1995;88:1185–1190.
26. Gifford RW Jr. An algorithm for the management of resistant hypertension. *Hypertension* 1988;11:II101–II105.
27. Kaplan NM. Management of hypertensive emergencies. *Lancet* 1994;344:1335–1338.
28. Murphy C. Hypertensive emergencies. *Emerg Med Clin North Am* 1995; 13:973–1007.
29. Bedoya LA, Vidt DG. Treatment of the hypertensive emergency. In: Jacobson HR, Striker GE, Klahr S, eds. *The Principles and Practice of Nephrology.* 15th ed. Philadelphia, PA: BC Decker; 1991:547–557.
30. Thach AM, Schultz PJ. Nonemergent hypertension. New perspectives for the emergency medicine physician. *Emerg Med Clin North Am* 1995;13:1009–1035.
31. Gales MA. Oral antihypertensives for hypertensive urgencies. *Ann Pharmacother* 1994;28:352–358.
32. Furberg CD, Psaty BM, Meyer JV. Nifedipine. Dose-related increase in mortality in patients with coronary heart disease. *Circulation* 1995;92:1326–1331.

33. Pahor M, Guralnik JM, Ferrucci L, et al. Calcium-channel blockade and incidence of cancer in aged populations. *Lancet* 1996;348:493–497.
34. Grossman E, Messerli FH, Grodzicki T, et al. Should a moratorium be placed on sublingual nifedipine capsules given for hypertensive emergencies and pseudoemergencies? *JAMA* 1996;276:1328–1331.
35. Hypertension Detection and Follow-up Program Cooperative Group. Five-year findings of the Hypertension Detection and Follow-up Program. II. Mortality by race, sex and age. *JAMA* 1979;242:2572–2577.
36. The Australian Therapeutic Trial in mild hypertension. Report by the Management Committee. *Lancet* 1980;1:1261–1267.
37. Amery A, Birkenhager W, Brixko P, et al. Mortality and morbidity results from the European Working Party on High Blood Pressure in the Elderly Trial. *Lancet* 1985;1:1349–1354.
38. Dahlof B, Lindholm LH, Hansson L, et al. Morbidity and mortality in the Swedish Trial in Old Patients with Hypertension (STOP-Hypertension). *Lancet* 1991;338:1281–1285.
39. MRC Working Party. Medical Research Council trial of treatment of hypertension in older adults: principal results. *Br Med J* 1992;304:405–412.
40. Thijs L, Fagard R, Lijnen P, et al. A meta-analysis of outcome trials in elderly hypertensives. *J Hypertens* 1992;10:1103–1109.

Chapter 3

Physical Activity and Coronary Heart Disease

Peter W.F. Wilson, MD

Introduction

The association of physical activity and fitness with lower coronary heart disease (CHD) incidence is of paramount interest in the prevention of heart disease. In the past most physical activity was associated with carrying out everyday activities, and many occupations involved manual labor. Over the past half century, however, American and European populations lost most of their agrarian roots; residents are more likely to live in the suburbs, now commuting to work and exercising little on the job. Modern conveniences facilitated this trend, and now there is greater time for jogging, walking, and other leisure activities.

This chapter provides a perspective for the impact of physical activity on CHD, drawing mostly from larger-scale investigations. The various types of activity will be discussed, their associations with known CHD risk factors will be demonstrated; and benefits, as well as potential adverse effects, will be presented. The data shown are largely observational and self-reported, as large-scale clinical trials that test the merits of physical activity fitness are lacking.

Definitions

Physical activity is "bodily movement produced by skeletal muscles that requires energy expenditure."[1] Taken most literally, the person who

From Robinson K, (ed): *Preventive Cardiology*. Armonk, NY: Futura Publishing Company, Inc. © 1998.

spends the entire day at bed rest demonstrated virtually no physical activity. Increments of activity above this basal level can be assigned energy equivalent scores. For instance, it is more arduous to sprint 100 m compared with jogging or walking the same distance. Exercise physiologists determined the energy level associated with each of these sorts of activities and graded them using a unit scale called metabolic equivalents, or METs, where one unit, the amount of energy spent for a person sitting at rest, is approximately 3.5 kcal per minute (Table 1).[2-4]

Exercise is defined as "physical activity that is planned, structured, and repetitive bodily movement done to improve or maintain one or more components of physical fitness."[1] Different types of physical activity have

Table 1
Physical Activity Rating Scale Examples of Metabolic Equivalents

Estimated Number of METs	Description	Type of Activity
1	Sleeping, reclining	Sunbathing, lying on a couch watching television
2	Sitting	Eating, reading, desk work
3	Very light exertion	Office work, driving in the city, standing in line
4	Light exertion, with normal breathing	Mopping, slow walking, shopping, bowling, golfing with a cart, gardening with power tools
5	Moderate exertion, with deep breathing	Normal walking, golfing on foot, slow biking, downhill skiing, calisthenics, raking leaves, slow dancing, light restaurant work
6	Vigorous exertion, with panting; overheating	Slow jogging, speed-walking, tennis, swimming, cross-country skiing, shoveling snow, fast biking, mowing with a push mower, heavy gardening, factory assembly work, softball, laying bricks
7	Heavy exertion, with gasping; much sweating	Running, fast jogging, nonstop racquetball, pushing a car stuck in snow, moving boulders, changing tires, shoveling heavy or deep snow, competitive basketball, touch football, ladder or stair climbing with a 23-kg load.
8	Extreme or peak exertion	Sprinting, fast running, jogging uphill, aggressive sports with frequent sprinting and no rest, pushing or pulling with all one's might, unusually extreme work

varying effects. Dynamic, isotonic exercise (muscular contraction of large muscle groups resulting in movement) is associated with increased cardiac output, greater oxygen consumption, and a fall in systemic vascular resistance. In contrast, isometric exercise (constant contraction of muscles without movement) is associated with a small increase in oxygen requirement, smaller increases in cardiac output, and an increase in systemic vascular resistance.[5] In general, long-duration isotonic exercise is associated with improved cardiovascular fitness determined by maximal oxygen consumption procedures.[6] For instance, a manual laborer may work long hours in the fields, a body builder may lift heavy weights, and a jogger may develop the endurance to complete a marathon. Each person developed a component of physical fitness, but different muscle groups were involved. The body builder may be quite strong in certain skeletal muscle groups, but he may not necessarily exhibit a high degree of cardiovascular fitness, as the maneuvers performed are often of very short duration and do not necessarily lead to an ability to exercise over prolonged periods. The manual laborer might be less strong, but more fit, and the jogger may have the least strength, but the greatest capacity to exercise, or perform work, over a prolonged period.

Early Studies

The first large studies that investigated the importance of physical activity and its potential impact on CHD were conducted in the 1950s and 1960s. The initial focus was on occupations, and investigations compared cardiovascular disease (CVD) risk and risk factor levels in occupational groups. An early study involved busmen in London, England. The investigators showed greater prevalence of CHD, a larger sum of skinfolds (a measure of obesity), higher cholesterol levels, and more hypertension in bus drivers compared with conductors who walked the aisles and collected the tickets on the two-story buses.[7,8] The authors concluded that conductors were more physically active, had better cardiovascular risk factors, and were less likely to develop CVD. Critics of these studies noted that a self-selection process might be operating, drivers may have been heavy when they started employment with the London Transit Authority, and conductors may have always been thin. Such criticism had merit, as a follow-up study showed that clothing sizes, determined from records kept of the uniforms worn, were greater for the drivers at the time of initial employment by the bus company. Other investigations involving physical activity associated with work concluded that active workers experienced less CHD. For example, farm workers experienced lower CHD rates in comparison with clerks, trade workers, and farm owners (Figure 1).[9] Similarly, longshoremen who loaded ships were shown to have better cardiovascular risk profiles and lower rates of CVD, even after statistical

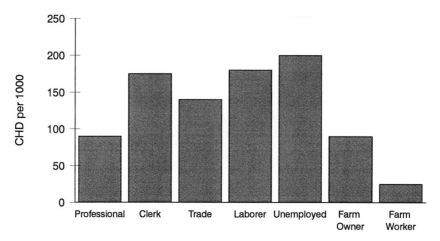

Figure 1. *Age-adjusted CHD incidence by occupation in the Evans County Study 1961–1968. Adapted with permission from Reference 9.*

adjustment for habits such as cigarette smoking, which tended to have an adverse effect on CHD rates.[10]

Population Studies Since 1970

The trend toward greater mechanization on the farm and in industry led to a new focus, starting in the 1960s, on leisure-time activity. Longitudinal cardiovascular investigations such as the Western Collaborative Study, the Framingham Heart Study, and the Minnesota Railroad Study gathered physical activity information.[4,11,12] For instance, persons reporting "regular exercise'" in the Western Collaborative Study experienced reduced rates of myocardial infarction (MI) and CHD, compared with other study participants who did not report such activity.[13] A simple physical activity index was used in the Framingham Heart Study and Honolulu Heart Study investigations, inquiring about the usual amount of time spent at rest and at various levels of activity over a 24-hour period. This weighted scale estimated the usual physical activity level of participants, and higher levels of reported activity were associated with a lower incidence of MI and CHD death over long-term follow-up (Figure 2).[12] A physical activity index, applied to longer follow-up in men and women from Framingham and men from Honolulu, was also associated with lower rates of cardiovascular mortality in general (Figure 3).[14,15]

Data from the United States and England showed that greater levels of current physical activity appeared to protect against CHD. The Harvard Alumni Study, based on the long-term experience of more than 17 000 men who attended Harvard College from 1962–1966, showed that phys-

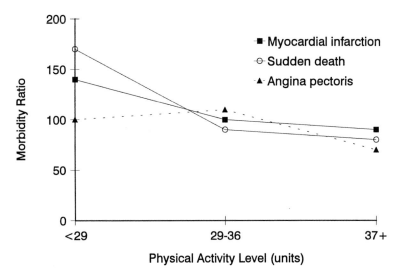

Figure 2. *CHD risk over 10 years according to physical activity level. Framingham men aged 38–70 years at baseline. Adapted with permission from Reference 12.*

ical activity in middle age was inversely associated with subsequent CVD, and the degree of this association was greater than for CVD and exercise undertaken while a college undergraduate (low- or high-frequency non-competitive intramural sports or competitive varsity athletics) (Figure 4).[16,17] Improved questionnaire survey methods allowed semiquantification of physical activity, and investigators demonstrated that greater

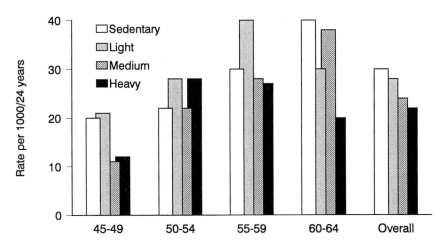

Figure 3. *Physical demands of work and CVD mortality in Framingham men followed for 24 years. Adapted with permission from Reference 14.*

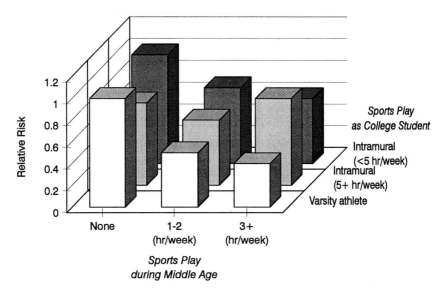

Figure 4. *Relative risk of first CHD attack during interval 1962–1972 according to alumnus vigorous sports play and college student sports play. Adapted with permission from Reference 17.*

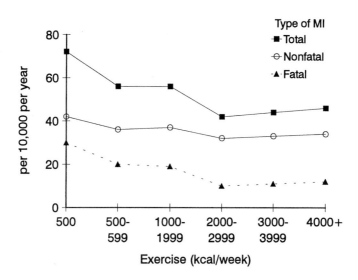

Figure 5. *Reported exercise and 8-year heart attack rate in the Harvard Alumni Study. Adapted with permission from Reference 18.*

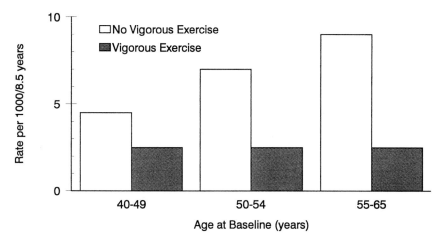

Figure 6. *Incidence of CHD over 8.5 years in 17 944 British civil servants according to whether persons reported vigorous exercise. Adapted with permission from Reference 70.*

amounts of regular activity during the week appeared to protect against CHD (Figure 5).[16,18] The overall estimate was that 2000 kcal of leisure time activity per week, roughly equivalent to 30 minutes of jogging three times a week, was highly associated with lower rates of CHD in middle-aged men. A comparable level of physical activity, "30 minutes or more of moderate-intensity physical activity on most, preferably all, days of the week" was recently recommended for all US adults.[19] Longer follow-up of a Harvard Alumni cohort recently showed that vigorous activities undertaken after college were associated with longevity.[20] Similar analyses from The Whitehall Study, conducted on more than 17 000 male British civil servants, and more vigorous physical activity (above 7.5 METs) was associated with one-half the risk of CHD (Figure 6).[21]

Physical Fitness and CHD

Self-reported physical activity suffered from inadequate classification of participants, and other measures were needed. Longer, more-detailed questionnaires were developed,[22–24] but there was a need for assessment of physical fitness in populations so its relation to CHD could be studied. Step tests, bicycle ergometry, and exercise treadmill protocols were used, building on the experience of exercise physiologists and cardiologists, to evaluate exercise performance in participants of large-scale studies to provide an objective measure of fitness.[25–27]

More than 4200 asymptomatic men in the Lipid Research Clinics Program underwent exercise testing. A lower heart rate after 6 minutes of

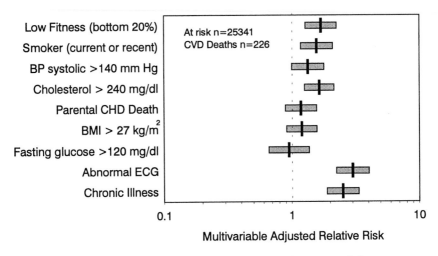

Figure 7. *CVD mortality in men for selected factor. Aerobics Center follow-up 1970–1989. Adapted with permission from Reference 71.*

exercise on a graded treadmill protocol and greater duration of exercise on the treadmill were associated with lower rates of CHD death during follow-up.[28] Similarly, approximately 10 000 men and 3000 women at the Aerobics Center in Dallas, Texas, were regularly evaluated with exercise testing and divided into quintiles of cardiovascular fitness according to time spent on a treadmill protocol without development of fatigue, an-

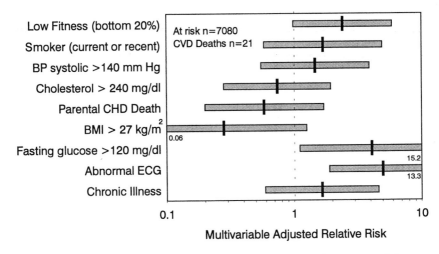

Figure 8. *CVD mortality in women for selected factor. Aerobics Center follow-up 1970–1989. Adapted with permission from Reference 71.*

gina, or ischemic changes on the electrocardiogram (ECG). Men and women at the lowest level of fitness in the Aerobics Center Study went on to develop the highest rates of CVD death. As the top four quintiles experienced relatively similar rates of CVD death, the authors concluded that low fitness (bottom quintile) in either sex placed persons at particularly high risk for disease, an effect that was statistically significant and independent of other risk factors in multivariate analyses. (Figures 7 and 8).[29,30] Comparable results were obtained in a total of 1960 middle-aged Norwegian men, and increasing time spent on a symptom-limited bicycle ergometer test was associated with reduced risk of cardiovascular death over 16 years.[31] Population studies therefore suggest that mild to moderate fitness is cardioprotective, and recent studies now show that multiple short bouts of moderate-intensity exercise appear to be associated with an increase in peak oxygen uptake, demonstrating that moderate fitness is achievable with 10-minute bouts of exercise several times a day.[32]

Physiological and Metabolic Effects of Physical Activity

Hematologic, Muscular, and Cardiac Changes

Increased levels of physical activity and training affect several physiological systems. Plasma volume, red cell mass, and hemoglobin are gen-

---

Table 2
Features that Occur more Commonly
in the Athlete's Heart

Left ventricle
    Increased diastolic cavity dimension
    Increased wall thickness
    Increased wall mass
    Electrocardographic LV hypertrophy
Rate, rhythm, and conduction
    Bradycardia
    Marked sinus arrhythmia
    First-degree heart block
    Second-degree heart block (Wenckebach)
Other ECG abnormalities
    Abnormal depolarization or repolarization
    ST segment with J-point elevation
    T-wave inversion in V1–3
    Loss of anterior forces or accentuated
        superior forces on ECG

---

erally increased with training, facilitating greater oxygen delivery to systemic tissues. Skeletal muscle responds to training with an increase in mitochondria and greater capillary formation. Musculoskeletal injury associated with exercise is associated with activity of greater intensity and may be more common in women.[33,34] With training the heart itself may undergo a variety of changes,[35,36] and individuals can develop an "athlete's heart." Several characteristics, including bradycardia, arrhythmias, conduction disturbances, biventricular hypertrophy, and thickening of the left ventricular (LV) wall may be present (Table 2). These adaptations are often observed in male and female athletes undergoing ECG and echocardiography.[35,37] Increased LV wall thickness and a nondilated LV cavity are likely to have primary forms of pathological hypertrophy.[38] Studies of elite athletes showed a greater prevalence of increased LV cavity dimension, wall thickness, and mass, and endurance sports tended to be associated with the greatest myocardial effects in women.[39]

Lipids

Regular physical activity, not necessarily at a high intensity, may also be associated with other differences, including higher high-density lipoprotein cholesterol (HDL-C) levels, lower cholesterol,[40] lower triglycerides and very-low-density lipoprotein cholesterol,[41] greater peak bone mass in women,[42] less obesity, less cigarette smoking, and a lower incidence of diabetes mellitus (DM) and stroke.[43-47] Lipids in physically active persons were particularly well studied. In a study of middle-aged men, mean levels of HDL-C were reported as approximately 43 mg/dL among those who were inactive, 58 mg/dL in joggers, and 65 mg/dL in marathon runners. In addition, the distance run was an excellent predictor of a more-favorable total/HDL-C ratio.[48] Data from studies of endurance involving moderate intensity exercise suggest that the time frame needed to achieve HDL-C change may exceed 2 years, a longer interval than that reported previously for younger populations.[49] Many other factors are important determinants of lipid levels, and HDL-C levels are especially likely to be increased in persons who take exercise regularly, are thin, and consume greater amounts of alcohol.[48,50,51]

Obesity and Diabetes Mellitus

Physical activity and fitness are also associated with lower blood pressure (BP) in most studies.[52-55] It is likely that the association of (BP) with physical activity is closely linked to the important finding of less obesity among persons who are active, and regular physical activity in middle-aged adults was consistently associated with a lower incidence of diabetes.[43,44,56-58]

Effects in the Elderly and in Women

Beneficial effects of physical activity were also found in studies of elderly persons who participated in training programs. A study that focused on walking in the elderly demonstrated an 8- to 10-mm Hg decrease in systolic BP (SBP) after 6 months.[53] Endurance time on a treadmill protocol, perceived exertion, minute ventilation, heart rate, and SBP decreased after 12-month training programs,[59] and conditioning effects, including increased levels of peak exercise achieved, were obtained consistently after coronary events.[60,61]

Favorable cardiovascular effects of exercise in women tended to focus on less-intense forms of exercise, as high-intensity exercise appears to be particularly associated with musculoskeletal injury.[33,34] As an example, the quantity and quality of walking showed to be associated with improved maximal oxygen uptake in a 24-week clinical trial of middle-aged women. The pace of walking was positively associated with aerobic capacity achieved at the end of the study, and participants tended to improve their HDL-C levels.[62]

Morbidity and Mortality Associated With Physical Activity

There is continued concern that physical activity may precipitate a MI or sudden death. Risk of cardiac arrest was shown to increase transiently during vigorous exercise, but habitual vigorous exercise was associated with an overall decreased risk of cardiac arrest.[63] The risk of MI was highest within 1 hour of heavy exercise (>6 METs) (Figure 9), the effect was graded, and persons who exercised at this level once a week experienced an MI at approximately 100 times the rate of persons who never performed such activities (Figure 10).[2]

Sudden cardiac death (SCD) is an infrequent, yet tragic event among young athletes. Pathology studies show that definite or probable hypertrophic cardiomyopathy is the most prevalent underlying disorder in young SCD victims[64]; a variety of other abnormalities appears to be responsible for sudden death in the remainder of the cases (Figure 11). The majority of SCD events in young athletes appears to occur in basketball and football players.[64]

Although exercise itself leads to a temporary increase in the risk of SCD, the overall impact in terms of absolute risk is relatively small. This phenomenon was recently well summarized by Thompson,[65] and Table 3 presents an adaptation of his findings, displaying the absolute risk for SCD in young adults according to their health and athletic status. Complementary to these data is the recently reported increased hazard of SCD during Armed Forces basic training in recruits with sickle cell trait (he-

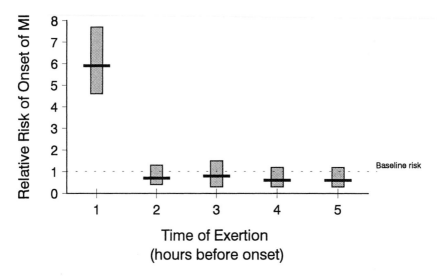

Figure 9. *Relative risk of myocardial infarction after an episode of heavy physical exertion. Adapted with permission from Reference 2.*

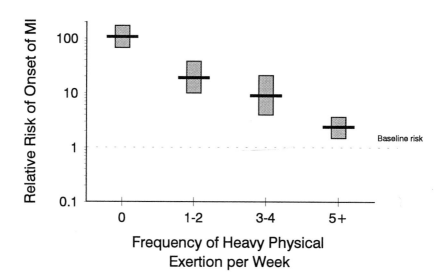

Figure 10. *Relative risk of myocardial infarction according to frequency of heavy exertion. Adapted with permission from Reference 2.*

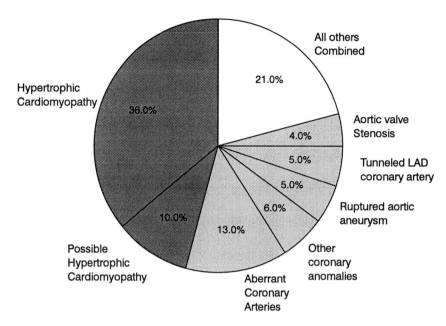

Figure 11. *Underlying pathological findings associated with sudden cardiac death in young competitive athletes aged 12–28 years. Adapted with permission from Reference 64.*

moglobin AS).[66] At present there are no universal standards for screening young athletes who participate in competitive sports, but an expert panel recently recommended that "some form of preparticipation cardiovascular screening for high school and collegiate athletes is justifiable and compelling, based on ethical, legal, and medical grounds."[67]

Recommendations

A recent statement for health professionals from the American Heart Association strongly endorsed regular aerobic physical activity to prevent initial and recurrent CVD and notes that risks of injury and SCD can be minimized with "medical evaluation, risk stratification, supervision, and education."[19] Patients and practitioners should recognize that much of the effect of regular physical activity is thought to operate via known mechanisms, exerting a favorable impact on blood lipids, arterial pressure, obesity, and DM. Cardiac rehabilitation programs can often meet such multidimensional needs, but such programs are not widely used.[68,69] The amount of regular physical activity is inversely associated with CVD in middle-aged and elderly populations, and benefits appear to be greatest for persons who were formerly inactive. Finally, mild to moderate levels

Table 3
Sudden Cardiac Death in Young Adults

Group	Risk (per 100 000 per year)
High school or college athletes	
Male	0.75
Female	0.13
College athletes—male	1.45
High school athletes—male	0.66
Healthy young adults (Seattle)	
Exercising	5.4
Not exercising	0.1
Healthy young adults (Rhode Island)	
Exercising	6.7
Not exercising	0.9

Adapted with permission from Reference 65.

of exertion are achievable by most persons, and moderate levels of fitness can be attained with multiple short bouts of exercise during the day.

References

1. National Institutes of Health Consensus Development Panel on Physical Activity and Cardiovascular Health. Physical activity and cardiovascular health. *JAMA* 1996;276:241–246.
2. Mittleman MA, Maclure M, Tofler GH, et al. Triggering of acute myocardial infarction by heavy physical exertion. Protection against triggering by regular exertion. Determinants of myocardial infarction onset study investigators. *N Engl J Med* 1993;329:1677–1683.
3. Taylor HL, Jacobs DR Jr, Schucker B, et al. A questionnaire for the assessment of leisure time physical activities. *J Chron Dis* 1978;31:741–755.
4. Folsom AR, Caspersen CJ, Taylor HL, et al. Leisure time physical activity and its relationship to coronary risk factors in a population-based sample. The Minnesota Heart Survey. *Am J Epidemiol* 1985;121:570–579.
5. Hanson P, Nagle F. Isometric exercise: cardiovascular responses in normal and cardiac populations. In: Hanson P, ed. *Exercise and the Heart, Cardiology Clinics.* Philadelphia, PA: WB Saunders; 1987:157–170.
6. Saltin B, Astrand PO. Maximal oxygen uptake in athletes. *J Appl Physiol* 1967;23:353–358.
7. Morris JN, Heady JA, Raffle PAB, et al. Coronary heart-disease and physical activity of work. *Lancet* 1953;2:1053–1057.
8. Morris JN, Kagan A, Pattison DC, et al. Incidence and prediction of ischaemic heart-disease in London busmen. *Lancet* 1966;2:553–559.
9. Cassel J, Heyden S, Bartel AG, et al. Incidence of coronary heart disease by ethnic group, social class, and sex. *Arch Intern Med* 1971;128:901–906.

10. Paffenbarger RS Jr, Laughlin ME, Gima AS, et al. Work activity of longshoremen as related to death from coronary heart disease and stroke. *N Engl J Med* 1970;282:1109–1114.
11. Rosenman RH, Bawol RD, Oscherwitz M. A 4-year prospective study of the relationship of different habitual vocational physical activity to risk and incidence of ischemic heart disease in volunteer male federal employees. *Ann N Y Acad Sci* 1977;301:627–641.
12. Kannel WB, Sorlie PD. Some health benefits of physical activity: The Framingham Study. *Arch Intern Med* 1979;139:857–861.
13. Rosenman RH, Brand RJ, Scholtz RI, et al. Multivariate prediction of coronary heart disease during 8.5-year follow-up in the Western Collaborative Group Study. *Am J Cardiol* 1976;37:903–910.
14. Kannel WB, Belanger AJ, D'Agostino RB, et al. Physical activity and physical demand on the job and risk of cardiovascular disease and death: the Framingham Study. *Am Heart J* 1986;112:820–825.
15. Rodriguez BL, Curb JD, Burchfiel CM, et al. Physical activity and 23-year incidence of coronary heart disease morbidity and mortality among middle-aged men. The Honolulu Heart Program. *Circulation* 1994;89:2540–2544.
16. Paffenbarger RS Jr, Hyde RT, Wing AL, et al. Physical activity, all-cause mortality, and longevity of college alumni. *N Engl J Med* 1986;314:605–613.
17. Paffenbarger RS Jr, Hyde RT, Wing AL, et al. The association of changes in physical-activity level and other lifestyle characteristics with mortality among men. *N Engl J Med* 1993;328:538–545.
18. Paffenbarger RS Jr, Wing AL, Hyde RT. Physical activity as an index of heart attack risk in college alumni. *Am J Epidemiol* 1978;108:161–175.
19. Fletcher GF, Balady G, Blair SN, et al. Statement on exercise: benefits and recommendations for physical activity programs for all Americans. *Circulation* 1996;94:857–862.
20. Lee IM, Hsieh CC, Paffenbarger RS Jr. Exercise intensity and longevity in men. The Harvard Alumni Health Study. *JAMA* 1995;273:1179–1184.
21. Morris JN, Clayton DG, Everitt MG, et al. Exercise in leisure time: coronary attack and death rates. *Br Heart J* 1990;63:325–334.
22. Blair SN, Haskell WL, Ho P, et al. Assessment of habitual physical activity by a seven-day recall in a community survey and controlled experiments. *Am J Epidemiol* 1985;122:794–804.
23. Sallis JF, Haskell WL, Wood PD, et al. Physical activity assessment methodology in the Five-City Project. *Am J Epidemiol* 1985;121:91–106.
24. Washburn RA, Montoye HJ. The assessment of physical activity by questionnaire. *Am J Epidemiol* 1986;123:563–576.
25. Eaton CB, Lapane KL, Garber CE, et al. Physical activity, physical fitness, and coronary heart disease risk factors. *Med Sci Sports Exerc* 1995;27:340–346.
26. Fletcher GF, Balady G, Froelicher VF, et al. Exercise standards. A statement for healthcare professionals from the American Heart Association Writing Group. *Circulation* 1995;91:580–615.
27. Detrano R, Froelicher VF. Exercise testing: uses and limitations considering recent studies. *Prog Cardiovasc Dis* 1988;31:173–204.
28. Ekelund LG, Haskell WL, Johnson JL, et al. Physical fitness as a predictor of cardiovascular mortality in asymptomatic North American men: the Lipid Research Clinics Mortality Follow-up Study. *N Engl J Med* 1988;319:1379–1384.
29. Blair SN, Kohl HW III, Paffenbarger RS Jr, et al. Physical fitness and all-cause mortality. A prospective study of healthy men and women. *JAMA* 1989;262:2395–2401.

30. Blair SN, Kohl HW, Barlow CE, et al. Changes in physical fitness and all-cause mortality. A prospective study of healthy and unhealthy men. *JAMA* 1995;273:1093–1098.
31. Sandvik L, Erikssen J, Thaulow E, et al. Physical fitness as a predictor of mortality among healthy, middle-aged Norwegian men. *N Engl J Med* 1993; 328:533–537.
32. DeBusk RF, Stenestrand U, Sheehan M, et al. Training effects of long versus short bouts of exercise in healthy subjects. *Am J Cardiol* 1990;65:1010–1013.
33. Pollock ML, Carroll JF, Graves JE, et al. Injuries and adherence to walk/jog and resistance training programs in the elderly. *Med Sci Sports Exerc* 1991;23:1194–1200.
34. Koplan JP, Powell KE, Sikes RK, et al. An epidemiologic study of the benefits and risks of running. *JAMA* 1982;248:3118–3121.
35. Huston TP, Puffer JC, Rodney WM. The athletic heart syndrome. *N Engl J Med* 1985;313:24–32.
36. Bryan G, Ward A, Rippe JM. Athletic heart syndrome. *Clin Sports Med* 1992;11:259–272.
37. Maron BJ, Pelliccia A, Spirito P. Cardiac disease in young trained athletes. Insights into methods for distinguishing athlete's heart from structural heart disease, with particular emphasis on hypertrophic cardiomyopathy. *Circulation* 1995;91:1596–1601.
38. Pelliccia A, Maron BJ, Spataro A, et al. The upper limit of physiologic cardiac hypertrophy in highly trained elite athletes. *N Engl J Med* 1991;324:295–301.
39. Pelliccia A, Maron BJ, Culasso F, et al. Athlete's heart in women: echocardiographic characterization of highly trained elite female athletes. *JAMA* 1996;276:211–215.
40. Tran ZV, Weltman A. Differential effects of exercise on serum lipid and lipoprotein levels seen with changes in body weight. A meta-analysis. *JAMA* 1985;254:919–924.
41. Dannenberg AL, Keller JB, Wilson PWF, et al. Leisure time physical activity in the Framingham Offspring Study. Description, seasonal variation, and risk factor correlates. *Am J Epidemiol* 1989;129:76–87.
42. Cooper C, Cawley M, Bhalla A, et al. Childhood growth, physical activity, and peak bone mass in women. *J Bone Miner Res* 1995;10:940–947.
43. Burchfiel CM, Sharp DS, Curb JD, et al. Physical activity and incidence of diabetes: The Honolulu Heart Program. *Am J Epidemiol* 1995;141:360–368.
44. Helmrich SP, Ragland DR, Leung RW, et al. Physical activity and reduced occurrence of non-insulin-dependent diabetes mellitus. *N Engl J Med* 1991;325:147–152.
45. Knowler WC, Narayan KM, Hanson RL, et al. Preventing non-insulin-dependent diabetes. *Diabetes* 1995;44:483–488.
46. Manson JE, Nathan DM, Krolewski AS, et al. A prospective study of exercise and incidence of diabetes among US male physicians. *JAMA* 1992;268:63–67.
47. Kiely DK, Wolf PA, Cupples LA, et al. Physical activity and stroke risk: the Framingham Study. *Am J Epidemiol* 1994;140:608–620.
48. Hartung GH, Foreyt JP, Mitchell RE, et al. Relation of diet to high-density-lipoprotein cholesterol in middle-aged marathon runners, joggers, and inactive men. *N Engl J Med* 1980;302:357–361.
49. King AC, Haskell WL, Young DR, et al. Long-term effects of varying intensities and formats of physical activity on participation rates, fitness, and lipoproteins in men and women aged 50 to 65 years. *Circulation* 1995;91:2596–2604.
50. O'Connor GT, Hennekens CH, Willett WC, et al. Physical exercise and reduced risk of nonfatal myocardial infarction. *Am J Epidemiol* 1995;142:1147–1156.

51. Hartung GH, Foreyt JP, Mitchell RE, et al. Effect of alcohol intake on high-density lipoprotein cholesterol levels in runners and inactive men. *JAMA* 1983;249:747–750.
52. Hagberg JM, Montain SJ, Martin WH III, et al. Effect of exercise training in 60- to 69-year-old persons with essential hypertension. *Am J Cardiol* 1989;64:348–353.
53. Braith RW, Pollock ML, Lowenthal DT, et al. Moderate- and high-intensity exercise lowers blood pressure in normotensive subjects 60 to 79 years of age. *Am J Cardiol* 1994;73:1124–1128.
54. Adner MM, Castelli WP. Elevated high-density lipoprotein levels in marathon runners. *JAMA* 1980;243:534–536.
55. Abbott RD, Levy D, Kannel WB, et al. Cardiovascular risk factors and graded treadmill exercise endurance in healthy adults: the Framingham Offspring Study. *Am J Cardiol* 1989;63:342–346.
56. Centers for Disease Control and Prevention. Prevalence of physical inactivity during leisure time among overweight persons—1994. *JAMA* 1996;275:905.
57. Bao W, Srinivasan SR, Berenson GS. Persistent elevation of plasma insulin levels is associated with increased cardiovascular risk in children and young adults. The Bogalusa Heart Study. *Circulation* 1996;93:54–59.
58. Helmrich SP, Ragland DR, Paffenbarger RS Jr. Prevention of non-insulin-dependent diabetes mellitus with physical activity. *Med Sci Sports Exerc* 1994;26:824–830.
59. Ades PA, Waldmann ML, Poehlman ET, et al. Exercise conditioning in older coronary patients. Submaximal lactate response and endurance capacity. *Circulation* 1993;88:572–577.
60. Ades PA, Grunvald MH. Cardiopulmonary exercise testing before and after conditioning in older coronary patients. *Am Heart J* 1990;120:585–589.
61. Ades PA, Hanson JS, Gunther PG, et al. Exercise conditioning in the elderly coronary patient. *J Am Geriatr Soc* 1987;35:121–124.
62. Duncan JJ, Gordon NF, Scott CB. Women walking for health and fitness: how much is enough? *JAMA* 1991;266:3295–3299.
63. Siscovick DS, Weiss NS, Fletcher RH, et al. The incidence of primary cardiac arrest during vigorous exercise. *N Engl J Med* 1984;311:874–877.
64. Maron BJ, Shirani J, Poliac LC, et al. Sudden death in young competitive athletes: Clinical, demographic, and pathological profiles. *JAMA* 1996;276:199–204.
65. Thompson PD. The cardiovascular complications of vigorous physical activity. *Arch Intern Med* 1996;156:2297–2302.
66. Kark JA, Posey DM, Schumacher HR, et al. Sickle-cell trait as a risk factor for sudden death in physical training. *N Engl J Med* 1987;317:781–787.
67. Maron BJ, Thompson PD, Puffer JC, et al. Cardiovascular preparticipation screening of competitive athletes: a statement for health professionals from the Sudden Death Committee (Clinical Cardiology) and Congenital Cardiac Defects Committee (Cardiovascular Disease in the Young), American Heart Association. *Circulation* 1996;94:850–856.
68. McNamara JR, Campos H, Ordovas JM, et al. Effect of gender, age, and lipid status on low density lipoprotein subfraction distribution: results from the Framingham Offspring Study. *Arteriosclerosis* 1987;7:483–490.
69. Thomas I, Gupta S, Sempos C, et al. Serum lipids of Indian physicians living in the US compared to US born physicians. *Atherosclerosis* 1986;61:99–106.
70. Morris JN, Pollard R, Everitt MG, et al. Vigorous exercise in leisure-time: Protection against coronary heart disease. *Lancet* 1980;2:1207–1210.
71. Blair SN, Kampert JB, Kohl HW III, et al. Influences of cardiorespiratory fitness and other precursors on cardiovascular disease and all-cause mortality in men and women. *JAMA* 1996;276:205–210.

Chapter 4

Diabetes Mellitus, Insulin Resistance, and Coronary Heart Disease

Peter W.F. Wilson, MD

Introduction

Although coronary heart disease (CHD) mortality declined over the past several decades in North America, a commensurate decline in coronary disease incidence did not ensue.[1] Over the same interval, the prevalence of diabetes mellitus (DM) and impaired glucose tolerance (IGT) appears to be rising.[2] These trends contribute to the continued burden of DM and heart disease in the United States. This chapter will include information related not only to DM and CHD but will also present data concerning hyperglycemia, insulin resistance, and CHD. The major focus will be on CHD, but other forms of heart disease, such as congestive heart failure (CHF), cardiomyopathy, conduction disease, and coronary risk factors will also be considered.

The greatest amount of information available is concerning DM and heart disease in middle-aged and older persons. For that reason, the majority of the discussion will focus on noninsulin-dependent DM (NIDDM) and heart disease. Where available, data will be given for heart disease and insulin-dependent DM (IDDM).

From Robinson K, (ed): *Preventive Cardiology*. Armonk, NY: Futura Publishing Company, Inc. © 1998.

Diabetes Prevalence

The prevalence of DM is best estimated from formal population surveys. Self-report of DM was commonly used in the past, but oral glucose tolerance testing (OGTT; typically 75-g oral load in adults) and diagnostic criteria introduced by the National Diabetes Data Group[3] in the late 1970s (Table 1) helped to standardize the approach and ensure more valid estimates.

The prevalence of NIDDM increases with age and approximately one-half of all persons with NIDDM are undetected if glucose tolerance testing is not performed (Figure 1).[2] The prevalence of IGT also increases with age in the United States. This intermediate level of abnormality is detected only by adminstering OGTT.[3–5] As seen in Figure 1, IGT in middle-aged adults typically equals the prevalence of NIDDM in populations

---

Table 1

Abbreviated Criteria for Diabetes Mellitus and Impaired Glucose Tolerance National Diabetes Data Group (NDDG) and World Health Organization (WHO) Criteria

---

Diabetes mellitus
- A. Presence of classic symptoms of diabetes with unequivocal elevation of plasma glucose, eg, postprandial or random plasma glucose ≥200 mg/dL
- B. Fasting glucose concentration elevation on more than one occasion; venous plasma <140 mg/dL
- C. Fasting glucose not elevated by sustained elevated glucose during oral glucose tolerance test
    - Venous plasma ≥200 mg/dL 2 h after 75-g glucose load and some other sample (NDDG)
    - Venous plasma ≥200 mg/dL 2 h after 75-g glucose load (WHO)

II. In an epidemiological setting
- A. Medical history of diabetes diagnosed by a physician
- B. Single fasting glucose concentration; venous plasma ≥140 mg/dL
- C. Single glucose concentration 2 h after ingesting a 75-g glucose load; venous plasma ≥200 mg/dL

Impaired glucose tolerance
- I. NDDG requires A, B, and C; WHO requires A and B
    - A. Fasting glucose concentration; venous plasma <140 mg/dL
    - B. Glucose concentration at 2 h after ingesting 75-g oral glucose; venous plasma ≥140 and <200 mg/dL
    - C. Glucose concentration at midtest (30, 60, or 90 min after 75-g load), venous plasma ≥200 mg/dL
- II. In an epidemiological setting or population screening
    - A. Glucose concentration at 2 h after ingesting 75-g oral glucose; venous plasma ≥140 and <200 mg/dL

Different cutoff values are obtained if sampling is by venous whole blood or capillary whole blood. For complete criteria, see References 3–5.

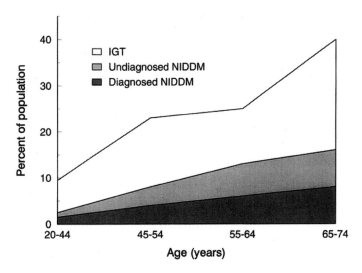

Figure 1. *Prevalence of NIDDM and IGT in the United States, 1976–1980. Adapted with permission from Reference 2.*

where the occurrence of diabetes is low to moderate.[2] Overall, approximately 10% of young adults have some degree of glucose intolerance, manifested by diabetes or IGT, and this proportion rises to >40% after age 65 (Figure 1).

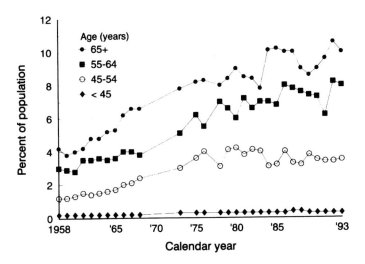

Figure 2. *Time trends in percent of the population with diagnosed diabetes, by age. US data from 1958–1993. Adapted with permission from Reference 2.*

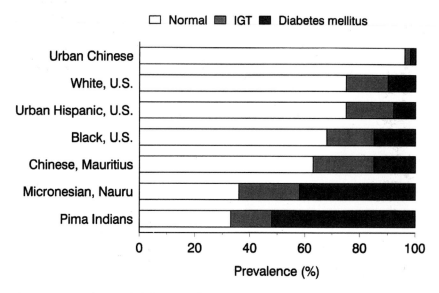

Figure 3. *Prevalence of diabetes and IGT in adults age 30–64. Adapted with permission from Reference 8.*

American data obtained as part of the National Health Interview Survey provide self-reported estimates of NIDDM prevalence across the adult age span. As seen in Figure 2, recent surveys estimate the prevalence of diabetes at <0.5% for young adults to >10% in the elderly. In comparison, IDDM is much less common. The pathological process leading to IDDM is largely immune based, obesity is less prevalent, and onset after age 30 is relatively uncommon.[6] Incidence of IDDM peaks at puberty, and the lifetime prevalence of IDDM is approximately 0.5%.[7]

As seen in Figure 3, the prevalence of NIDDM varies according to the group studied.[8] Occurrence is low in underdeveloped and developing countries, ranges from 10% to 15% in the Americas and Europe, and in a few regions affects >50% of middle-aged adults. Examples of the latter include the Pima Indians in Arizona and Nauru Islanders from the South Pacific. It does not necessarily follow, however, that areas of increased prevalence of DM experience high rates of CHD.

Diabetes and Death

Adults with DM are at a high risk to die prematurely. For instance, in a 25-year follow-up study of adults from Rochester, Minnesota, the 10-year mortality rate was approximately 40% among diabetics versus 30% among an age- and sex-matched comparison group, and the excess mortality was largely attributable to coronary disease.[9] In a similar study,

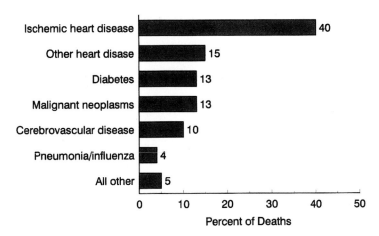

Figure 4. *Approximate distribution of causes of death in persons with diabetes, based on US studies. Adapted with permission from Reference 136.*

based on the 14-year follow-up experience of Rancho Bernardo partici-pants 40–79 years at baseline, CHD death rates were increased among diabetics, with a risk-factor-adjusted relative odds of 3.3 in women and 1.9 in men, suggesting that NIDDM may be particularly lethal among women.[10] A recent summary analysis reported that about 65% of all deaths among diabetics are secondary to vascular or heart disease (ische-mic heart disease, cerebrovascular disease, and other heart disease), 13% are due to diabetes itself, 13% are from neoplasms, and the remaining 9%

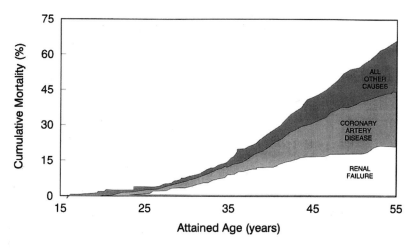

Figure 5. *Cumulative mortality due to CAD and other causes of death among patients with IDDMN followed 20–40 years. Adapted with permission from Reference 14.*

are from other causes (Figure 4).[11] In addition, the duration of diabetes was linked to shorter survival in a 20-year study of 10 000 diabetics from the United States.[12] Although much of the adult information related to death and diabetes is based on patients with NIDDM, data from cohort studies of IDDM patients show that risk of premature death is highly associated with diabetes duration, and the major causes of death are renal failure and coronary artery disease (CAD) (Figure 5).[13–15]

The overall impact of diabetes on life expectancy was estimated in an Iowa study. In an analysis that included men to age 80 and women to age 75, largely measuring the population impact of NIDDM, the estimated life expectancy was 59.7 years at birth for diabetic men and 69.8 years for diabetic women. The authors estimated that diabetic men lived 9.1 fewer years and diabetic women lived 6.7 fewer years than the nondiabetic Iowa population.[16]

Angina and Ischemia

Diabetes is associated with an increased risk of angina pectoris (recognized ischemia).[17,18] Approximately 30% to 50% of ischemic episodes occur without symptoms (unrecognized),[19] a phenomenon that occurs with similar frequency in NIDDM and nondiabetics. An increased prevalence of unrecognized (painless) ischemia was generally reported for NIDDM subjects in population-based studies located in Rancho Bernardo (both sexes), San Luis Valley (non-Hispanic white women), and King County (men).[11] Electrocardiographic (ECG) evidence of ischemia is more common among diabetics,[20] whereas a clinical history of angina pectoris may be less reliable among diabetics with thallium-positive exercise tests.[21] An outpatient study of 58 men with DM showed that silent myocardial ischemia, diagnosed by ≥ 1 mm of ST-segment depression on exercise testing or ambulatory ECG monitoring, was associated with autonomic dysfunction of the heart and exercise-induced reversible defects on thallium scintigraphy.[22] An arteriographic study of 24 diabetics and 31 nondiabetics suggested that reduced coronary vasodilatation occurs in diabetics after submaximal increases in myocardial demand. Such abnormalities might help to explain clinical syndromes of silent ischemia in diabetics.[23]

Myocardial Infarction

Myocardial infarction (MI) rates are increased among diabetics at all ages. Among middle-aged adults, MI rates are typically twice that of the nondiabetic population among men and triple that of nondiabetics among women (Figure 6). More extensive coronary atherosclerosis at the time of the MI may limit efficacy of thrombolytic therapy

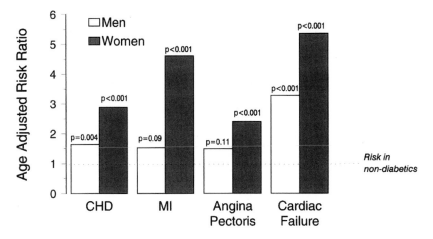

Figure 6. *Diabetes and heart disease risk. Thirty-year experience of the Framingham cohort, men and women aged 35–64. Adapted with permission from Reference 137.*

in diabetics, and thrombolysis is relatively contraindicated in the presence of proliferative retinopathy.[24] Therapeutic concerns at the time of MI should include control of glycemica, acidosis, and severe hypertriglyceridemia (>1000 mg/dL).

Although infarction size is usually not increased in diabetics compared to nondiabetics, complications such as early mortality, cardiogenic shock, myocardial rupture, and acute arrhythmias appear to occur more frequently among diabetics.[25–28] Location of the MI appeared to make a difference in a Duke study, and significantly higher mortality was experienced in men and women with anterior MIs compared to other infarction sites (47% vs 13%) over 12 years of follow-up, and fatalities were more common among diabetics. Furthermore, the 60-day mortality after anterior MI was significantly greater in diabetic (55%) than in nondiabetic subjects (31%).[29] The overall 1-, 2-, and 5-year survival post-MI in a population-based Swedish cohort study of 73 diabetics and 1229 nondiabetics was approximately 94%, 92%, and 82% in nondiabetics and 82%, 78%, and 58% in diabetics, respectively. The corresponding 1-, 2-, and 5-year reinfarction rates were 12%, 17%, and 27% in nondiabetics and 18%, 28%, and 46% in diabetics, respectively (Figure 7).[30] In the Framingham Study a recurrent MI was more common among women, especially if CHF supervened.[31] β-Blockade after MI appears to benefit diabetics, as shown in the Norwegian Timolol Multicenter Study, which demonstrated that β-blockade in diabetics was associated with reduced rates of nonfatal reinfarction, cardiac death, and all-cause mortality.[32,33]

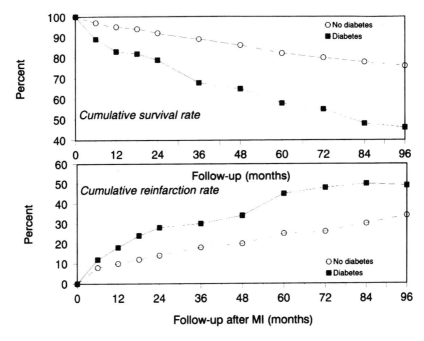

Figure 7. *Cumulative survival and reinfaction post-MI in diabetics and nondiabetics. Adapted with permission from Reference 30.*

Angiography, Angioplasty, and Revascularization

Pathological data suggest that CAD and myocardial lesions are more extensive in diabetics compared to nondiabetics,[34] and hearts from diabetics have low capillary densities.[35] Studies over the past decade demonstrated that diabetes is associated with higher rates of restenosis after angioplasty.[36] Other reports showed that more severe diabetes and worse glycemic control may adversely affect long-term outcome following coronary artery bypass grafting (CABG).[37] The Bypass Angioplasty Revascularization Investigation compared the merits of CABG versus percutaneous transluminal coronary angioplasty (PTCA) in diabetics with coronary ischemia and at least two obstructions in major coronary arteries.[38] After 5 years the patients with diabetes who were on hypoglycemic medication (insulin or oral agents) had a significantly lower death rate with CABG (19% deaths) compared with PTCA (34% deaths). For patients without diabetes and those with diabetes but who were not on drug therapy, the 5-year death rates for CABG and PTCA were approximately 9%. The results of this trial suggest that CABG is the preferred procedure for initial revascularization among diabetics with multivessel coronary disease who are taking hypoglycemic medication.

Congestive Heart Failure and Cardiomyopathy

Diabetes is an important precursor of CHF, and, among Framingham participants aged 45–74, the frequency was increased twofold for men with diabetes and fivefold for women.[39] Deterioration into CHF occurred particularly in diabetic women who experienced an MI.[25,31] A specific etiology of CHF among diabetics is often unclear, and multiple causes, such as MI, infarct size, long-standing hypertension, and microvessel disease, may contribute.[40] The actual impact of microvessel disease on CHF occurrence in diabetics is unknown, but diabetic persons dying of CHF were reported to show myocardial lesions that are typical of diabetes, such as arteriolar thickening, microaneurysms, and basement membrane thickening.[35]

Diastolic dysfunction, characterized by an increased left ventricular end diastolic pressure (LVEDP), a reduced LV end diastolic volume, and normal ejection fraction, may be more common in diabetics than in non-diabetics.[25] Among patients with clinical CHF, a restrictive or dilated cardiomyopathy may be present.[41,42] Abnormalities in myosin isozyme content, myocardial cell calcium homeostasis, sarcolemma sodium exchange, and a decrease in Na-K-ATPase activity appear to underlie the diabetic cardiomyopathy, and insulin resistance was suggested as a possible mechanism.[40] Echocardiographic evidence of increased LV wall thickness and LV mass was evident among Framingham Heart Study participants with NIDDM.[43] Other investigators reported depressed LV function (ejection fraction <50%), and a subnormal increase in LV ejection fraction in response to exercise (<5% increase) was more common in NIDDM subjects.[44] In a study of 40 nondiabetic obese subjects, insulin resistance was a determinant of LV mass.[45,46] Therapy with angiotensin-converting enzyme (ACE) inhibitors post-MI was associated with a lowered risk of CHF and cardiovascular death, a result that can presumably be extended to therapy of CHF among diabetics.[47]

Conduction Disorders, Atrial Fibrillation, and Heart Rate Variability

Left bundle-branch block (LBBB) and atrial fibrillation appear to be more common among diabetics.[48,49] Aging and diabetes are associated with a cardiac autonomic neuropathy that may be reflected by abnormalities such as increased heart rate after 15 minutes of rest, less beat-to-beat variability in the heart rhythm, and orthostatic hypotension.[50,51] Studies showed that diabetics with cardiac autonomic neuropathy experience a lower 5-year survival compared to an age- and sex-matched population sample.[52,53]

Risk Factors in Diabetics

Glycemic Control

Control of glycemia to prevent diabetic complications was the focus of several clinical trials. The first of these, the University Group Diabetes Program (UGDP), was conducted in the 1960s to "determine the efficacy of various forms of treatment for recent maturity-onset diabetes." The results were unexpected, as persons taking the oral hypoglycemic agent tolbutamide during the trial experienced more cardiovascular deaths than persons taking a placebo.[54,55] The trial underwent severe criticism after completion. The protocol was not up to modern standards, and case definitions of diabetes and trial entry criteria were not scrupulously adhered to during the course of recruitment. Information that would likely be related to cardiovascular death, such as smoking history and duration of diabetes, was not collected during the study. The UGDP trial also included an insulin therapeutic arm that was compared to placebo, and no favorable effect of insulin therapy on cardiovascular mortality was observed.[56,57]

The cardiovascular experience of diabetics with poor glycemic control compared to diabetics with good control was difficult to assess until glycosylated hemoglobin, a test that reflects the average glycemic control over the previous 6 weeks, came into regular use during the 1980s.[58] A single glycosylated hemoglobin level was not associated with CHD in young adults with IDDM who were followed over 4 years.[59] A similar tendency, higher glycosylated hemoglobin levels and later CHD, was observed in studies of middle-aged and elderly Finnish persons with NIDDM.[60,61]

Clinical trials of metabolic control among diabetics focused on blood sugar control and followed participants for small vessel complications of the eye and kidney.[62] The most comprehensive study to date, the Diabetes Control and Complication Trial, compared intensive therapy with multiple daily injections of insulin to conventional control of glycemia among more than 1400 persons age 13–39 with IDDM. Efficacy was monitored with glycosylated hemoglobin levels. Intensive therapy was associated with a decreased rate of retinopathy and renal disease progression in this trial.[63] The study was not specifically designed to test whether assiduous glycemic control was associated with a decrease in cardiovascular morbidity or mortality, but improved lipids, lower blood pressure (BP), and fewer macrovascular complications (statistical significance $P = 0.08$) were

Table 2
Recommended Glycemic Control for People with Diabetes

Biochemical Index	Nondiabetic	Diabetic Goal
Preprandial glucose (mg/dL)	<115	80–120
Bedtime glucose (mg/dL)	<120	100–140
HbA$_{1c}$ (%)	<6	<7

Adapted with permission from Reference 67.

found over the 6.5-year course of the trial for the intensive therapy group compared to conventional treatment.[64]

A recent 27-month pilot study of glycemic control compared intensive insulin therapy to conventional insulin therapy in 153 men who were US veterans. Preliminary results suggested a favorable effect ($P = 0.10$) of intensive therapy on cardiovascular disease (CVD) incidence, and a larger trial is planned.[65] A multicenter, randomized trial of glycemic control in NIDDM from the United Kingdom is in its ninth year and nearing completion.[66] This investigation includes 4209 asymptomatic patients with newly diagnosed NIDDM, intensive glycemic therapy using sulfonylureas, insulin or metformin, and glycemic monitoring with fasting blood glucose levels and glycosylated hemoglobin.

More intensive glycemic control can be achieved with a variety of regimens. Often a stepped-care approach is adopted and always includes diet and exercise. Stepped-care for medications can follow, with oral hypoglycemic agents, insulin once or twice a day, and finally insulin three or more times a day.[67,68] Oral hypoglycemic agents such as the biguanides and α-glucosidase inhibitors hold promise as single agents, combined with sulfonylureas or with insulin therapy. The biguanides in particular appear to suppress hepatic glucose, lower free fatty acid levels in plasma, and inhibit lipid oxidation.[69] The goal of intensive therapy is glycemic control, and recent recommendations for target levels of glucose control appear in Table 2.[67,68]

Blood Pressure, Renal Disease, and Microalbuminuria

Hypertension in diabetics is associated with increased rates of small vessel disease of the kidney and eye and appears to foster greater CHD risk. Arterial pressure, particularly systolic pressure level, is typically greater in subjects with NIDDM compared to persons without diabetes.[17,70] Although BP tends to fall during sleep in nondiabetics, higher BP levels may persist throughout the night among diabetics.[71] Treatment of diabetics with hypertension was associated with less microalbuminuria and probably a slower decline in renal function compared to untreated diabetics.[72-76] Use of ACE inhibitors is currently recommended for diabetics with microalbuminuria, but the situation is less clear for diabetics with hypertension and no proteinuria. In this instance, no single BP medication appears to be "renoprotective."[76] Fewer data are available related to the impact of hypertension control on CHD among diabetics,[77,78] and BP elevation in diabetics is associated with a greater degree of albuminuria and CHD, especially in the presence of dyslipidemia.

Current recommendations for antihypertensive therapy for patients with diabetes separate medications into three major groups. The first group includes agents that may have a special advantage in diabetics: ACE inhibitors, α-1-receptor blockers, calcium antagonists, and thiazides in low doses. The second group includes agents that should be used with caution in diabetics: α- and β-blockers, β-blockers, centrally acting α_2-agonists, potassium-sparing agents, and sympatholytic agents. The third group includes agents in which the presence of diabetes does not modify their use: direct vasodilators and loop-acting diuretics.[78]

Lipids

Lipid measures were compared in diabetics, prediabetics, and non-diabetics.[70,79-81] Mean levels of total cholesterol and low-density lipoprotein cholesterol (LDL-C) often do not usually differ in diabetics and non-diabetics, but high-density lipoprotein cholesterol (HDL-C) levels are typically lower and triglycerides are usually higher in diabetics.[79] Representative mean levels for cholesterol, LDL-C, HDL-C, and triglycerides appear in Table 3 for persons with undiagnosed NIDDM and IGT and normal persons aged 20-74 years.[82,83] In both sexes there is a tendency for mean cholesterol and triglyceride levels to be increased in NIDDM and IGT subjects compared to those without. In addition, a greater proportion of NIDDM and IGT subjects have elevated cholesterol, elevated triglycerides, and low HDL-C, as seen at the bottom of Table 3.

Apolipoprotein (apo) levels tend to parallel the results for the cholesterol fractions. Apo-B, largely contained in LDL and VLDL particles, is often increased in diabetics, but not always. On the other hand, apo-A, found in HDL particles, is typically decreased in most studies of diabetics.[84] Lipoprotein (a) [Lp(a)] is another potentially atherogenic particle. It is composed of an LDL moiety that has an attached protein called apoprotein (a). Concentrations were reported to vary according to glycemic control in IDDM and are no different in NIDDM subjects compared to nondiabetic controls; data are scarce relating Lp(a) to CHD incidence among diabetics.[85,86]

Table 3

Mean Lipid Levels in Persons Age 20–74 by Diabetes Status
(US 1976–1980)

Lipid Measure or Category (mg/dL)	Men			Women		
	Undiagnosed NIDDM	IGT	Normal	Undiagnosed NIDDM	IGT	Normal
Lipid mean						
Cholesterol	222	227	209	245	229	208
LDL-C	141	144	139	158	149	131
HDL-C	44	42	45	50	52	55
Triglycerides	175	167	126	182	149	108
Lipid Category						
Cholesterol ≥240	36.6%	35.8%	24.3%	52.5%	36.8%	23.7%
LDL-C ≥160	30.9%	31.6%	27.6%	43.8%	34.6%	23.0%
HDL-C <35	30.1%	27.9%	14.6%	10.6%	10.4%	5.3%
Triglycerides ≥250	13.9%	16.8%	5.6%	22.2%	10.8%	2.4%

Adapted with permission from References 82 and 83.

The size of LDL particles varies in plasma. Originally characterized as pattern B (small and dense) and pattern A (large and buoyant),[87,88] it is now apparent that at least four to seven LDL particles of different sizes may be present in plasma.[89] The major determinant of small, dense LDL particles is the triglyceride level.[90] Patients with NIDDM typically have an increased concentration of the small, dense LDL particles, but the same patients usually have elevated triglyceride concentrations. Genetic markers associated with lipoprotein metabolic pathways are beginning to investigate interactions with DM. For instance, restriction fragment polymorphisms of the lipoprotein lipase gene were associated with altered risk of CHD in diabetics,[91] and the ϵ2 allele was associated with diminished risk of macrovascular complications of NIDDM in a study of Finnish men and women.[92]

Table 4

Recommended Lipid Levels for Adults with Diabetes

Risk for Adult Diabetic Patients	Cholesterol (mg/dL)	HDL-C (mg/dL)	LDL-C (mg/dL)	Triglycerides (mg/dL)
Acceptable	<200	—	<130	<200
Borderline	200–239	—	130–159	200–399
High	≥240	≤35	≥160	≥400

Adapted with permission from Reference 93.

Current recommendations for lipid levels in adult diabetics, put forward by the National Cholesterol Education Panel Adult Treatment Panel and the American Diabetes Association, are given in Table 4.[93] Ensuring that LDL-C <100 mg/dL, HDL-C <35 mg/dL, and triglycerides <200 mg/dL are key to these guidelines. A more aggressive recommendation, LDL-C <100 mg/dL, was taken for diabetics and nondiabetics with macrovascular disease.[94]

Other Factors

Lens opacities and retinal disease, both evidence for microvascular disease in diabetics, were associated with an increased risk of CHD among NIDDM subjects participating in the Framingham Heart Study.[95,96] Elevated levels of fibrinogen[97,98] and increased platelet adhesiveness[99–101] were associated with diabetes and greater atherosclerotic risk for atherosclerosis in population studies. Higher fibrinogen concentrations were associated with vascular conditions such as CHD, stroke, and carotid atherosclerosis.[102,103] Plasminogen activator inhibitor also appears to be elevated in diabetics, and abnormal fibrinolysis may contribute to CHD in diabetics.[104] Specific interventions to improve hemostatic function in diabetics were not studied extensively. A study that utilized short-term intensive glycemic control in diabetics did demonstrate less tendency for platelets to aggregate.[105]

Total Risk Factor Burden

The impact of risk factors and diabetes on CHD can be estimated from the experience of an observational investigation such as the Framingham Heart Study, where risk factors were measured regularly and persons followed for the occurrence of disease. Using multivariate formulations it is possible to estimate the risk of CHD for diabetics with various combinations of risk factors.[106] Figure 8 presents estimated CHD risk for Framingham men and women according to various combinations of risk factors, including diabetes, systolic pressure level, cigarette smoking, total cholesterol, HDL-C, and LV hypertrophy. Similarly, Figure 9 shows that risk of CVD death was increased according to smoking habits, hypertension, and elevated cholesterol among more than 347 000 diabetic and nondiabetic male screenees for the Multiple Risk Factor Intervention Trial (MRFIT).[107] Although less extensively studied, IDDM subjects with lower lipids and BP experienced fewer macrovascular complications over a 25-year period.[15] Diabetes among Asian immigrants to Europe seems to be particularly associated with lower HDL-C levels, higher triglyceride concentrations, and CHD.[26]

Although attention particularly focused on glycemic control in diabetics, diabetics and practitioners should work together to reduce the

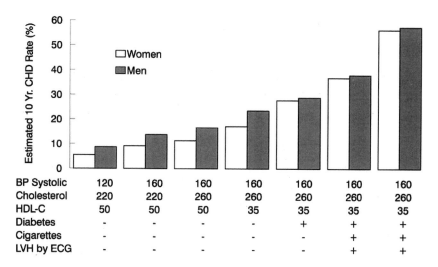

BP Systolic	120	160	160	160	160	160	160
Cholesterol	220	220	260	260	260	260	260
HDL-C	50	50	50	35	35	35	35
Diabetes	-	-	-	-	+	+	+
Cigarettes	-	-	-	-	-	+	+
LVH by ECG	-	-	-	-	-	+	+

Figure 8. *Estimated 10-year CHD rate according to combinations of risk factors. Adapted with permission from Reference 106.*

overall burden of risk factors. Diet and exercise programs, smoking cessation, BP control, and lipid reductions are important issues to lower the risk of CHD in diabetics.[108]

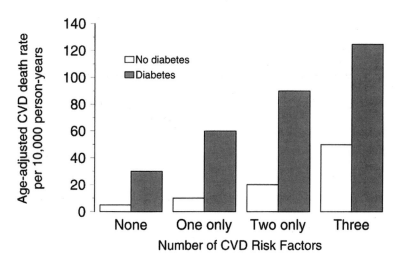

Figure 9. *CVD death rates for MRFIT screenees according to number of risk factors (elevated cholesterol, smoking, hypertension). Adapted with permission from Reference 107.*

Insulin-Resistance Syndrome

Insulin

Studies of Helskinki policeman and residents of Busselton, Australia, showed insulin level as a risk factor for CHD as early as 1979.[109–111] In the Helsinki study OGTT was performed; glucose and insulin concentrations were determined at 0, 1, and 2 hours.[112] Persons at the top of population sample distribution for the 1- and 2-hour insulin levels, but not the fasting values, experienced an increased risk of CHD over the course of the follow-up (Figure 10).[112] In Busselton data the plasma insulin levels at 1 hour after a glucose load were associated with greater risk of CVD during follow-up.[111] Approximately one-half of subsequent reports confirmed an association between fasting insulin and subsequent CHD among nondiabetic men, but data are less supportive of an association between insulin levels and CHD in women (Table 5).[79,109,111–124] Complementary data on asymptomatic hyperglycemia support an association between elevated glucose levels during OGTT and subsequent CHD in men from the Honolulu, Whitehall, and Chicago Peoples Gas Studies.[125–127]

Elevated insulin levels, typically measured in a basal state, were also noted to be a marker for progression from the nondiabetic state to NIDDM in San Antonians, Pima Indians, and British civil servants.[80,128–130] Pro-

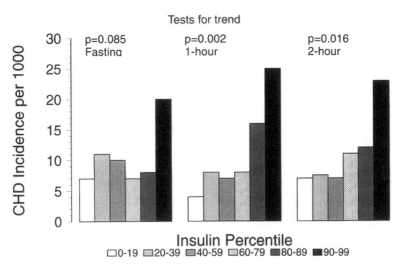

Figure 10. *Blood insulin level and CHD risk in a Finnish male cohort. Insulin-sampled fasting and at 1 and 2 hours after an oral glucose load. Higher insulin levels at the 1- and 2-hour sampling were significantly associated with CHD risk. Adapted with permission from Reference 122.*

Table 5

Prospective Association of Endogenous Insulin and Heart Disease in Nondiabetic Adults

Reference	Population	Diabetics Excluded	Years Follow-up	Sex	No.	End Points	Insulin	Multivariate Association
111	Busselton, Australia (1966, age ≥21)	? ?	12 12	M F	1634 1697	CHD/CVD CHD/CVD	1 h 1 h	$P < 0.05/.01$ (positive) ns/ns
113	Busselton, Australia (1966, age 40–74)	? ?	13 13	M F	840 724	CHD/CVD CHD/CVD	1 h 1 h	ns/ns ns/ns
109	Helsinki, Finland (1971–1972, age 35–64)	Known	5	M	1042	MI/CHD	Fasting 1 h 2 h	ns $P < 0.01/ns^*$ (positive) $P < 0.01/.01$ (positive)
112	Helsinki, Finland (1971–1972, age 35–64)	Known	9.5	M	982	MI and CHD	Fasting 1 h 2 h	ns $P < 0.05$ (positive) $P < 0.01$ (positive)
114	Paris, France (1968–1973, age 43–54)	Known	5	M	7246	MI and CHD	Fasting 2 h	$P < 0.01$ (positive)
115	Paris, France (1968–1973, age 43–54)	Insulin treated	15	M	7028	CHD	Fasting 2 h	ns $P < 0.01^{**}$ (positive)

continues

Table 5 Continued

Reference	Population	Diabetics Excluded	Years Follow-up	Sex	No.	End Points	Insulin	Multivariate Association
116	Caerphilly, South Wales (1979–1983, age 45–59)	Known and borderline	5	M	2022	MI and CHD	Fasting	$P = 0.04$ (positive)[+]
117	Gothenburg, Sweden (1980, age 67)	Known	8	M	563	MI and CHD	Fasting / 1 h	ns* / ns*
118	Pima Indians, US (1975, age ≥25)	New and known	15 (mean 6.7)	M and F	589	Abnormal ECG	Fasting / 2 h	ns / ns
119	MRFIT, US (1973–1976, age 35–57)	Known	7–10 / 7–10	M / M (Apo E 3/2)	622 / 58	MI and CHD / MI and CHD	Fasting / Fasting	ns / $P = 0.02$ (positive)
120	San Luis Valley, US (1984–1988, age 25–74)	New and known	4	M and F	626	MI and CHD	Fasting / Area	ns / ns
121	Rancho Bernardo, US (1984–1987, age 50–89)	New and known	5	M	538	CHD/CVD	Fasting / 2 h	ns/ns / ns/$P = 0.01$ (negative)
		New and known	5	F	705	CHD/CVD	Fasting / 2 h	ns/ns / ns/ns
124	Quebec City, Canada (1985–1990, age 45–76)	New and known	5	M	2103	CHD	Fasting	$P < 0.001$ (positive)

MRFIT, Multiple Risk Factor Intervention Trial; MI, nonfatal myocardial infarction; CHD, fatal coronary heart disease; CVD, fatal cardiovascular disease; ns, not statistically significant. [+] Known, previously diagnosed diabetics; new, NIDDM by OGTT according to WHO criteria; * univariate analysis; ** highest quantile vs. lower quantiles;

Reproduced with permission from Reference 11.

spective studies revealed that obesity, particularly abdominal adiposity, low HDL-C, and high triglycerides often cluster.[80,130] Persons with such tendencies usually have insulin resistance, if studied with metabolic ward techniques to assess insulin resistance.[131] A critical component of the latter is insulin sensitivity, which is defined as the increase of the fractional turnover of glucose per unit increase of insulin concentration. As seen in Figure 11, several factors appear to reduce insulin sensitivity, including female sex, obesity, and oral contraceptive use. Other factors associated with greater insulin resistance and decreased insulin sensitivity are currently under active investigation. Abnormalities in carbohydrate metabolism, lipoprotein lipase activity and myocardial cell function may all occur in tandem.[132–134] Although insulin resistance was classically studied using metabolic studies and clamp techniques, newer adaptations are being developed to study persons participating in large outpatient studies.[135]

Obesity, particularly abdominal adiposity, appears to underlie the insulin-resistance syndrome (IRS). Various components of IRS were proposed, including the elements obesity, abnormal HDL-C, and elevated triglycerides and VLDL concentrations, and an abnormal insulin measure appears to be key (Table 6). It appears less likely that hypertension is actually part of the syndrome.[129] The actual population impact of such definitions will not be known until a definition is developed and applied to cohort studies to assay the overall impact on heart disease in the population.

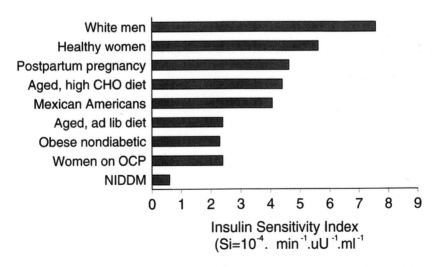

Figure 11. *Typical levels of insulin sensitivity in various groups. Insulin sensitivity determined using the minimal model technique according to Bergman. Reproduced with permission from Reference 131.*

Table 6
Insulin Resistance Syndrome

Resistance to insulin-stimulated glucose uptake
Hyperinsulinemia
Hypertension (?)
Glucose intolerance
Increased VLDL triglyceride
Decreased HDL-C
Abdominal adiposity

References

1. Higgins M, Thom TJ. Trends in CHD in the United States. *Int J Epidemiol* 1989;18(suppl):58–66.
2. Harris MI, Hadden WC, Knowler WC, et al. Prevalence of diabetes and impaired glucose tolerance and plasma glucose levels in U.S. Population aged 20–74 yr. *Diabetes* 1987;36:523–534.
3. National Diabetes Data Group. Classification and diagnosis of diabetes mellitus and other categories of glucose intolerance. *Diabetes* 1979;28:1039–1057.
4. World Health Organization. Report of the Expert Committee on Diabetes. WHO Technical Report Series. Geneva: World Health Organization; 1980:646.
5. World Health Organization. Diabetes Mellitus. Report of a Study Group. WHO Technical Report Series. Geneva: World Health Organization; 1985:727.
6. Kahn CR. Banting lecture. Insulin action, diabetogenes, and the cause of type II diabetes. *Diabetes* 1994;43:1066–1084.
7. Atkinson MA, Maclaren NK. The pathogenesis of insulin-dependent diabetes mellitus. *N Engl J Med* 1994;331:1428–1436.
8. King H, Rewers M. Global estimates for prevalence of diabetes mellitus and impaired glucose tolerance in adults. WHO Ad Hoc Diabetes Reporting Group [see Comments]. *Diabetes Care* 1993;16:157–177.
9. Palumbo PJ, Elveback LR, Chu CP, et al. Diabetes mellitus: incidence, prevalence, survivorship, and causes of death in Rochester, Minnesota, 1945–1970. *Diabetes* 1976;25:566–573.
10. Barrett-Connor EL, Cohn BA, Wingard DL, et al. Why is diabetes mellitus a stronger risk factor for fatal ischemic heart disease in women than in men? *JAMA* 1991;265:627–632.
11. Wingard DL, Barrett-Connor EL. Heart disease and diabetes. In Harris MI, ed. *Diabetes in America*. Bethesda, MD: National Institutes of Health; 1995:429–448.
12. Goodkin G. Mortality factors in diabetes. A 20 year mortality study. *J Occup Med* 1975;17:716–721.
13. Krolewski AS, Kosinski EJ, Warram JH, et al. Magnitude and determinants of coronary artery disease in juvenile-onset, insulin-dependent diabetes mellitus. *Am J Cardiol* 1987;59:750–755.
14. Krolewski AS, Warram JH, Rand LI, et al. Epidemiologic approach to the etiology of type I diabetes mellitus and its complications. *N Engl J Med* 1987;317:1390–1398.

15. Orchard TJ, Dorman JS, Maser RE, et al. Factors associated with avoidance of severe complications after 25 yr of IDDM: Pittsburgh Epidemiology of Diabetes Complications Study I. *Diabetes Care* 1990;13:741–747.
16. Bale GS, Entmacher PS. Estimated life expectancy of diabetics. *Diabetes* 1977;26:434–438.
17. Kannel WB, McGee DL. Diabetes and cardiovascular risk factors: the Framingham Study. *Circulation* 1979;59:8–13.
18. Kannel WB, McGee DL. Diabetes and glucose tolerance as risk factors for cardiovascular disease: the Framingham Study. *Diabetes Care* 1979;2:120–126.
19. Kannel WB, Abbott RD. Incidence and prognosis of unrecognized myocardial infarction. An update on the Framingham Study. *N Engl J Med* 1984;311:1144–1147.
20. Scheidt-Nave C, Barrett-Connor E, Wingard DL. Resting electrocardiographic abnormalities suggestive of asymptomatic ischemic heart disease associated with non-insulin-dependent diabetes mellitus in a defined population. *Circulation* 1990;81:899–906.
21. Nesto RW, Phillips RT, Kett KG, et al. Angina and exertional myocardial ischemia in diabetic and nondiabetic patients: assessment by exercise thallium scintigraphy [Erratum *Ann Intern Med* 1988;108:646]. *Ann Intern Med* 1988;108:170–175.
22. Langer A, Freeman MR, Josse RG, et al. Detection of silent myocardial ischemia in diabetes mellitus. *Am J Cardiol* 1991;67:1073–1078.
23. Nahser PJ Jr, Brown RE, Oskarsson H, et al. Maximal coronary flow reserve and metabolic coronary vasodilation in patients with diabetes mellitus. *Circulation* 1995;91:635–640.
24. Granger CB, Califf RM, Young S, et al. Outcome of patients with diabetes mellitus and acute myocardial infarction treated with thrombolytic agents. The Thrombolysis and Angioplasty in Myocardial Infarction (TAMI) Study Group. *J Am Coll Cardiol* 1993;21:920–925.
25. Stone PH, Muller JE, Hartwell T, et al. The effect of diabetes mellitus on prognosis and serial left ventricular function after acute myocardial infarction: contribution of both coronary disease and diastolic left ventricular dysfunction to the adverse prognosis. The MILIS Study Group. *J Am Coll Cardiol* 1989;14:49–57.
26. Woods KL, Samanta A, Burden AC. Diabetes mellitus as a risk factor for acute myocardial infarction in Asians and Europeans. *Br Heart J* 1989;62:118–122.
27. Herlitz J, Malmberg K, Karlson BW, et al. Mortality and morbidity during a five-year follow-up of diabetics with myocardial infarction. *Acta Med Scand* 1988;224:31–38.
28. Hands ME, Rutherford JD, Muller JE, et al. The in-hospital development of cardiogenic shock after myocardial infarction: incidence, predictors of occurrence, outcome and prognostic factors. The MILIS Study Group [see Discussion 47–48]. *J Am Coll Cardiol* 1989;14:40–46.
29. Weitzman S, Wagner GS, Heiss G, et al. Myocardial infarction site and mortality in diabetes. *Diabetes Care* 1982;5:31–35.
30. Ulvenstam G, Aberg A, Bergstrand R, et al. Long-term prognosis after myocardial infarction in men with diabetes. *Diabetes* 1985;34:787–792.
31. Abbott RD, Donahue RP, Kannel WB, et al. The impact of diabetes on survival following myocardial infarction in men versus women: the Framingham Study. *JAMA* 1988;260:3456–3460.

32. Pedersen TR. Six-year follow-up of the Norwegian Multicenter Study on Timolol After Acute Myocardial Infarction. *N Engl J Med* 1985;313:1055–1058.
33. Gundersen T, Kjekshus J. Timolol treatment after myocardial infarction in diabetic patients. *Diabetes Care* 1983;6:285–290.
34. Burchfiel CM, Reed DM, Marcus EB, et al. Association of diabetes mellitus with coronary atherosclerosis and myocardial lesions. An autopsy study from the Honolulu Heart Program. *Am J Epidemiol* 1993;137:1328–1340.
35. Yarom R, Zirkin H, Stammler G, et al. Human coronary microvessels in diabetes and ischaemia. Morphometric study of autopsy material. *J Pathol* 1992;166:265–270.
36. Stein B, Weintraub WS, Gebhart SP, et al. Influence of diabetes mellitus on early and late outcome after percutaneous transluminal coronary angioplasty. *Circulation* 1995;91:979–989.
37. Lawrie GM, Morris GC Jr, Glaeser DH. Influence of diabetes mellitus on the results of coronary bypass surgery. Follow-up of 212 diabetic patients ten to 15 years after surgery. *JAMA* 1986;256:2967–2971.
38. Anonymous. Comparison of coronary bypass surgery with angioplasty in patients with multivessel disease. The Bypass Angioplasty Revascularization Investigation (BARI) Investigators. *N Engl J Med* 1996;335:217–225.
39. Kannel WB, Hjortland MC, Castelli WP. Role of diabetes in congestive heart failure. The Framingham Study. *Am J Cardiol* 1974;34:29–34.
40. Schaffer SW. Cardiomyopathy associated with noninsulin-dependent diabetes. *Mol Cell Biochem* 1991;107:1–20.
41. Zarich SW, Nesto RW. Diabetic cardiomyopathy. *Am Heart J* 1989;118:1000–1012.
42. Bouchard A, Sanz N, Botvinick EH, et al. Noninvasive assessment of cardiomyopathy in normotensive diabetic patients between 20 and 50 years old. *Am J Med* 1989;87:160–166.
43. Galderisi M, Anderson KM, Wilson PWF, et al. Echocardiographic evidence for the existence of a distinct diabetic cardiomyopathy (the Framingham Heart Study). *Am J Cardiol* 1991;68:85–89.
44. Mustonen JN, Uusitupa MI, Laakso M, et al. Left ventricular systolic function in middle-aged patients with diabetes mellitus. *Am J Cardiol* 1994;73:1202–1208.
45. Sasson Z, Rasooly Y, Bhesania T, et al. Insulin resistance is an important determinant of left ventricular mass in the obese. *Circulation* 1993;88:1431–1436.
46. Reid DD, Hamilton PJS, McCartney P, et al. Smoking and other risk factors for coronary heart-disease in British civil servants. *Lancet* 1976;2:979–984.
47. Pfeffer MA, Braunwald E, Moye LA, et al. Effect of captopril on mortality and morbidity in patients with left ventricular dysfunction after myocardial infarction. Results of the survival and ventricular enlargement trial. The SAVE Investigators [see Comments]. *N Engl J Med* 1992;327:669–677.
48. Schneider JF, Thomas HE Jr, Sorlie PD, et al. Comparative features of newly acquired left and right bundle branch block in the general population: the Framingham Study. *Am J Cardiol* 1981;47:931–940.
49. Benjamin EJ, Levy D, Vaziri SM, et al. Independent risk factors for atrial fibrillation in a population-based cohort. The Framingham Heart Study. *JAMA* 1994;271:840–844.
50. Straub RH, Thum M, Hollerbach C, et al. Impact of obesity on neuropathic late complications in NIDDM. *Diabetes Care* 1994;17:1290–1294.
51. Consensus statement: standardized measures in diabetic neuropathy. *Diabetes Care* 1996;19(suppl):72–92.

52. Ewing DJ, Borsey DQ, Travis P, et al. Abnormalites of ambulatory 24-hour heart rate in diabetes mellitus. *Diabetes* 1983;32:101–105.
53. Ewing DJ, Campbell IW, Clarke BF. The natural history of diabetic autonomic neuropathy. *Q J Med* 1980;49:95–108.
54. Skyler JS. The UGDP and insulin therapy. Editorial. *Diabetes Care* 1978;1:328–329.
55. Anonymous. American diabetes association policy statement: the UGDP controversy. *Diabetes Care* 1979;2:1–3.
56. Knatterud GL, Klimt CR, Levin ME, et al. Effects of hypoglycemic agents on vascular complications in patients with adult-onset diabetes. VII. Mortality and selected nonfatal events with insulin treatment. *JAMA* 1978;240:37–42.
57. Genuth S. Exogenous insulin administration and cardiovascular risk in non-insulin-dependent and insulin-dependent diabetes mellitus. *Ann Intern Med* 1996;124:104–109.
58. Nathan DM, Singer DE, Hurxthal K, et al. The clinical information value of the glycosylated hemoglobin assay. *N Engl J Med* 1984;310:341–346.
59. Orchard TJ. From diagnosis and classification to complications and therapy. DCCT. Part II. Diabetes Control and Complications Trial. *Diabetes Care* 1994;17:326–338.
60. Kuusisto J, Mykkanen L, Pyorala K, et al. NIDDM and its metabolic control predict coronary heart disease in elderly subjects. *Diabetes* 1994;43:960–967.
61. Laakso M. Glycemic control and the risk for coronary heart disease in patients with non-insulin-dependent diabetes mellitus: the Finnish Studies. *Ann Intern Med* 1996;124:127–130.
62. Godine JE. The relationship between metabolic control and vascular complications of diabetes mellitus. *Med Clin North Am* 1988;72:1271–1284.
63. Anonymous. The effect of intensive treatment of diabetes on the development and progression of long-term complications in insulin-dependent diabetes mellitus. The Diabetes Control and Complications Trial Research Group [see Comments]. *N Engl J Med* 1993;329:977–986.
64. Anonymous. Effect of intensive diabetes management on macrovascular events and risk factors in the Diabetes Control and Complications Trial. *Am J Cardiol* 1995;75:894–903.
65. Colwell JA. The feasibility of intensive insulin management in non-insulin-dependent diabetes mellitus: implications of the Veterans Affairs Cooperative Study on Glycemic Control and Complications in NIDDM. *Ann Intern Med* 1996;124:131–135.
66. Turner R, Cull C, Holman R. United Kingdom prospective diabetes study 17: a 9-year update of a randomized, controlled trial on the effect of improved metabolic control on complications in non-insulin-dependent diabetes mellitus. *Ann Intern Med* 1996;124:136–145.
67. Consensus statement: the pharmacological treatment of hyperglycemia in NIDDM. *Diabetes Care* 1996;19(suppl):54–61.
68. Henry RR, Genuth S. Forum One: current recommendations about intensification of metabolic control in non-insulin-dependent diabetes mellitus. *Ann Intern Med* 1996;124:175–177.
69. Perriello G, Misericordia P, Volpi E, et al. Acute antihyperglycemic mechanisms of metformin in NIDDM. Evidence for suppression of lipid oxidation and hepatic glucose production. *Diabetes* 1994;43:920–928.
70. Wilson PWF, Anderson KM, Kannel WB. The epidemiology of diabetes mellitus in the elderly: the Framingham Study. *Am J Med* 1986;80:3–9.

71. Nielsen FS, Rossing P, Bang LE, et al. On the mechanisms of blunted nocturnal decline in arterial blood pressure in NIDDM patients with diabetic nephropathy. *Diabetes* 1995;44:783–789.
72. Mogensen CE, Christensen CK, Vittinghus E. The stages in diabetic renal disease: with emphasis on the stage of incipient diabetic nephropathy. *Diabetes* 1983;32(suppl):64–78.
73. Mogensen CE, Keane WF, Bennett PH, et al. Prevention of diabetic renal disease with special reference to microalbuminuria. *Lancet* 1995;346:1080–1084.
74. Rossing P, Rossing K, Jacobsen P, et al. Unchanged incidence of diabetic nephropathy in IDDM patients. *Diabetes* 1995;44:739–743.
75. Parving HH, Rossing P. Calcium antagonists and the diabetic hypertensive patient. *Am J Kidney Dis* 1993;21:47–52.
76. Consensus statement: diagnosis and management of nephropathy in patients with diabetes mellitus. *Ann Intern Med* 1996;19(suppl):103–106.
77. Parving HH, Gall MA, Nielsen FS. Dyslipidaemia and cardiovascular disease in non-insulin-dependent diabetic patient with and without diabetic nephropathy. *J Intern Med* 1994;736(suppl):89–94.
78. Consensus statement: treatment of hypertension in diabetes. *Diabetes Care* 1996;19(suppl):107–113.
79. Howard BV, Lee ET, Cowan LD, et al. Coronary heart disease prevalence and its relation to risk factors in American Indians. The Strong Heart Study. *Am J Epidemiol* 1995;142:254–268.
80. Haffner SM, Stern MP, Hazuda HP, et al. Cardiovascular risk factors in confirmed prediabetic individuals: does the clock for coronary heart disease start ticking before the onset of clinical diabetes? *JAMA* 1990;263:2893–2898.
81. Laakso M, Ronnemaa T, Pyorala K, et al. Atherosclerotic vascular disease and its risk factors in non-insulin-dependent diabetic and nondiabetic subjects in Finland. *Diabetes Care* 1988;11:449–463.
82. Harris MI. Hypercholesterolemia in diabetes and glucose intolerance in the US population. *Diabetes Care* 1991;14:366–374.
83. Cowie CC, Harris MI. Physical and metabolic characteristics of persons with diabetes. In Harris MI, ed. *Diabetes in America.* Bethesda, MD: National Institutes of Health; 1995:117–164.
84. Howard BV. Lipoprotein metabolism in diabetes mellitus. *J Lipid Res* 1987;28:613–628.
85. Haffner SM, Tuttle KR, Rainwater DL. Decrease of Lp(a) with improved glycemic control in subjects with insulin-dependent diabetes mellitus. *Diabetes Care* 1991;14:302–307.
86. Haffner SM. Lipoprotein (a) and diabetes. An update. *Diabetes Care* 1993;16:835–840.
87. Krauss RM, Burke DJ. Identification of multiple subclasses of plasma low density lipoproteins in normal humans. *J Lipid Res* 1982;23:97–104.
88. Austin MA, Breslow JL, Hennekens CH, et al. Low density lipoprotein subclass patterns and risk of myocardial infarction. *JAMA* 1988;260:1917–1921.
89. Campos H, Genest JJ Jr, Blijlevens E, et al. Low density lipoprotein particle size and coronary artery disease. *Arterioscler Thromb* 1992;12:187–195.
90. McNamara JR, Jenner JL, Li Z, et al. Change in LDL particle size is associated with change in plasma triglyceride concentration. *Arterioscler Thromb* 1992;12:1284–1290.
91. Ukkola O, Savolainen MJ, Salmela PI, et al. DNA polymorphisms at the lipoprotein lipase gene are associated with macroangiopathy in type 2 (non-insulin-dependent) diabetes mellitus. *Atherosclerosis* 1995;115:99–105.

92. Ukkola O, Kervinen K, Salmela PI, et al. Apolipoprotein E phenotype is related to macro- and microangiopathy in patients with non-insulin-dependent diabetes mellitus. *Atherosclerosis* 1993;101:9–15.

93. Consensus statement: detection and management of lipid disorders in diabetes. *Ann Intern Med* 1996;19(suppl):96–102.

94. Expert Panel on Detection Evaluation and Treatment of High Blood Cholesterol in Adults. Summary of the second report of the National Cholesterol Education Program (NCEP) expert panel on detection, evaluation, and treatment of high blood cholesterol in adults (Adult Treatment Panel II). *JAMA* 1993;269:3015–3023.

95. Podgor MJ, Kannel WB, Cassel GH, et al. Lens changes and the incidence of cardiovascular events among persons with diabetes. *Am Heart J* 1989;117:642–648.

96. Hiller R, Sperduto RD, Podgor MJ, et al. Diabetic retinopathy and cardiovascular disease in type II diabetics. The Framingham Heart Study and the Framingham Eye Study. *Am J Epidemiol* 1988;128:402–409.

97. Kannel WB, Wolf R, Castelli WP, et al. Fibrinogen and risk of cardiovascular disease. The Framingham Study. *JAMA* 1987;258:1183–1186.

98. Kannel WB, D'Agostino RB, Wilson PWF, et al. Diabetes, fibrinogen, and risk of cardiovascular disease: the Framingham experience. *Am Heart J* 1990;120:672–676.

99. Colwell JA, Halushka PV, Sarji K, et al. Altered platelet function in diabetes mellitus. *Diabetes* 1976;25(suppl):826–831.

100. Sowers JR, Standley PR, Ram JL, et al. Hyperinsulinemia, insulin resistance, and hyperglycemia: contributing factors in the pathogenesis of hypertension and atherosclerosis. *Am J Hypertens* 1993;6(suppl):260–270.

101. Eldwood PC, Beswick AD, Sharp DS, et al. Whole blood impedance platelet aggregometry and ischemic heart disease. the Caerphilly Collaborative Heart Disease Study. *Arteriosclerosis* 1990;10:1032–1036.

102. Ernst E, Resch KL. Fibrinogen as a cardiovascular risk factor: a meta-analysis and review of the literature. *Ann Intern Med* 1993;118:956–963.

103. Folsom AR, Wu KK, Shahar E, et al. Association of hemostatic variables with prevalent cardiovascular disease and asymptomatic carotid artery atherosclerosis. The Atherosclerosis Risk in Communities (ARIC) Study Investigators. *Arterioscler Thromb* 1993;13:1829–1836.

104. Yudkin JS. Coronary heart disease in diabetes mellitus: three new risk factors and a unifying hypothesis. *J Intern Med* 1995;238:21–30.

105. Davi G, Averna M, Catalano I, et al. Platelet function in patients with type 2 diabetes mellitus: the effect of glycaemic control. *Diabetes Res* 1989;10:7–12.

106. Anderson KM, Wilson PWF, Odell PM, et al. An updated coronary risk profile. A statement for health professionals. *Circulation* 1991;83:357–363.

107. Stamler J, Vaccaro O, Neaton JD, et al. Diabetes, other risk factors, and 12-yr cardiovascular mortality for men screened in the Multiple Risk Factor Intervention Trial. *Diabetes Care* 1993;16:434–444.

108. Savage PJ. Cardiovascular complications of diabetes mellitus: what we know and what we need to know about their prevention. *Ann Intern Med* 1996;124:123–126.

109. Pyorala K. Relationship of glucose tolerance and plasma insulin to the incidence of coronary heart disease: results from two population studies in Finland. *Diabetes Care* 1979;2:131–141.

110. Pyorala K, Savolainen E, Lehtovirta E, et al. Glucose tolerance and coronary heart disease: Helsinki policemen study. *J Chron Dis* 1979;32:729–745.

111. Welborn TA, Wearne K. Coronary heart disease incidence and cardiovascular mortality in Busselton with reference to glucose and insulin concentrations. *Diabetes Care* 1979;2:154–160.
112. Pyorala K, Savolainen E, Kaukola S, et al. Plasma insulin as coronary heart disease risk factor: relationship to other risk factors and predictive value during 9.5 year follow-up of the Helsinki Policemen Study population. *Acta Med Scand* 1985;701(suppl):38–52.
113. Cullen K, Stenhouse NS, Wearne KL, et al. Multiple regression analysis of risk factors for cardiovascular disease and cancer mortality in Busselton, Western Australia—13-year study. *J Chron Dis* 1983;36:371–377.
114. Fieback NH, Viscoli CM, Horwitz RI. Differences between women and men in survival after myocardial infarction: biology of methodology? *JAMA* 1990;263:1092–1096.
115. Feinleib M. Summary of a workshop on cholesterol and noncardiovascular disease mortality. *Prev Med* 1982;11:360–367.
116. Yarnell JW, Sweetnam PM, Marks V, et al. Insulin in ischaemic heart disease: are associations explained by triglyceride concentrations? The Caerphilly prospective study. *Br Heart J* 1994;71:293–296.
117. Welin L, Eriksson H, Larsson B, et al. Hyperinsulinaemia is not a major coronary risk factor in elderly men. The study of men born in 1913. *Diabetologia* 1992;35:766–770.
118. Liu QZ, Knowler WC, Nelson RG, et al. Insulin treatment, endogenous insulin concentration, and ECG abnormalities in diabetic Pima Indians. Cross-sectional and prospective analyses. *Diabetes* 1992;41:1141–1150.
119. Orchard TJ, Eichner J, Kuller LH, et al. Insulin as a predictor of coronary heart disease: interaction with apolipoprotein E phenotype. A report from the Multiple Risk Factor Intervention Trial. *Ann Epidemiol* 1994;4:40–45.
120. Rewers M, Shetterly SM, Baxter J, et al. Insulin and cardiovascular disease in Hispanics and non-Hispanic white (NHW): the San Luis Valley Diabetes Study. *Circulation* 1992;85:865.
121. Ferrara A, Barrett-Connor EL, Edelstein SL. Hyperinsulinemia does not increase the risk of fatal cardiovascular disease in elderly men or women without diabetes: the Rancho Bernardo Study, 1984–1991. *Am J Epidemiol* 1994;140:857–869.
122. Donahue RP, Barrett-Connor EL, Orchard TJ, et al. Endogenous insulin and sex hormones in atherosclerosis and coronary heart disease. *Arteriosclerosis* 1988;8:544–548.
123. Fontbonne AM, Eschwege EM. Insulin and cardiovascular disease. Paris Prospective Study. *Diabetes Care* 1991;14:461–469.
124. Despres JP, Lamarche B, Mauriege P, et al. Hyperinsulinemia as an independent risk factor for ischemic heart disease. *N Engl J Med* 1996;334:952–957.
125. Donahue RP, Abbott RD, Reed DM, et al. Postchallenge glucose concentrations and coronary heart disease in men of Japanese ancestry. The Honolulu Heart Program. *Diabetes* 1987;36:689–692.
126. Fuller JH, McCartney P, Jarrett RJ, et al. Hyperglycaemia and coronary heart disease: the Whitehall Study. *J Chron Dis* 1979;32:721–728.
127. Vaccaro O, Ruth KJ, Stamler J. Relationship of postload plasma glucose to mortality with 19-yr follow-up. Comparison of one versus two plasma glucose measurements in the Chicago Peoples Gas Company Study. *Diabetes Care* 1992;15:1328–1334.
128. Haffner SM, Stern MP, Hazuda HP, et al. Hyperinsulinemia in a population at high risk for non-insulin-dependent diabetes mellitus. *N Engl J Med* 1986;315:220–224.

129. Saad MF, Knowler WC, Pettitt DJ, et al. Insulin and hypertension. relationship to obesity and glucose intolerance in Pima Indians. *Diabetes* 1990;39:1430–1435.
130. Perry IJ, Wannamethee SG, Walker MK, et al. Prospective study of risk factors for development of non-insulin dependent diabetes in middle aged British men [see Comments]. *Br Med J* 1995;310:560–564.
131. Bergman RN. Lilly lecture 1989. Toward physiological understanding of glucose tolerance. Minimal-model approach. *Diabetes* 1989;38:1512–1527.
132. Ahn YI, Ferrell RE, Hamman RF, et al. Association of lipoprotein lipase gene variation with the physiological components of the insulin-resistance syndrome in the population of the San Luis Valley, Colorado. *Diabetes Care* 1993;16:1502–1506.
133. Marshall JA, Hoag S, Shetterly S, et al. Dietary fat predicts conversion from impaired glucose tolerance to NIDDM. The San Luis Valley Diabetes Study. *Diabetes Care* 1994;17:50–56.
134. Robillon JF, Sadoul JL, Jullien D, et al. Abnormalities suggestive of cardiomyopathy in patients with type 2 diabetes of relatively short duration. *Diabetes Metab* 1994;20:473–480.
135. Anderson RL, Hamman RF, Savage PJ, et al. Exploration of simple insulin sensitivity measurements derived from frequently sampled intravenous glucose tolerance (FSIGT) tests. The Insulin Resistance Atherosclerosis Study. *Am J Epidemiol* 1995;142:724–732.
136. Geiss LS, Herman WH, Smith PJ. Mortality in non-insulin-dependent diabetes. In: Harris MI, ed. *Diabetes in America.* Bethesda, MD: National Institutes of Health; 1995:233–258.
137. Kannel WB, Wolf, PA, Garrison, RJ. Section 34: some risk factors related to the annual incidence of cardiovascular disease and death using pooled repeated biennial measurements: Framingham Heart Study, 30-year followup. Springfield, VA: National Technical Information Service; 1987:1–459.

Chapter 5

Nutrition and Dietary Factors in Cardiovascular Disease

Patricia J. Elmer, PhD

Introduction

Diet and nutrition continue to be a focus of ongoing efforts to reduce heart disease and other chronic conditions. Scientific advances, public health policies, and cultural and lifestyle changes over the past decades provide the current context for a heightened national interest in diet and nutrition. Clinical guidelines and public health recommendations emphasize diet as a key element for cardiovascular health. Public awareness and action regarding diet and health increased, and the nation's food producers and manufacturers responded by providing new food options.[1,2] Recently, national efforts underscored the roles of obesity and physical activity in cardiovascular disease (CVD) and health promotion as well as their interrelations with diet.[3-6]

Understanding the role of diet in the development and treatment of heart disease advanced through significant developments in the fields of education and epidemiology and in the biological studies of atherosclerosis, lipoprotein and apolipoprotein metabolism, thrombosis and hemostasis, vessel wall biology, and cell and molecular biology. Subsequently, a renewed interest in vitamins and other dietary components led

From Robinson K, (ed): *Preventive Cardiology.* Armonk, NY: Futura Publishing Company, Inc. © 1998.

to important new diet- and nutrition-related research and clinical activities. This chapter will review the current nutrition and dietary guidelines for CVD prevention and treatment and will address topics of recent interest—fatty acids, dietary patterns, antioxidants, and obesity.

Fifty years of epidemiological data and clinical trial evidence support both aggressive treatment of the modifiable risk factors and population-wide intervention to prevent disease. Epidemiological studies comparing the relation between diet and disease identified dietary factors that play a key role in the etiology of coronary heart disease (CHD). The classic epidemiological investigation, the Seven Countries Study, provided evidence for the association among the type of dietary fat, total cholesterol (TC) level, and incidence of CHD[7] and a notably strong positive association between saturated fatty acid (SFA) intake and total blood cholesterol levels. These findings prompted well-controlled clinical trials that investigated the role of the type and amount of dietary fat and cholesterol on CHD risk factors as well as diet and pharmacologic studies aimed at reducing blood cholesterol and CHD risk. The studies of Keys et al[8] and Hegsted et al[9] established the effect of the fatty acid classes on blood cholesterol levels. As a result, equations to predict these effects of different fats on serum lipids were developed. Current efforts focus on furthering our understanding of the effect of fatty acid classes on other metabolic parameters and their interactions with plasma lipids, lipoproteins, and hemostasis. This combined body of evidence provides the background for current dietary recommendations.

Guidelines for Treatment of Elevated Cholesterol

Guidelines for the treatment of elevated cholesterol in adults as well as population guidelines to prevent high blood cholesterol were established as a part of the National Cholesterol Education Program (NCEP).[10–12] Dietary treatment is a major focus of these clinical guidelines. The guidelines are evidence based and were reviewed, endorsed, and adopted by scientific groups and medical societies throughout the United States. They were designed to be practical and provide information for clinical use, patient education, and counseling. The NCEP guidelines provide a systemic approach for the assessment of lipid levels, diagnosis of hypercholesterolemia including consideration of the other risk factors, and treatment and follow-up recommendations.

Diet therapy is considered the first line of treatment for cholesterol management and is an integral part of the treatment approach. Table 1 shows patient profiles and the corresponding low-density lipoprotein cholesterol (LDL-C) levels at which dietary treatment is initiated. The aim of dietary change is to lower elevated blood cholesterol while maintaining

Table 1
NCEP Guidelines: LDL Levels for Dietary Treatment

Patient Profile	LDL Initiation Level (mg/dL)	LDL Treatment Goal (mg/dL)
Without CHD and with fewer than two risk factors	≥160	<160
Without CHD and with two or more risk factors	≥130	<130
With CHD	>100	≤100

Reproduced with permission from Reference 11.

a nutritionally adequate eating pattern. The recommendations provide a two-step approach where dietary fat, saturated fats, and cholesterol are progressively reduced. Table 2 lists the recommended macronutrient levels for these two diets (step I and step II). Emphasis is placed on reducing saturated fat through reductions in total fat by reducing foods that are major sources of saturated fats and by including fruits, vegetables, and grains. Dietary cholesterol is also progressively reduced. The dietary rec-

Table 2
NCEP Recommended Macronutrient Levels for Dietary Treatment of High Blood Cholesterol

Nutrient	Step I Diet Recommendations	Step II Diet Recommendations
Total fat	30% or less of total calories	Less than 30% of total calories
Saturated fatty acids	10% or less of total calories	Less than 7% of total calories
Polyunsaturated fatty acids	Up to 10% of total calories	Up to 10% of total calories
Monounsaturated fatty acids	10% to 15% of total calories	10% to 15% of total calories
Carbohydrate	50% to 60% of total calories	50% to 60% of total calories
Protein	10% to 20% of total calories	10% to 20% of total calories
Cholesterol	Less than 300 mg/day	Less than 200 mg/day
Total calories	To achieve and maintain desirable weight	To achieve and maintain desirable weight
Fruits and vegetables	≥5 servings/day	≥5 servings/day

Reproduced with permission from Reference 11.

ommendations incorporate recent research findings regarding CVD risk and the beneficial effects of various foods and nutrients and emphasize the importance of calorie balance and weight reduction for the successful management of hyperlipidemia.

Today more than ever, consumers and patients are interested in nutrition and are attempting dietary changes to improve their health.[1] Consumers recognize that dietary fat and cholesterol are related to blood cholesterol and heart disease; more than one-half of US adults have had their cholesterol levels measured, and many report reducing fat in their diet.[2,13] The reported fat intake for adults in the United States by the Third National Health and Nutrition Examination Survey (NHANES III, 1988–1991) was 34% kcal from total fat and 12% kcal from saturated fat,[14] a decline from the 37% kcal from the total fat reported in the previous survey. Consumption of red meat declined whereas intake of poultry and fish and low-fat dairy products increased.[15] Meat, dairy, and baked products are the major sources of saturated fat. The number of meals eaten away from home also increased; this may result in higher fat intakes and lower intakes of fruits and vegetables. Nutrition labels provide information on the fat and saturated fat content of food, which can help individuals with food choices.

Saturated Fatty Acids

SFAs are the major dietary determinants of LDL-C. Predictive equations show that for every 1% of calories consumed from saturated fat there is an approximate 2.7 mg/dL increase in TC.[15] The cholesterolemic effects of dietary fatty acids vary. The longer-chain SFAs, mainly lauric (C12:0), myristic (C14:0), and palmitic (C16:0), raise cholesterol, whereas the short-chain fatty acids (C3:0-10) and stearic acid (C18:0) were shown to be neutral.[16] Collectively, the evidence available from well-controlled feeding studies shows that C12:0, C14:0, and C16:0 raise TC, LDL-C, and high-density lipoprotein cholesterol (HDL-C) compared to carbohydrate and the unsaturated fatty acids.[15,17] Palmitic acid (C16:0) is the major SFA in the food supply, contributing 50% to 60% of the dietary SFA intake. Major sources of SFA in the diet are animal fats and certain vegetable oils— palm, palm kernel, and coconut—and cocoa butter. Beef fat is high in SFA—both palmitic and stearic—whereas pork has relatively less stearic acid. Trimming external fat and selecting lower-fat cuts and cooking methods all reduce saturated fat intake. Although cocoa butter is relatively high in stearic acid, related feeding studies demonstrated little cholesterol-raising effect.[18] Butter and tropical oils and coconut, palm, and palm kernel oil cause the largest increases in LDL-C due to their high saturated fat content.[19] The recognition that some SFAs do not raise cholesterol provides opportunities for engineering fat blends and food products with more-desirable fat profiles.

There is emerging evidence that saturated fats may contribute to thrombosis through effects on hemostatic factors. Factor VII levels were related to saturated fat intake and decrease when saturated fat is decreased.[20]

trans-Fatty Acids

Hydrogenation is a process used in food manufacturing to convert vegetable oils to more solid fats. Hydrogenated fats are then used to manufacture solid margarine and vegetable shortening. Through this process, the saturated fat content of the product is increased by increasing stearic acid. Hydrogenation also converts some polyunsaturated fat to monounsaturated fatty acids (MUFAs) of two types—oleic acid (*cis*-fatty acid) and *trans*-fatty acid.[21,22] Concerns were raised regarding the health effects of *trans*-fatty acids. In a prospective cohort study, women with the highest intakes of *trans*-fatty acids had the highest risk of myocardial infarction (MI).[23] Recent metabolic studies showed that *trans*-fatty acids lower HDL-C and raise LDL-C to levels somewhat intermediate to the effects observed for saturated fats. However, the exact amount of cholesterol raising and HDL lowering continues to be debated.[24,25] It was suggested that *trans*-fatty acids may have effects on CVD through mechanisms other than LDL. *trans*-Fatty acids were reported to raise levels of lipoprotein (a), a potential risk factor for CHD; however, the data are limited for this effect.[24,26] In the American diet, *trans*-fatty acids contribute from 2% to 5% of total calories.[24] Because there is considerable debate regarding *trans*-fatty acids and the health effects are not totally known, the NCEP guidelines suggest that it may be wise to limit *trans*-fatty acid intake, particularly in very high-risk individuals.[11] This can be accomplished by lowering the intake of solid vegetable shortening and stick margarine. Soft margarines contain lower amounts of *trans*-fatty acids, and future advances in food technology may be able to further reduce the level of *trans*-fatty acids.

Low-Fat Diets and Unsaturated Fats

Polyunsaturated fatty acids (PUFAs), those from the ω-3 and ω-6 groups, include polyunsaturated (linoleic and linolenic), monounsaturated (oleic), and the ω-3 eicosapentanoic acid (EPA) dicosahexanoic acids (DHAs). Linoleic acid is the major PUFA in the diet; vegetable oils (corn, soybean, canola, and sunflower) are the major sources.[19] PUFAs decrease TC and LDL-C when they replace carbohydrate.[27] The NCEP report estimated that linoleic acid (C18:2) will decrease TC by approximately 1.4 mg/dL for each 1% decrease in calories from fat. In addition to lipid-lowering properties of PUFA, it was suggested that polyunsaturated fats (n-6) may protect from sudden death by increasing the electrical threshold for ventricular fibrillation.[28,29] The ω-3 fatty acids may have a variety of effects on thrombosis by affecting platelet function and aspects of hemostasis.[30,31] However, the optimal amount of PUFA in the diet remains unclear. From a practical perspective, questions were raised. What is the best replacement for saturated fat? What is the optimal diet for lipid lowering? Large intakes of polyunsaturated fats (>10% kcal) are no longer recommended due to concerns about the potential for oxidation and tumor promotion in animals.[15] It is clear that, when calories are kept constant and saturated fats are reduced by replacing them with carbohydrate as in the step I diet, triglyceride (TG) levels increase and HDL-C levels decline.[11,32] However, there is evidence to show that, in the long term (20–40 weeks), TG and HDL-C may return to near baseline levels.[33,34] Alternate diets of differing composition that would prevent a fall in HDL-C were proposed. High-monounsaturated diets may not result in decreased HDL-C. When individuals are placed on a step I diet and reduce weight, TGs fall and HDL-C increases.[35,36] Response of both LDL and HDL-C to a low-fat diet was correlated with body weight. A recent trial of a low-fat diet in premenopausal women found that only lean women had a fall in LDL, whereas obese women showed little change in LDL-C.[34]

Monounsaturated Fatty Acids

Oleic acid is the primary MUFA in the United States. Its major sources are meat and dairy foods. For many years, it was believed that oleic acid was neutral in its effects on serum cholesterol.[9,15,37,38] Recent data show that oleic acid reduces TC nearly as much as the PUFA linoleic acid when it replaces saturated fat. The recognition that HDL-C levels decline and TG levels increase when dietary saturated fats are replaced with carbohydrate led to many metabolic studies evaluating the effects of high-monounsaturated fat diets on lipids.[37,39,40] It was proposed that diets that maintain higher percentages of total calories from fat (35% to 37%) by replacing SFA with monounsaturated fat may be preferable to a low-fat step I diet because oleic acid may result in a better HDL profile. In several short-term studies, substitution of olive oil for carbohydrate resulted in either little change or a slight increase in HDL-C. However, these findings are not totally consistent, as others reported a fall in HDL-C levels with a diet high in MUFAs. A recent large, tightly controlled metabolic feeding study, Dietary Effects on Lipoprotein and Thrombogenic Activity (DELTA),[42–44] compared the effects of a high-monounsaturated fat diet (37% total fat, 22% MUFA) with those of the step I diet (30% total fat, 15% MUFA) when switching from a usual American diet (37% total fat, 14% MUFA). LDL-C was similarly reduced on both diets (−6%). HDL-C levels were reduced to a lesser degree with the MUFA diet (−4%) compared to the step I diet (−7.6%). TG levels increased on the step I diet (6.9%) but were reduced on the MUFA diet (−4.6%). Factor VIIc levels were reduced on both diets.[42] It was also proposed that high-monounsaturated fat diets, when compared to low-fat diets, may have a more favorable effect on postprandial lipids or glucose and insulin response. Although the data are limited and not entirely consistent, the DELTA study found that these two diets had equal effects on these parameters.[43,44]

There are concerns about widely recommending the higher-fat MUFA diet when high-fat consumption may contribute to obesity. High-fat foods are readily overeaten. This may be due to increased palatability or to the higher caloric density of fat. High-fat foods are also not very satiating. Satiation is the process involved in termination of a meal; satiety refers to the effects of a food or meal after eating ended.[45] It appears that appetite-control systems have only weak mechanisms to prevent the overconsumption of dietary fat.[46] Whereas carbohydrate intake may suppress appetite for some time following a meal, fat may have little effect on appetite suppression. The dramatic increase in the prevalence of obesity during the past decade (Figure 1), underscores concern about this problem and the need for diet approaches to combat it. The current evidence is inconclusive regarding the overall benefits of substituting MUFA for SFA rather than increasing carbohydrate in the diet. For individuals with CVD and high blood cholesterol, it remains unresolved whether attempting to minimize the reduction in HDL-C by partial substitution of SFA with MUFA is more beneficial than increasing carbohydrate intake.

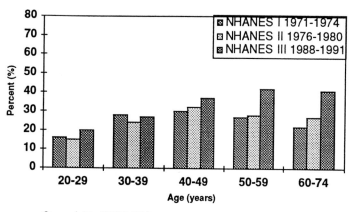

Overweight = BMI ≥ 27.8
Source: Kuczmarski, et al (127)

Figure 1. *Prevalence of overweight US men, NHANES 1971–1991. Reproduced with permission from Reference 47.*

To date, no study showed that the reductions in HDL-C due to dietary modification are deleterious. The use of MUFA to replace carbohydrate can provide an alternative for some patients.

Fish, Fish Oils, and ω-3 Fatty Acids (C18:3)

There was great interest in the potential health benefits of fish oil and fish intake, particularly EPA and DPA. Despite the early promises of many beneficial effects on CVD risk factors, the primary effect of the ω-3 fatty acids is to lower TGs.[30] They act by reducing secretion of very-low-density lipoprotein (VLDL) TG. Although early studies with very high doses of fish oil suggested a lowering of total and LDL-C, more recent studies showed small but significant increases in LDL-C.[48] Speculation that large intakes of fish may be protective for heart disease stemmed from early observations of low rates of CHD in natives of Japan and Greenland.[30,49] Some epidemiological studies support an inverse association between fish intake and CHD.[50-52] In the Zutphen study, compared to those who did not eat fish, Dutch men who consumed 30 g of fish per day had nearly half the risk of CHD mortality, although these findings are not entirely consistent among prospective cohort studies.[15,53] Mechanisms proposed for the benefits of fish intake include reduced VLDL and TGs, reduced thrombotic tendencies and blood viscosity, and increased fibrinolytic activity. Reduced tendencies for arrhythmias and blood pressure (BP) were also proposed; however, recent reviews of the numerous trials of fish oil supplementation revealed relatively small and clinically insignificant effects on BP.[54,55]

Currently available data do not support the use of fish oil supplements as a routine preventive measure. Despite the lack of clinical benefit for fish oil supplementation on lipids and BP, it is proposed that the antithrombotic mechanisms may yet be important aspects responsible for beneficial effects of fish consumption.[56] It is possible that other components in fish may confer benefit, or fish intake may be a marker for other beneficial diet and lifestyle patterns.[50] Although fish oil supplements provide no apparent benefit, increased fish intake can be a part of the dietary pattern for lipid lowering.

Expected Response to Recommended Diets

Numerous metabolic and free-living studies evaluated the effects of and compliance with low-fat and fat-modified diets.[32,37,40,57] These diets reduce serum cholesterol levels from 3% to 14%.[11] Variability in response reflects differences in initial lipid levels, underlying metabolic abnormalities and inherent biological responsiveness, baseline diet, and individual compliance. Those with a higher initial cholesterol are likely to have greater reductions following the step I diet. Currently, dietary saturated fat intake contributes about 11% to 12% of calories to the US diet, which also contains from 220 mg to 340 mg of cholesterol per day (Table 3). Given these intakes, dietary equations[9,15,38] predict that a step I diet will reduce TC levels in men from 5% to 7%. It was suggested that women may have a slightly lower response to reductions in unsaturated fat.[11] Those that progress to the step II diet (lower SFA) should receive another 3% to 7% reduction in cholesterol levels. Reduction in weight can also significantly lower cholesterol levels, and obesity may be an important predictor of cholesterol response.[61] Increased dietary fiber may also provide additional cholesterol reductions. Although there is considerable research into genetic determinants of cholesterol response, it is not possible to determine an individual's inherent responsiveness. For patient populations, the lack of dietary adherence accounts for a large amount of the difference between the predicted and observed changes in cholesterol. Continued support and reinforcement for dietary change in the clinical setting are essential for assisting patients with long-term compliance.

Table 3

Mean Daily Dietary Intake for Men and Women, Aged 40–49 Years in the US Population, NHANES III, 1990–1994.

Nutrients	Men	Women
Kilocalories	2545	1764
Protein (% kcal)	16	16
Fat (% kcal)	34	35
SFA (% kcal)	11	12
PUFA (% kcal)	7	8
MUFA (% kcal)	13	13
Cholesterol (mg)	338	235
Carbohydrate (% kcal)	47	49
Fiber (gm)	18	13
Calcium (mg)	834	685
Potassium (mg)	3263	2388
Magnesium (mg)	349	251
Sodium (mg)[a]	3960	2919
Vitamin E (IU)	10	8
Vitamin C (mg)	115	88
Folate (μg)	317	220
Fruit and vegetable servings	3.3	3.9

[a] May not include added salt.

Reproduced with permission from References 58–60.

Diet Interventions for
Secondary Prevention

In addition to studies of the step I diet and metabolic studies, results from several relatively large diet trials for the secondary prevention of CVD were reported. These trials modified fat, fiber fruits and vegetables, and fish—with the underlying hypothesis that dietary components may act through mechanisms related to oxidation or thrombosis. The Lyon Diet Heart study evaluated the effect of a Mediterranean diet rich in α-linolenic acid for the secondary prevention of CHD.[62] The primary end points were cardiovascular death and nonfatal MI. Patients ($n = 605$) were randomized to either control (low-fat diet advice) or treatment (Mediterranean diet). The Mediterranean diet recommended more bread, fish, root and green vegetables, fruit every day, less meat, use of olive or canola oil in place of other oils, and replacement of butter and cream with the margarine supplied by the study (made from canola oil, containing 48% oleic acid and 16% linolenic acid). The control group received standard post-MI clinical dietary advice for fat modification. Mean follow-up was 27 months (range 1–4 years). Compared to controls, patients receiving the Mediterranean diet significantly increased consumption of bread, fruit, and margarine, showed a trend toward increases in vegetables and legumes, and decreased meat, cream, and butter consumption. The diet group consumed less total and saturated fat and cholesterol but more oleic and α-linolenic acids, which were confirmed by serum measures. Blood lipids, BP, and body weight were not different between the two groups. There were 16 cardiovascular deaths in the control group versus 3 in the treatment group, and 17 versus 5 nonfatal MIs, respectively. Dramatic reductions in risk were observed. The risk ratios after adjustment for these two end points were 0.27 [97% confidence interval (CI): 0.12–0.59, $p = 0.001$] and 0.30 (95% CI: 0.11–0.82, $p = 0.02$). The rationale for the use of the α-linolenic acid-enriched (an ω-3 fatty acid) margarine was based on observations that this fatty acid was relatively high in the Cretan and Japanese diets (populations with extremely low CVD mortality) and that this fatty acid was associated with decreased platelet reactivity.[63] The lack of a difference in blood lipid levels between the two groups and the rapid protective effect observed suggests that, in high-risk patients, this diet may act through antithrombotic or antiarrhythmic effects rather than effects on atherosclerosis.

In another randomized secondary prevention trial conducted in India, the effects of adding fruits and vegetables to a low-fat step I diet was evaluated in 505 men and women who had a previous MI.[64] Follow-up was for 1 year; the primary end points were CHD mortality. All patients (treatment and control) received dietary counseling for a low-fat diet (30% kcal, polyunsaturated to saturated fat ratio [P/S] 1) and replacement of animal fat with vegetable oils. The treatment group also increased intake of fruits and vegetables (>400 g/day), lentils, nuts, and fish. The treatment group reported slightly larger reductions in total fat and saturated fats when compared to the control group. Serum TC and LDL, TGs, and glucose were significantly lower in the treatment group. CHD mortality and cardiac events were reduced by approximately 40% in the treatment group. A previous study by this research group showed that, after stabilizing individuals with existing coronary artery disease on a low-fat diet, the additions of fruits, vegetables, and lentils for 12 additional weeks resulted in a further 6.5% reduction in TC. Although HDL-C levels fell in both the treatment and control group during the initial low-fat diet period, the HDL levels returned to baseline levels when fruits and vegetables were added in the group; TGs and glucose were also further reduced.[65] This trials provides evidence that increasing fruits, vegetables, and legumes may be beneficial in the treatment approach for those with existing CHD.

The Diet and Reinfarction Trial evaluated the effects of changes in fat, fish, and fiber on total mortality and recurrent MI using a factorial design in 2033 men.[56] The diets were fat advice (reduce fat to 30% kcal, increase the P/S ratio to 1.0), fish advice (eat at least two servings of fatty fish per week), and fiber advice (increase cereal fiber to 18 g/day). Follow-up was 2 years. Diet intakes following treatment for each diet advice group compared to controls were fat intake, 33.3% kcal versus 35% kcal/day; fish, 2.4 servings versus 0.6 servings per week; fiber, 17 g versus 9 g of cereal fiber per day. The fish advice group experienced a significant 29% reduction in all-cause mortality. However, the fat and fiber groups did not experience any benefits in total mortality. The fat advice resulted in a 3% to 4% reduction in TC; compliance with this dietary component was less than anticipated. The modest dietary changes may not have been large enough for an effect.

These studies each provide a somewhat different but overlapping perspective on the benefits of dietary modifications on CVD risk reduction. They suggest that α-linolenic acid, fruits and vegetables, and fish may yield protection on top of modest fat reductions. However, saturated fat intakes were also lower in each of the treatment groups compared to the control groups in the above studies. Given the nature of dietary change—reduction of one food component usually results in a concomitant increase in another—it is difficult to sort out the independent effects of dietary components. However, two of these trials that focused on foods and dietary patterns with high intakes of fruit and vegetables yielded impressive results. These findings support further research into comprehensive diet pattern changes and their effects on prevention of CVD.

Diet Patterns and Cardiovascular Disease

Extensive epidemiological evidence indicates that diets high in plant foods, particularly fruits and vegetables, and grains are protective for CVD and cancer.[65–69] Several populations from Mediterranean countries and some areas of Asia where traditional intakes are high in plant foods exhibit low rates of many chronic diseases. Worldwide, Japan has the lowest documented rates of CVD, followed by France.[70] The "French Paradox" received considerable scientific and media attention. In this paradoxical situation, the diet in some parts of France is relatively high in total fat and saturated fat, and yet France experiences some of the lowest rates of CVD in the world.[70,71] Several other Mediterranean countries with low rates of CVD also have relatively high total fat intakes, although the source of fat is predominantly from olive oil.[15,72] Table 4 shows a comparison of dietary characteristics of the United States, Greece, and Japan in the 1960s. Intakes in the United States show high consumption of fat, saturated fat, meat, and eggs. In contrast, Japan had low consumption of fat, saturated fat, meat, and fruit. Greece had high intakes of fat, but a low intake of saturated fat and meat. Meat intake was traditionally low in these populations. Intake of red meat was associated with increased risks of CHD and colon and other cancers. Possible mechanisms may involve saturated

Table 4

Estimated Daily Intake of Nutrients and Foods in the United States, Greece, and Japan in the 1960s

Dietary Characteristics[a]	United States	Greece	Japan
Fat (% of kcal)	39	37	11
Saturated fat (% of kcal)	18	8	3
Vegetables (g/day)	171	191	198
Fruits (g/day)	233	463	34
Legumes (g/day)	1	30	91
Breads and cereals (g/day)	123	453	481
Potatoes (g/day)	124	170	65
Meat (g/day)[3]	273	35	8
Fish (g/day)	3	39	150
Eggs (g/day)	40	15	29
Alcohol (g/day)	6	23	22

[a] Dietary information from the Seven Countries Study. Means of data from Crete and Corfu were averaged for Greece, and means of data from Tanushimaru and Ushibuka were averaged for Japan. Since 1960, consumption of red meat and animal fat greatly increased in Greece and Japan.
[b] Includes poultry.
Reproduced with permission from Reference 73.

fat, dietary cholesterol, heme iron, and the presence of carcinogens formed during cooking.[74]

Fruits, vegetables, grains, antioxidant vitamins, and red wine, in addition to monounsaturated fats, fish, and fiber were all suggested as potential protective factors in these diets.[65–68,71,72,75] A dominant hypothesis was that antioxidants contribute significantly to lower CVD risk through effects on both atherosclerosis and thrombosis.[63,76–78]

Antioxidants

Epidemiological findings such as those noted above and metabolic and clinical studies provided a synergistic research focus on the hypothesis that dietary antioxidants—particularly Vitamin E, Vitamin C, and β-carotene—prevent CVD.[79] Substantial evidence from laboratory, animal, and human studies suggests that oxidation of LDL-C is a critical step in the development of atherosclerosis.[80] Extensive reviews were published on the pathogenesis of atherosclerosis and the role of the modification of LDL in this process.[81] It is believed that oxidized LDL-C accumulates in the cells that line the blood vessels and, through the actions of proliferative and chemotactic mechanisms, leads to fatty streaks and atherosclerotic lesions. A number of in vivo findings supports this hypothesis. Oxidized LDL-C is found in atherosclerotic plaques and appears to increase uptake of LDL by macrophages, enhancing foam cell formation and development of fatty streaks. Increased titers of autoantibodies against modified LDL are also seen in patients with atherosclerosis. Modified LDL may also promote atherosclerosis by other mechanisms.[82]

It is believed that antioxidants in the form of vitamins and other compounds can inhibit LDL oxidation, and this was also extensively reviewed.[83–85] The inhibition of atherosclerosis in animals by antioxidants such as probucol, butylated hydroxytoluene, and α-tocopherol supports this hypothesis.[86] Presumably, antioxidant compounds and vitamins act through protection of oxidation; however, these nutrients may also preserve endothelial function, affect hemostasis by reducing platelet aggregation, and lower both LDL-C levels and BP.[87,88]

The major lipid-soluble antioxidant vitamins are Vitamin E (α-tocopherol) and β-carotene, a precursor of Vitamin A; the major water-soluble antioxidant vitamin is Vitamin C (ascorbic acid). Many other dietary constituents, including folate and the flavonoids, are thought to have antioxidant properties.[89] Vitamin E is important in preventing oxidation of cholesterol. In vitro studies showed that this process does not begin until oxidative stress depletes the host Vitamin E content; β-carotene may prevent oxidation of cholesterol, although this finding is inconsistent. Vitamin C was also shown to prevent oxidation of LDL-C and to preserve Vitamin E and β-carotene levels during oxidative stress.[85,88,90,91]

Observational Epidemiological Studies

The epidemiological data suggest that a high intake of Vitamin E, either from diet or from vitamin supplementation, is associated with a reduced risk for fatal and nonfatal CVD.[79,92–97] Data from large cohort studies contributed greatly to our understandings of these associations. In the Nurses' Health Study (NHS), the largest observational study to examine this hypothesis, more than 87 000 women were followed for 8 years.[96] Women in the highest Vitamin E quintile had a 34% lower risk of major coronary disease (nonfatal MI and fatal CHD) (p for trend = 0.02) and a 24% lower risk of ischemic stroke (p for trend = 0.07) compared to those in the lowest quintile after adjustment for age, CVD risk factors, and Vitamin C and β-carotene intake. The benefit was found primarily in those individuals who consumed high levels of Vitamin E provided by supplements and not diet. The Health Professionals Follow-Up Study (HPFS), a cohort of 39 910 male health professionals, also showed that Vitamin E intake from supplements was associated with a lower risk for CHD.[95] For these two studies, the benefit of Vitamin E was mainly found in those who used a dose of 100 IU/day or more for at least 2 years. In contrast, the Iowa Women's Health Study, a cohort of 34 486 postmenopausal women, reported a relative risk of 0.38 for CHD mortality among women in the highest quintile of dietary intake of Vitamin E (p for trend = 0.004).[93] Use of Vitamin E supplements was not associated with reduced risk of CVD. Because the benefits of Vitamin E correlated with intake from food but not supplements, this study suggests that food-derived Vitamin E might be a marker for other beneficial substances in these foods. However, in this cohort relatively few women took Vitamin E supplements, and information on the duration of use was not available. These factors could explain the lack of association between CVD and supplement use. A recent report from the Established Populations for Epidemiologic Study of the Elderly found that use of Vitamin E supplements reduced the risk of all-cause mortality, relative risk (RR) = 0.66 (95% CI: 0.53–0.83), and CHD mortality, RR = 0.53 (95% CI: 0.34–0.84).[94] The strongest association was found for those who used supplements at two points compared to those who did not them. This is consistent with the finding in the NHS. Information on dose, overall duration, and dietary Vitamin E intake was not available in this study.

It is not clear if these beneficial effects on CVD are directly derived from Vitamin E or are related to other dietary constituents or lifestyle factors. In the United States, major sources of Vitamin E intake includes margarine and salad dressings (which are also high in polyunsaturated fats), nuts and seeds (which contain unique fats, proteins, and other compounds), and whole grains (which are high in fiber and supply other potentially protective compounds).[69] Higher Vitamin E intakes and the use of supplements are also associated with more healthful behaviors and a more healthful cardiovascular risk factor profile.[93,96]

The relation between β-carotene intake and CVD was also examined in large prospective cohort studies. Protective trends were observed in several studies,[95,96,98,99] although only two studies, the HPFS and the Massachusetts Health Care Panel Study,[100] achieved statistical significance. The Iowa Women's Health Study did not find a protective association between β-carotene intake and CVD.[93] Although many studies examined the relation between Vitamin C intake and the incidence of heart disease, the results are inconsistent. Protective effects from high Vitamin C intake were observed,[79,98] while in other studies, protective associations were no longer significant after adjustment was made for intake of Vitamin E or multivitamins.[93-96] The Iowa Women's Health Study[96] found trends (although nonsignificant) toward an increase in risk with the highest levels of Vitamin C, after multivariate adjustments were made. Although the data from prospective studies of both dietary intake and biological markers suggest benefit from antioxidant vitamins, numerous questions remain about the multicollinearity of nutrients and the doses that may be protective as well as possible explanations for findings that indicate increased risk. Uncontrolled confounding inherent in observational studies could account for the observed benefit.

The suggestion of substantial protective effects from antioxidant vitamins prompted the initiation of clinical trials to definitively test their efficacy in the primary and secondary prevention of cancer and CVD. Results were recently reported from several of these trials, although most of the trials focused primarily on cancer end points (Table 5).

The Linxian Chinese Cancer Prevention Trial randomized 29 584 men and women to one of eight treatment arms that provided nutrient supplements of various combinations of nine vitamins and minerals (retinol, zinc, riboflavin, niacin, Vitamin C, molybdenum, β-carotene, Vitamin E, and selenium).[102] The study population was poorly nourished and at high risk for developing cancer. Primary end points were total mortality and cause-specific mortality. A marginally significant reduction in total mortality was reported among those assigned to the combined treatment with β-carotene (15 mg/day), α-tocopherol (30 mg/day), and selenium (50 μg/day). The reduction was largely due to a reduction in cancer mortality and, specifically, stomach cancer mortality. Ischemic heart disease accounted for <9% of the total deaths, and cerebrovascular mortality comprised 26% of the total deaths. There was an apparent, though nonsignificant, reduction in the risk of cerebrovascular mortality (RR = 0.90, 95% CI: 0.76–1.07). In this population, most strokes are likely to be hemorrhagic rather than thromboembolic. No significant effects on mortality rates from all causes were found for any of the other supplement combinations. With this trial design, using combinations of nutrients, the ef-

Table 5

Randomized, Large-Scale, Double-Blind, Placebo-Controlled Trials of Antioxidants—Vitamin E, β-carotene, Retinol, and Selenium in the Treatment or Prevention of Cardiovascular Disease

Trial	Type[a]	Population	Treatment	Endpoints	Results
DeMaio et al 1992[101]	S	100 patients following angioplasty	Vitamin E (400 IU/day) for 4 months	Restenosis by angiogram or exercise test	Nonsignificant trend toward reduction
Blot et al 1993; Linxian China Study[102]	P	29 584 Chinese men and women at high risk for gastric cancer	Combined supplement of β-carotene (15 mg), α-tocopherol (30 mg), and selenium (50 µg) daily for 5 years	Gastric cancer, disease-specific mortality	Nonsignificant trend toward reduction
The ATBC Cancer Prevention Study Group, 1994[103]	P	29 133 Finnish male smokers	Factorial design: synthetic β-carotene (20 mg/day) and synthetic α-tocopherol (50 mg/day) for 5 years	Lung cancer and cause-specific mortality	Increased lung cancer and total mortality for β-carotene No reduction for CVD mortality for either antioxidant alone or in combination

Study	Type[a]	Intervention	Endpoints	Results
Rapola et al, 1996[104]				Marginally reduced incidence of angina for vitamin E
Omenn et al, 1996, CARET[105]	P	β-carotene (30 mg) and retinol (25,000 IU) daily for 4 years	Lung cancer incidence, cause-specific mortality	Trial stopped early; increased incidence and risk of death from lung cancer; no reduction for cardiovascular endpoints; nonsignificant trend for increased CVD mortality
Hennekens et al, 1996 Physician's Health Study[106]	P	β-carotene (50 mg) on alternate days for 12 years	Malignant neoplasm, MI, stroke, CVD events, total mortality	Trial stopped early; no reduction for any end-point CVD or cancer
Stephens et al, 1996, CHAOS[107]	S	α-tocopherol (400 IU/day or 800 IU/day) for 1.4 years	Combined CV death and nonfatal MI; nonfatal MI; CV death	Decrease in combined CV endpoints and nonfatal MI; nonsignificant increase in total CV deaths

[a] S = secondary prevention; P = primary prevention.

fects of individual nutrients could not be determined. In this population, CHD rates were too low to determine the effect of these interventions on this end point.

The α-Tocopherol, β-Carotene Cancer Prevention Trial was a large-scale randomized trial of antioxidant vitamins in a well-nourished population.[103] This trial tested, in a 2 × 2 factorial design, the effect of β-carotene (20 mg/day) and α-tocopherol (50 mg/day) in the prevention of lung cancer among 29 133 Finnish male smokers.[103] β-Carotene led to a significant increase in lung cancer incidence and total mortality. There was a nonsignificant increase in ischemic heart disease deaths (RR = 1.12, 95% CI: 1.00–1.25) and a nonsignificant increase in the incidence of angina.[104] For Vitamin E, there was no clear reduction in the risk of ischemic heart disease of ischemic stroke mortality; however, an increased risk of fatal hemorrhagic stroke (RR = 1.50, 95% CI: 1.03–2.20) was found, which was no longer significant after adjustment for multiple testing. The cumulative risk of developing angina was slightly lower among those assigned to Vitamin E (RR = 0.97, 95% CI: 0.85–1.10, p = 0.63) compared to placebo.[104] It was suggested that the lack of benefit from Vitamin E on CHD mortality may be due to the relatively low supplemental dose; however, this trial was not designed to specifically evaluate CVD.

With these mixed and even disappointing results, the scientific community wondered whether larger trials with longer follow-up or those with CVD as a primary end point would demonstrate benefits of β-carotene or Vitamin E. Results from two additional randomized trials also showed negative or no beneficial effects for β-carotene. The Physicians' Health Study showed no effect of β-carotene supplementation for the prevention of CVD or cancer.[106] Here, 22 071 US male physicians took either β-carotene (50 mg) or placebo every other day for an average of 12 years. The 12-year rates of MI, stroke, CVD death, malignancy, and total death were identical in both groups, and there was no effect on the incidence of any specific neoplasm.

β-Carotene was also tested in the β-Carotene and Retinol Efficacy Trial (CARET) among 18,314 men and women who were either current or former smokers or were exposed to asbestos.[105] CARET tested a combined treatment of β-carotene (30 mg/day) and retinol (25 000 IU/day); the primary end point was lung cancer incidence. Based on projections that there would be no ability to detect a benefit over the planned follow-up period and the observance of a trend toward increased lung cancer (RR = 1.28, 95% CI: 1.04–1.57) and total mortality (RR = 1.17, 95% CI: 1.03–1.33) in the treatment group, this trial was stopped early, after 4 years of active supplementation. Nonfatal CVD events were not reported, whereas a trend toward excess CVD mortality (RR = 1.26, 95% CI: 0.99–1.61) was observed.

To date, only limited data are available from randomized trials of Vitamin E supplementation, which were specifically for the treatment or primary prevention of CVD. Several early, short-term trials tested the efficacy of Vitamin E in patients with angina, claudication, and angioplasty. Three trials that examined the effects of Vitamin E supplementation on claudication, after 1–3 years of follow-up, had results that suggested some clinical benefit.[108–110] Findings for short-term trials that studied angina using high doses of Vitamin E (1600 and 3200 IU/day) demonstrated no benefit.[78,83] A more-recent trial of Vitamin E (400 IU/ day) supplementation in patients who underwent angioplasty found a nonsignificant 30% reduction in the rate of restenosis after 4 months.[101] These trials had a variety of limitations, including small sample size, high dropout rates, and short duration. Since the mechanisms proposed for the beneficial effects of Vitamin E are related to the progression of atherosclerosis, the short duration of these trials may have limited the ability to observe effects. Nevertheless, these trials provided an encouraging perspective for Vitamin E supplementation in individuals at high risk for subsequent CVD morbidity and mortality.

The Cambridge Heart Antioxidant Study, also a secondary prevention trial, recently reported results of Vitamin E supplementation in 2002 patients with angiographically defined atherosclerosis.[107] The treatments were 800 IU or 400 IU of Vitamin E or placebo; average follow-up was 17 months. Those assigned to Vitamin E had a significant reduction in nonfatal MI (RR = 0.23, 95% CI: 0.011–0.47) and in the combined end point of CVD death plus nonfatal MI (RR = 0.53, 95% CI: 0.34–0.83). However, a nonsignificant excess of CVD deaths (RR = 1.18, 95% CI: 0.62–2.27) was also observed. These results regarding nonfatal events are promising; however, the disparity in the treatment effects for MI and CVD death is of concern. A larger trial with greater power for these end points is critically needed to help clarify these effects.

Thus far, the completed randomized trials do not provide conclusive evidence that antioxidant vitamins beneficially affect total mortality or mortality from CVD. The randomized trials do provide clear evidence that β-carotene provides no benefit for the primary prevention of CVD, despite previous promising observational data. The available data do not yet offer a clear answer regarding the benefits of Vitamin E supplementation.

Clinical trial evidence currently does not support the use of antioxidant vitamins for the prevention or treatment of CVD. The disappointing results from trials of β-carotene reaffirm the need for a rigorous clinical trial to establish clinical and public policies. Ongoing randomized trials addressing the efficacy of antioxidants—Vitamins E and C and β-carotene—for the primary and secondary prevention of CVD[79,111] should help to resolve the uncertainties regarding the safety and efficacy of these nutrient supplements.

Flavonoids

Interest in antioxidants led to the search for other protective food compounds. Many common foods contain nonnutritive components that may provide protection against chronic diseases including CVD and some forms of cancer.[112–114] Historically, plants were known to have many pharmacologic effects, but the mechanisms by which plant-derived compounds act are still being elucidated. Among the most-investigated compounds, in addition to the antioxidant vitamins, are plant polyphenols, flavonoids, and sulfer-containing compounds.[89] Fruits, grains, garlic, onions, soybeans, tea, and red wine are the major sources of these compounds.[115]

The flavonoids include two major groups of related compounds, the anthocyanins and the anthoxanthins. The anthoxanthins include various flavones, flavonols, and flavonones, which influence the color and flavor of foods. Flavonols have a number of antioxidant characteristics, including scavenging of superoxide anions, singlet oxygen, and lipid peroxyradicals. In addition, they are known to bind metal ions. The most common flavonol is quercetin, which was reported to inhibit oxidation and cytotoxicity of LDLs in vitro.[89] Flavonols and flavones may affect platelet aggregation and reduce thrombotic tendencies through modification of eicosanoid biosynthesis by inhibition of cyclooxygenase and promoting relaxation of cardiovascular smooth muscle with the potential for antihypertensive and antiarrhythmic effects. Flavonoids were also shown to exhibit antiviral and anticarcinogenic properties.[89,112]

Epidemiological studies support the hypothesis that these compounds may be protective for CVD. The Zutphen Elderly Study, a longitudinal study of risk factors for chronic disease in elderly Dutch men[116] determined the flavonoid content of the common foods in the Dutch diet. Dietary intakes of flavonoids were then calculated; the mean intake was 25 g/day. Tea, onions, and apples were the major sources of flavonoids.[117] Flavonoid intake was significantly inversely associated with CHD mortality. The adjusted relative risk of CHD mortality in the highest quintile of flavonoid intake versus the lowest was 0.32 (95% CI).[34] In this population, intake of flavonoids was also associated with a reduced risk of stroke.[118] In the United States, onions, apples, broccoli, and tea are major sources of flavonoid intake, which, for adults, is estimated to range from 12 mg/day to 40 mg/day. As with all observational studies, it is not clear if flavonoids are the protective factor or if they serve as a marker for fruit and vegetable intake or other healthful behaviors.

Although this is a promising field, further studies are needed to determine conclusively whether flavonoids inhibit development of atherosclerotic plaques or affect thrombosis. The available evidence again supports the increased intake of fruits and vegetables. Phenolic compounds or derivatives may hold particular promise in the development of pharmacologic agents for a variety of therapeutic purposes.[119]

Fiber

Over the past 20 years, dietary fiber emerged as an important dietary factor in the prevention and treatment of chronic diseases.[69] High-fiber intakes are associated with lower serum cholesterol levels, reduced BP, enhanced weight control, increased insulin sensitivity and better glycemic control, and decreased factor VIIc as well as reduced risk of CHD.[15,120,121]

Dietary fiber includes fibrous, insoluble substances such as cellulose as well as water-soluble amorphous gels and gums including pectin. Insoluble dietary fiber passes through the small intestine to the colon where it is fermented to some degree by the gastrointestinal bacteria. Soluble dietary fiber exerts its main effect in the small intestine where its viscosity can affect digestion or absorption.[122] High intakes of dietary fiber, particularly soluble fiber, were shown to decrease TC and LDL-C with little effect on HDL.[120] Soluble fibers include oat bran, pectin, guar gum, and psyllium. Legumes, barley, rice bran, and several other types of gum may also reduce cholesterol levels.[122,123] A recent meta-analysis estimated that soluble fiber from oats may lower cholesterol from 0.5% to 2%/gram of soluble fiber intake.[124] The analysis also showed that individuals with higher initial cholesterol levels have a greater response to fiber. Adding approximately 3 g of soluble fiber per day could lower cholesterol from 5 to 6 mg/dL. Observational data support the relation between fiber intake and CHD. Recently, the HPFS reported that fiber intake was associated with a decreased risk of CHD for men in the highest quintile of dietary fiber intake (median 28.9 g/day) compared with men in the lowest group (12.4 g/day).[67] The age-adjusted relative risk was 0.59 (95% CI: 0.46–0.76). These results were independent of fat and other nutrient intakes. Among the three main contributors to total fiber—vegetables, fruit, and cereal—cereal was most strongly associated with reduced risk of total MI. The authors noted that the substantial reduction in risk from cereal fiber (29%) was larger than the benefit predicted for reductions in serum cholesterol due to fiber intake, suggesting that several mechanisms may act together to confer protection. The findings support the national guidelines for increasing intakes of fiber to 25–30 g/day. Currently, middle-aged US adults have relatively low fiber and fruit and vegetable intakes (Table 3). Major dietary changes are still needed in order to achieve these national goals, given the low fiber intakes of 13–18 g daily and consumption of only three servings of fruits and vegetables per day. Investigations are ongoing to determine the effects of whole grains on disease based on the belief that whole grains contain many nutrients and nonnutrients (including, but not limited to fiber), which act synergistically to reduce risk of many diseases.[69,125]

Soy

The consumption of vegetable protein in place of animal protein was associated with a lower risk of CHD.[7,126] Soy is a major source of vegetable protein in the Japanese diet and in the diets of several vegetarian groups.[77,127,128] Soy protein may contribute to the protective effects of these dietary patterns. Numerous clinical investigations attempted to determine the health effects of soy in relation to heart disease, cancer, and osteoporosis. To date, the most conclusive evidence regarding soy and CVD is its effect on serum cholesterol. A recent meta-analysis of 38 controlled clinical studies of soy intake demonstrated that intakes of 31–47 g of soy protein per day were effective in lowering serum cholesterol.[129] Dietary fat intakes were generally similar between the treatment and control diets in these trials. Individuals with higher initial serum cholesterol experienced the greatest reductions in LDL; those in the highest quartile of TC at baseline (>335 mg/dL) experienced, on average, a 24% reduction in LDL-C. Overall, consumption of 25 g of soy protein per day decreased TC by 8.9 mg/dL.[129]

Individuals could achieve an intake of 25 g by consuming two to three servings of soy products daily. The amounts of soy protein found in available soy products are 4 oz of tofu: 8–13 g, 8 oz of soy milk: 4–10 g, 4 oz of textured soy protein: 11 g, and 3.2 oz of meat analog: 18 g.

Although the mechanisms responsible for lipid lowering are unknown, soy may affect bile acids or cholesterol absorption, glucagon and insulin levels, or hepatic cholesterol synthesis.[129] Soy estrogens (isoflavones and phytoestrogens) may contribute to the lipid-lowering effects.[20,129,130] The use of estrogen replacement therapy and the synthetic antiestrogen drug tamoxifen decrease serum LDL-C levels; it is believed that soy estrogens may have similar actions.[129,131] The intake of soy may also affect CVD risk through antioxidant properties and by reducing platelet aggregation. Soy products are widely available, and new products are continually being developed. Increased soy consumption may be a feasible dietary modification that could provide significant benefits in the prevention of CVD.

Obesity

Overweight and obesity constitute one of the most prevalent health problems in the United States.[47] Although obesity may be defined in several ways, body mass index (BMI) (weight/height^2) is a commonly used standard that allows for comparisons among individuals who differ greatly by weight and height. Overweight is defined as a BMI of 24–27.8

for men and 23–27.3 for women; obesity is defined by a BMI of 27.8–40 for men and 27.3–40 for women; morbid obesity is defined as a BMI of ≥40 for both sexes.[132]

Despite a cultural preoccupation with body weight and weight loss, the prevalence of obesity continues to rise for both adults and children. The most recent data from the NHANES III (1988–1991) show an alarming trend—for adults, the prevalence of obesity increased from 25% to 33% during the past decade.[47] The age-adjusted prevalences of obesity for men and women, respectively, are 32% and 35% compared to a prevalence of 24 and 27% from the NHANES II (1976–1980) survey (Figures 1 and 2). Obesity is particularly prevalent among women and minorities.[133] Forty percent or more or Mexican American, Native American, and black women are obese and, among Native Hawaiians, the prevalence exceeds 60% for both men and women.[47]

Obesity contributes to the development and morbidity associated with chronic diseases including CVD, cancer, diabetes, and degenerative bone disease.[134] Obesity is recognized both as an independent[135,136] and a contributing risk factor for CVD,[134] whereby its effects are partially mediated through effects on established risk factors. Obesity is associated with an increased risk for hypertension, diabetes, hypercholesterolemia, hypertriglyceridemia, and lower levels of HDL-C.[132,134,137–139] The majority of individuals with non-insulin-dependent diabetes mellitus (NIDDM) are obese. NIDDM increases with increasing BMI, and obesity is predictive of the subsequent development of NIDDM.[132,140] Obesity is associated with a two- to threefold increased risk for hypertension, and obese indi-

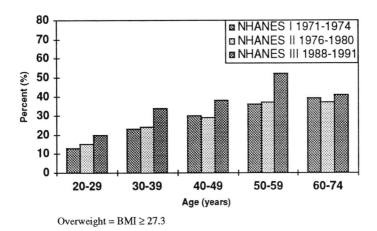

Overweight = BMI ≥ 27.3

Figure 2. *Prevalence of overweight US women, NHANES 1971–1991. Reproduced with permission from Reference 47.*

viduals commonly have elevated LDL-C and lower HDL-C levels.[139,141] Even in young adults, overweight and weight gain has a pronounced effect on BP and lipids.[139] Recent reports point out that, clinically, obesity was relatively unrecognized or underemphasized as a major contributor to high blood cholesterol and that it may, in part, explain the lack of responsiveness to dietary saturated fat modifications for treatment of moderate hypercholesterolemmia.[34,142] Obesity may also increase cardiovascular morbidity and mortality through effects on cardiac function including left ventricular hypertrophy and the associated risks of arrhythmia and sudden death.[143–145] Recently, increased levels of thrombogenic factors were also been linked to obesity.[146–148]

Weight gain over time is a risk factor for development of CHD risk factors and for CHD morbidity and mortality.[140,141] In men participating in the Framingham Heart Study, each 10% increase in relative weight was associated with an 11-mg/dL increase in serum cholesterol as well as a 2.5-mg/dL increase in serum glucose and a 6.6-mm Hg increase in systolic blood pressure (SBP).[141] In the United States, weight increases with age; women are at the greatest risk for weight gain during early to middle adulthood. The 10-year NHANES I follow-up study revealed that, between ages 25 and 54, women gained, on average, 7.3 kg.[149,150] Very large weight gains were also common among women; pregnancy and menopause were periods of potential risk for large weight gains. In the Coronary Artery Risk Development in Young Adults Study, the first pregnancy was associated with a weight gain compared to nulliparous women.[151–153]

The effects of obesity on cardiovascular risk factors and the risk of CHD also reflect its strong association with insulin resistance. Central obesity, a common form of obesity characterized by accumulation of adipose tissue in the abdomen, is closely related to insulin resistance. Insulin resistance, hyperinsulinemia, and central obesity are associated with hypertension, elevated glucose, TGs, factor VII and fibrinogen, and lower HDL-C as well as increased CVD mortality.[154–157] Central obesity is commonly characterized by the waist-to-hip ratio; desirable ratios are <0.9 for men and <0.8 for women. The effects of central obesity are generally shown to be independent of BMI. However, BMI itself is strongly predictive of CVD risk factors and disease, and it accounts for a substantial proportion of excess risk. Weight loss should be recommended for all overweight patients.

The relation of weight and weight loss to mortality is a complex issue. The effect of lower levels of obesity on total mortality and CVD risk not clear. Although many cohort studies reported linear associations in both men and women between obesity and CHD,[136,138,140,156,158,159] J-shaped mortality curves were reported for total mortality and CHD,[160,161] where those with moderate obesity experience the lowest mortality, and those with the highest and lowest weight have the greatest mortality. Examination of these reports suggest that the risks associated with lower body weights may be the result of confounding factors.[162] Preexisting illness, cigarette smoking, and alcoholism may explain the low baseline weights and also result in mortality. Failure to account for these factors could cause a distortion of the true obesity and mortality relation.

Obesity clearly confers an increased risk for CVD and for other chronic illnesses. However, due to the moderate progression of obesity over time, the chronic nature of this condition, and limitations in the long-term treatment success, obesity is often overlooked or left untreated. Weight reduction is a component of current clinical practice guidelines for the treatment of hypertension, diabetes, and hypercholesterolemia.[11,163,164] Clinical trials clearly demonstrated that even modest weight loss can result in important reductions in BP, lipids, and glucose.[35,165–168] A recent meta-analysis of the effects of weight loss on lipids estimated that, for each kilogram of weight lost, TC is reduced by 1.93 mg/dL, LDL-C by 0.77 mg/dL, and HDL-C is increased by 0.35 mg/dL.[36] Whereas individual patients may experience even greater reductions depending on weight loss, BP may fall, on average, from 2 mm Hg to 10 mm Hg.[165] Improvements in measures of quality of life in patients with hypertension and hyperlipidemia were also reported following weight loss.[169,170]

Thousands of individuals who attempt weight loss are often unsuccessful over the long term. Data suggest that many individuals may regain from one-third to two-thirds of the weight lost within 1 year and may regain all of the initial weight lost within 5 years.[171] "Weight cycling" is the repeated loss and regain of weight over a period of years. Although concerns were raised about possible negative health effects from this cycling, the data are inconsistent.[172–176] Mechanisms suggested for the adverse effects of weight cycling include a lower resting metabolic rate, which could make future weight loss more difficult, and increased fat preference, which could lead to excess fat and calorie consumption or a change in body fat distribution to be more abdominal, which would result in detrimental effects on BP, lipids, and glucose tolerance. Some observational studies reported that weight cycling is associated with CVD mortality, but these findings were not consistently demonstrated.[171,173–175,177] Unfortunately, methodologic limitations of these studies make conclusions difficult. Commonly, the reasons for weight loss are unavailable. Unintentional weight loss due to disease could effect mortality and distort the association. Use and change in use of alcohol, tobacco, and other drugs and medications, depression and other mental disorders, and change in physical activity are also potential confounders. Standard definitions of "weight cycling" were difficult to establish; many studies have inadequate data thus limiting comparison across studies.

Currently, there is no consensus that weight cycling results in adverse effects. A recent report on this topic issued by the National Task Force on the Prevention and Treatment of Obesity concluded that weight cycling does not significantly alter metabolism and that data on long-term health effects are lacking.[177] Concern about weight cycling should not prevent recommendations for weight loss in the clinical setting. The challenge is to develop better methods for sustaining weight loss and ultimately preventing weight gain.

The problems of overweight and obesity that include diet and exercise are multifaceted and involve complex questions that have no simple solutions.[178–180] A focus on both safe and effective treatments as well as strategies for prevention are needed. In order to guide patients, weight loss methods should be evaluated by criteria that include effectiveness (expected amount of short-term weight loss and long-term weight maintenance), improvements in CVD risk factors, safety, and anticipated level of patient compliance and burden and cost.[181]

The most widely accepted weight-loss approaches include dietary modification from combined caloric reduction and nutrient modification, behavioral therapy, increased physical activity, and pharmacologic agents (not reviewed here). Caloric restriction, diet pattern, and diet composition modifications are the cornerstones of obesity treatment. Recommendations stress that caloric levels should not be less than 1200 kcal/day for women and 1500 kcal/day for men.[181,182] A reasonable weight-reduction plan for many individuals is one that reduces caloric intake by about 500 calories per day. The goal is to achieve a realistic caloric restriction and weight reduction; a loss from one-half to 2 lb/week is appropriate. Recommendations include reduction of total fat and saturated fat with an increase in fiber and nutrient-rich foods, including fruits and vegetables and whole grains. Table 6 illustrates recommended levels of total fat and saturated fat by calorie level to achieve the guidelines of the step I and step II diets.

A review of controlled trials of weight loss indicated an average weight loss of 8.5 kg over 20 weeks of behavioral diet treatment. Clinical trials that employed weight loss for the treatment or prevention of hypertension demonstrated average weight losses of 3–7 kg when 12- to 24-week diet and behavioral programs were used.[35,166–168,183] Weight loss and weight maintenance in both of these settings improved with greater supervision of the participant, longer programs, use of behavioral and cognitive approaches including self-monitoring and specific skills training, and increase in physical activity.[180,184] A moderate increase in physical activity was shown to reduce weight regain, although men and women may show differential response. This may be partially due to lower levels of physical activity adopted by women, underlying metabolic differences, or to compliance with exercise and diet changes. Increased energy expen-

Table 6

NCEP Guidelines for Dietary Intake of Fat and Saturated Fatty Acids by
Calorie Level to Achieve the Step I and Step II Diets[a]

	Caloric Level							
	1600	1800	2000	2200	2400	2600	2800	3000
Total fat (g)[b]	53	60	67	73	80	87	93	100
Step I diet, saturated fat (g)[c]	18	20	22	24	27	29	31	33
Step II diet, saturated fat (g)[c]	12	14	16	17	19	20	22	23

[a] The average daily energy intake for women is about 1800 calories; for men, about 2500 calories

[b] Total fat of both diets = 30% of calories (estimated by multiplying calorie level by 0.3 and dividing the product by 9 calories/per gram).

[c] The recommended intake of saturated fat for the step I diet is 8–10% of total calories, and less than 7% for the step II diet.

Reproduced with permission from Reference 11.

diture through regular physical activity is an integral component of weight reduction and maintenance. Although many studies showed that increased physical activity alone may not be sufficient to produce significant weight loss, regular moderate activity was associated with weight maintenance following weight loss.[185–187]

It was suggested that a greater weight loss may be achieved by altering dietary composition—substantially lowering fat or increasing fiber rather than caloric reduction. This is based on the belief that compliance with caloric restriction is difficult to achieve and sustain. However, the efficacy of these approaches is largely unsubstantiated. Recent studies indicate that reducing fat while total calories are presumably unchanged can result in modest weight losses of 1–2 kg.[188–190] This approach is perhaps most applicable to the prevention of weight gain and is a major component of recommendations for maintaining weight loss.

Fad diets such as the Eat-All-You-Want Diet, the Cabbage Diet, the Fat Burner Diet, and the Grapefruit Diet are popular commercial versions of these approaches. These diets recommend eating large amounts of specific foods purported to increase fat metabolism and require rigid food consumption patterns. Despite the "eat all you want" claims, most of these diets are accompanied by large reductions in caloric intake. Fad diets are often nutritionally imbalanced, do not promote changes in eating patterns and behavior consistent with a long-term healthful dietary pattern, are associated with a rapid regain in weight, and may be harmful for individuals with medical conditions.[191]

A variety of "alternative weight loss" approaches are commercially available. Diet pills, appetite suppressants, vitamin supplements, and herbal and nutritional preparations account for a billion dollar consumer market.[185] Alleged benefits of these products include rapid and simple weight loss, increased metabolic rate, appetite suppression, decreased fat absorption, increased fat metabolism, elimination of "cellulite," cell activation, and body detoxification.[61,192] Although product advertisements rely on consumer testimonials citing dramatic weight loss, these weight loss results are rarely substantiated by scientifically conducted trials. The Food and Drug Administration ordered numerous product manufacturers to discontinue unsubstantiated claims regarding weight loss efficacy and other benefits of such products. Patients who use these approaches may not seek appropriate medical care or may discontinue medical therapy in hopes of rapid results. These methods and products may exacerbate existing medical conditions and produce side effects related to toxicities or other negative health consequences. Health care providers need to be aware of the numerous problems associated with these approaches. Patients may have a decreased motivation for future weight loss due to negative experiences and the rapid regain of weight often associated with these approaches.

Blood Pressure

Diet and lifestyle modifications are recommended for both the primary prevention and treatment of hypertension.[163,164] Controlled clinical trials clearly demonstrated that antihypertensive therapy reduces CVD in individuals with diastolic blood pressure (DBP) levels ≥90 mm Hg and in those with SBP levels ≥160 mm Hg and DBP ≤90 mm Hg. Even those who derive optimal BP lowering from antihypertensive therapy are likely to have a higher risk of CVD morbidity and mortality than normotensive individuals at similar BPs.[193] Control of hypertension usually requires lifetime therapy since treatment reduces risk but does not cure the condition. Antihypertensive medications may be associated with side effects and can be accompanied by significant patient burden and medical costs.[163] Diet and lifestyle modifications are used as definitive and adjunctive therapy for hypertension. These approaches may reduce BP levels enough to avoid initiation of medication, and, even when BP is not lowered sufficiently to avoid medication, reduced doses of antihypertensive medication are often adequate for BP control.[163] Diet and lifestyle modifications are particularly important in the large proportion of hypertensive patients who also have dyslipidemia or diabetes.[194]

Weight reduction, sodium reduction, moderation of alcohol intake, and increased physical activity are the major components of intervention for BP control. In addition, a low-fat, low-saturated fat diet is recommended for overall cardiovascular risk reduction. The numerous benefits of weight reduction on CVD risk factors are well established. Due to the potential for significant BP-lowering effect through weight loss, the Joint National Committee on the Detection, Diagnosis and Treatment of Hypertension V recommends that initial therapy for all hypertensive patients who are above ideal weight should focus on weight loss combined with lifestyle modifications for 3–6 months before initiating pharmacologic therapy. Generally, the degree of BP lowering is related to the amount of weight loss and the initial BP level, but even modest reductions in weight can have a favorable effect on hypertension.[163]

Intervention Studies

The efficacy of nutritional nonpharmacologic approaches for the treatment and prevention of hypertension were addressed in many clinical trials,[164,170] and several were recently reported.[195,196] Single-component interventions as well as combined lifestyle approaches including weight loss, sodium reduction, physical activity, and nutrient supplementation were evaluated. Overall, the diet-lifestyle trials demonstrated very favorable results in terms of both the amount of lifestyle changes that could be achieved and the resulting BP reductions. The Treatment of Mild Hypertension Study was a randomized, double-blind 4-year study evaluating the BP effects of combining nonpharmacologic treatment and medications in 902 individuals with stage 1 hypertension.[35,197] All study participants received nonpharmacologic intervention for weight loss, sodium reduction, alcohol modification, and increased physical activity as well as one of five active BP medications or placebo. If BP went above specified levels, individuals had medications increased or, in the case of the placebo group, medication initiated. After 4 years of follow-up, mean weight loss was 6 lb, 70% of participants remained below their baseline weight, 34% maintained a weight loss of greater than 10 lb, and physical activity was increased 50% above baseline levels. Over 4 years, a substantial proportion (59%) of participants in the diet plus placebo group was able to achieve BP control without the addition of antihypertensive medications. Mean DBP was reduced 8.6 mm Hg in the lifestyle intervention plus placebo group.

The Primary Prevention of Hypertension Study also tested the efficacy of a multifactorial intervention (weight, sodium and alcohol reduction, and increased physical activity) for preventing hypertension in individuals with high-normal BP. After 5 years, weight reduction in the intervention group was 5.9 lb compared to the usual care group. Participants who received the multifactorial intervention experienced a 50% lower 5-year incidence of hypertension.[166] The Trials of Hypertension Prevention Study was a randomized multicenter study that tested seven interventions, in parallel fashion, for the prevention of hypertension in individuals with high-normal BP.[183] The interventions included weight loss, sodium reduction, stress reduction, or supplementation with fish oil, magnesium, potassium, or calcium. After 18 months, the mean weight loss in the weight intervention group was 8.5 lb, which resulted in reductions in SBP and DBP of 2.9 mm Hg and 2.3 mm Hg, respectively. Additionally, weight loss was associated with a 51% reduction in the incidence of hypertension. Sodium reduction also resulted in a significantly lower BP and a trend toward decreased incidence of hypertension. Stress management and the nutrient supplementation arms did not show any apparent benefit for BP reduction.

Little information was available regarding efficacy of nonpharmacologic therapy for BP control in the elderly. It was suggested that usual approaches may not be feasible or effective in this population. The Trial of Nonpharmacologic Interventions in the Elderly tested weight loss (WL), sodium reduction (Na), and a combination of weight loss and sodium (WLNa) for the control of BP in 975 hypertensive individuals, 60–80 years of age, who had their antihypertensive medications withdrawn by study protocol.[198] Mean weight loss after 36 months in the WL intervention was 10 lb and 8 lb with WLNa. Study end points were the return to BP of <150/90. The end points were significantly reduced in both the WL and the Na groups compared to the control. Compliance was high, as was attendance at clinic visits. These results underscore the value and feasibility of weight loss and sodium reduction in the elderly hypertensive population.

Epidemiological studies suggest that a variety of foods and nutrients may provide protection for the development of hypertension. Dietary patterns characterized by high intakes of fiber, antioxidants, fish, calcium, magnesium, zinc, potassium, protein, and fruits and vegetables were associated with lower BP and lower risk of stroke.[66,118,199] Despite the promising epidemiological evidence, numerous clinical trials of supplementation with individual nutrients failed to show apparent benefits for clinically meaningful BP reductions.[55,164,183] These findings suggest that the effect observed in the epidemiological situations might be due to other components in foods or due to the combined effects of foods and nutrients. The Dietary Approaches to Stop Hypertension Study was a multicenter, randomized, parallel arm controlled feeding trial in individuals with high-normal BP that tested the effects on BP of two modified dietary patterns compared to a control diet.[200,202] The diets tested were eaten for 8 weeks and included a typical American diet (control), a diet pattern that was high in fruits and vegetables, and a combination diet pattern that was high in fruits, vegetables, and low-fat dairy and whole grain products but that was also low in total fat and saturated fat. Results revealed significant BP changes over the 8 weeks. Both experimental diets resulted in significant BP reductions. The fruit and vegetable diet showed an effect some-what intermediate to the low-fat combination diet where SBP and DBP fell by approximately 5 mm Hg and 3 mm Hg, respectively.[202] These results suggest that dietary patterns that maximize overall nutrient content through emphasis on whole foods and large amounts of fruits and vegetables and a decrease in fat may have a substantial impact on the prevention of hypertension. Given that this was a controlled feeding study, the maximal effect of these diets could be observed, and these results may indicate that a lack of compliance could account for modest effects observed in some previous diet intervention trials.

Alcohol

An association between alcohol consumption and BP levels was observed in over 60 population studies worldwide.[41] The relation is generally linear, although some studies observed a threshold effect at two or three standard drinks a day. Alcohol intake may contribute substantially to the daily caloric intake; excess intake may lead to obesity. Replacement of food calories with alcohol calories may also negatively affect nutritional status. The few controlled trials in this area showed that reducing alcohol consumption lowers BP in both treated and untreated hypertensives.[164] Despite predisposing to hypertension, there are extensive data indicating that regular light to moderate drinking (one to four drinks a day) protects against CHD deaths and ischemic strokes. Heavier drinking increases the risk of hemorrhagic stroke and heart disease. Light drinkers have lower mortality than nondrinkers; those drinking more than two alcohol drinks per day show a rising mortality as well as an increased risk of hypertension. It is believed that confounding may account for some of these findings. The low- or no-alcohol group may suffer from preexisting illness or may have been former heavy drinkers. Smoking and former smoking may be associated with previous heavy alcohol use. There was some suggestion that wine consumption may be associated with lower cardiovascular risks, potentially from antioxidants found in red wine or by reducing platelet aggregation.[71] As previously discussed, these and numerous other factors may account for the observed affects in the Mediterranean countries where red wine intake is high. Beverage preference and drinking patterns correlated strongly with diet habits and physical activity, smoking, education, and socioeconomic status, factors that may confound the interpretation of epidemiological association suggesting favorable cardiovascular effects to a particular beverage.[41] Alcohol appears to provide cardiovascular benefits at moderate levels; however, there are negative aspects to alcohol intake including increased risk of hypertension and cancer. Evaluation of the individual or patient's needs and status is needed when making recommendations for alcohol intake.

Summary

Nutrition plays a key role in the reduction of risk for CVD. The effects of diet on CVD act through numerous biological mechanisms that include not only effects on lipids and atherosclerosis but also a host of emerging effects on thrombosis and arrhythmias as well as energy metabolism and cellular function. Despite the focus of clinical trials on supplementation with various nutrients (antioxidant vitamins, fish oils, fiber, and minerals) there is, to date, little evidence to support use above levels established by the Recommended Dietary Allowances for reduction of risk factors and treatment of existing CHD.[201] In contrast, clinical trials of diet modification, weight loss, and physical activity demonstrated clinically important reductions in risk factors, with dietary patterns that are high in fruits, vegetables, and grain products being consistently related to beneficial effects for prevention of CVD. Evidence does support the role of maintaining overall adequate nutritional status. This may be particularly important in elderly populations that have a reduced food intake and physiologic functions related to nutrient absorption and metabolism that may be compromised by aging or disease.

Nutrition intervention is a cornerstone of the treatment approach for high blood cholesterol level, hypertension, and obesity and the treatment of individuals with existing CHD. The dietary guidelines of the NCEP and National High Blood Pressure Education Program, in addition to reducing dietary fat and saturated fat, include recommendations for increased intakes of fruits, vegetables, and grain products. In light of current evidence, a substantially increased emphasis on these components is warranted in diet counseling. Weight reduction and prevention of weight gain are critical for alleviating the underlying metabolic abnormalities associated with CVD. Caloric reduction, alteration in diet patterns, and physical activity are essential for control of body weight. These findings have implications for clinical interventions, public education, and the formulation of new food products, which may assist in providing optimal levels of these foods and nutrients.

References

1. ABT Associates Inc, eds. *Trends in the United States.* Washington, DC: Food Marketing Institute; 1996.
2. Food Marketing Institute. *Trends 1989: Consumer Attitudes and the Supermarket.* Washington, DC: Food Marketing Institute; 1989.
3. Godfrey Meisler J, St. Jeor S. Summary and recommendations from the American Health Foundation's Expert Panel on Healthy Weight. *Am J Clin Nutr* 1996;63(suppl):474–477.
4. Hirsch J, Bell CH, Dwyer JT, et al. Health implications of obesity: summary. National Institutes of Health Consensus Development Conference Statement 1985;5:1–7.

5. NIH Consensus Development Panel on Physical Activity and Cardiovascular Health. Physical activity and cariovascular health. *JAMA* 1996;276:241–246.
6. US Department of Health and Human Services. *Physical Activity and Health: A Report of the Surgeon General.* Washington, DC: US Department of Health and Human Services; 1996.
7. Keys A, Menotti J, Karvonen MJ. The diet and 15-year death rate in the Seven Countries Study. *Am J Epidemiol* 1986;124:903–915.
8. Keys A, Anderson JT, Grande F. Serum cholesterol response to changes in the diet. II. The effect of cholesterol in the diet. *Metabolism* 1965;14:759–765.
9. Hegsted DM, McGandy RB, Myers ML, et al. Quantitative effects of dietary fat on serum cholesterol in man. *Am J Clin Nutr* 1965;17:281–295.
10. Expert Panel on Detection, Evaluation and Treatment of Elevated Cholesterol. *Report of the Expert Panel on Detection, Evaluation, and Treatment of High Blood Cholesterol in Adults.* Washington, DC; 1989. US Dept of Health, Education, and Welfare publication NIH 89-2925.
11. Expert Panel on Detection Evaluation and Treatment of High Blood Cholesterol. Summary of the Second Report of the National Cholesterol Education Program (NCEP) Expert Panel on Detection, Evaluation, and Treatment of High Blood Cholesterol in Adults (Adult Treatment Panel II). *JAMA* 1993; 269:3015–3023.
12. Expert Panel on Blood Cholesterol Levels in Children and Adolescents. *Report of the Expert Panel on Blood Cholesterol Levels in Children and Adolescents.* Washington, DC; 1991. US Dept of Health, Education, and Welfare publication NIH 91-2732.
13. Schucker B, Bailey K, Heimbach JT. Change in public perspective on cholesterol and heart disease: results from two national surveys. *JAMA* 1987; 258:3527–3531.
14. McDowell MA, Briefel R, Alaimo K, et al. Energy and macronutrient intakes of persons ages 2 months and over in the United States: Third National Health and Nutrition Examination Survey, Phase 1, 1988–1991. *Advance Data* 1994;255:1–24.
15. Committee on Diet and Health Food and Nutrition Board; Commision on Life Sciences; National Research Council, eds. *Diet and Health: Implications for Reducing Chronic Disease Risk.* Washington, DC: National Academy Press; 1989.
16. Bonanome A, Grundy SM. Effect of dietary stearic acid on plasma cholesterol and lipoprotein levels. *N Engl J Med* 1988;318:1244–1248.
17. Brook RH. Using scientific information to improve quality of health care. *Ann N Y Acad Sci* 1993;703:74–85.
18. Kris-Etherton PM, Mitchell DC, Mustad VA, et al. The role of fatty acid saturation on plasma lipids, lipoproteins, and apolipoproteins. I. Effects of whole food diets high in cocoa butter, olive oil, soybean oil, dairy butter, and milk chocolate on the plasma lipids of young men. *Metabolism* 1993;42:121–128.
19. Grundy SM. Influence of stearic acid on cholesterol metabolism relative to other long-chain fatty acids. *Am J Clin Nutr* 1994;60(suppl):986–990.
20. Miller GJ, Cruickshank JK, Ellis LJ, et al. Fat consumption and factor VII coagulant activity in middle-aged men: an association between a dietary and thrombogenic coronary risk factor. *Atherosclerosis* 1989;78:19–24.
21. Booyens J, Van Der Merwe CF. Margarines and coronary artery disease. *Med Hypotheses* 1992;37:241–244.
22. Emken EA. Nutrition and biochemistry of trans and positional fatty acid isomers in hydrogenated oils. *Ann Rev Nutr* 1984;339–376.

23. Willett WC, Stampfer MJ, Colditz GA. Intake of trans fatty acids and risk of coronary heart disease among women. *Lancet* 1993;341:581–585.
24. Kris-Etherton, PM, Nicolosi RJ. *Trans Fatty Acids and Coronary Heart Disease Risk.* Washington, DC: ILSI Press; 1995.
25. Willett W, Ascherio A. Response to the International Life Sciences Institute report on trans fatty acids. *Am J Clin Nutr* 1995;62:524–526.
26. Nestel P, Noakes M, Belling B. Plasma lipoprotein lipid and Lp[a] changes with substitution of elaidic acid for oleic acid in the diet. *J Lipid Res* 1992;33:1029–1036.
27. Williamson DF, Kahn HS, Remington PL, et al. The 10-year incidence of overweight and major weight gain in US adults. *Arch Intern Med* 1990;150:665–672.
28. Charnok JS, McLennan PL, Abeywardena MY. Dietary modulation of lipid metabolism and mechanical performance of the heart. *Mol Cell Biochem* 1992;116:19–25.
29. Hetzel BS, Charnock JS, Dwyer T, et al. Fall in coronary disease mortality in USA and Australia due to sudden death: evidence for the role of polyunsaturated fat. *J Clin Epidemiol* 1989;42:885–893.
30. Leaf A, Weber PC. Cardiovascular effects of n-3 fatty acids. *N Engl J Med* 1988;318:549–557.
31. Renaud S, de Lorgeril M. Dietary lipids and their relation to ischaemic heart disease: from epidemiology to prevention. *J Intern Med* 1989;225:39–46.
32. Grundy SM. Comparison of monounsaturated fatty acids and carbohydrates for lowering plasma cholesterol. *N Engl J Med* 1986;314:746–748.
33. Truswell AS. Food carbohydrates and plasma lipids—an update. *Am J Clin Nutr* 1994;59(suppl):710–718.
34. Cole TG, Bowen PE, Schmeisser D, et al. Differential reduction of plasma cholesterol by the American Heart Association Phase 3 Diet in moderately hypercholesterolemic, premenopausal women with different body mass indexes. *Am J Clin Nutr* 1992;55:385–394.
35. Elmer PJ, Grimm R, Laing B, et al. Lifestyle intervention in the Treatment of Mild Hypertension Study (TOMHS): final intervention results. *Prev Med* 1995;24:378–388.
36. Dattilo AM, Kris-Etherton M. Effects of weight reduction on blood lipids and lipoproteins: a meta-analysis. *Am J Clin Nutr* 1992;56:320–328.
37. Mattson FH, Grundy SM. Comparison of effects of dietary saturated, monounsaturated, and polyunsaturated fatty acids on plasma lipids and lipoproteins in man. *J Lipid Res* 1985;26:194–202.
38. Hegsted DM, Ausman LM, Johnson JA, et al. Dietary fat and serum lipids: an evaluation of the experimental data. *Am J Clin Nutr* 1993;57:875–883.
39. Mensink RP, Katan MB. Effect of monounsaturated fatty acids versus complex carbohydrates on high-density lipoproteins in healthy men and women. *Lancet* 1987;1:122–125.
40. Mensink RP, Katan MB. Effects of dietary fatty acids on serum lipids and lipoproteins: a meta-reviews analysis of 27 trials. *Arterioscler Thromb* 1992; 12:911–919.
41. Moore RD, Pearson TA. Moderate alcohol consumption and coronary artery disease: a review. *Medicine* 1986;65:242–267.
42. Elmer PJ. Effects of a step 1 diet and a high monounsaturated (MUFA) fat diet on hemostatic factors in individuals with markers for insulin resistance. *FASEB J* 1996;10:2667.
43. Ginsberg HN. The step 1 diet and a high monounsaturated fat diet have equal effects on postprandial triglyceride, glucose and insulin levels in individuals with markers for insulin resistance. *FASEB J* 1996;10:2668.

44. Kris-Etherton PM. Effects of replacing saturated fat (SFA) with monoun-saturated fat (MUFA) or carbohydrate (CHO) on plasma lipids and lipopro-teins in individuals with markers for insulin resistance. *FASEB J* 1996;10:2666.
45. Rolls BJ, Hammer VA. Fat, carbohydrate, and the reguation of energy intake. *Am J Clin Nutr* 1995;62(suppl):1086–1095.
46. Blundell JE, Burley VJ, Cotton JR, et al. Dietary fat and the control of energy intake: evaluating the effects of fat on meal size and postmeal satiety. *Am J Clin Nutr* 1993;57(suppl):772–778.
47. Kuczmarski RJ, Flegal KM, Campbell SM, et al. Increasing prevalence of over-weight among US adults: the National Health and Nutrition Examination Surveys, 1960 to 1991. *JAMA* 1994;272:205–211.
48. Failor RA, Childs MT, Bierman EL. The effects of ω-3 and ω-6 fatty acid-enriched diets on plasma lipoproteins and apoproteins in familial combined hyperlipidemia. *Metabolism* 1988;37:1021–1028.
49. Bang HO, Dyerberg J, Sinclair HM. The composition of the Eskimo food diet in north western Greenland. *Am J Clin Nutr* 1980;33:2657–2661.
50. Kromhout D, Bosscheiter EB, de Lezenne Coulander C. The inverse relation between fish consumption and 20-year mortality from coronary heart dis-ease. *N Engl J Med* 1985;312:1205–1209.
51. Dolecek TA. Epidemiological evidence of relationships between dietary poly-unsaturated fatty acids and mortality in the Multiple Risk Factor Intervention Trial. *Proc Soc Exp Biol Med* 1992;200:177–182.
52. Shekelle RB, Missell L, Paul O, et al. Fish consumption and mortality from coronary heart disease. *N Engl J Med* 1985;313:820.
53. Curb JD, Reed DM. Fish consumption and mortality from coronary heart disease. Letter. *N Engl J Med* 1985;313:821.
54. National High Blood Pressure Education Program Working Group. National High Blood Pressure Education Program. Working Group report on primary prevention of hypertension. *Arch Intern Med* 1993;153:86–208.
55. Morris MC, Sacks FM, Rosner B. Does fish oil lower blood pressure? A meta-analysis of controlled trials. *Circulation* 1993;88:523–533.
56. Burr ML, Gilbert JF, Holliday RM, et al. Effects of changes in fat, fish, and fibre intakes on death and myocardial reinfarction: Diet and Reinfarction Trial (DART). *Lancet* 1989;334:757–761.
57. Caggiula AW, Watson JE. Characteristics associated with compliance to cho-lesterol lowering eating patterns. *Patient Ed Counsel* 1992;19:33–41.
58. Alaimo K, McDowell MA, Briefel R, et al. Dietary intake of vitamins, min-erals, and fiber of persons ages 2 months and over in the United States: Third National Health and Nutrition Examination Survey, Phase 1, 1988–1991. *Ad-vance Data* 1994.
59. McDowell MA, Briefel R, Alaimo K, et al. Energy and macronutrient intakes of persons ages 2 months and over in the United States: Third National Health and Nutrition Examination Survey, Phase 1, 1988–1991. *Advance Data* 1994;1–24.
60. Subar AF, Heimendinger J, Patterson BH, et al. Fruit and vegetable intake in the United States: the baseline survey of the Five A Day for Better Health Program. *Am J Health Promot* 1995;9:352–360.
61. Koff RS. Herbal hepatotoxicity: revisiting a dangerous alternative. *JAMA* 1994;273–502.
62. de Lorgeril M, Renaud S, Mamelle N, et al. Mediterranean α-linolenic acid-rich diet in secondary prevention of coronary heart disease. *Lancet* 1994; 343:1454–1459.

63. Renaud SC. What is the epidemiologic evidence for the thrombogenic potential of dietary long-chain fatty acids? *Am J Clin Nutr* 1992;56(suppl):823–824.
64. Singh RB, Rastogi S, Verma R. Randomised controlled trial of cardioprotective diet in patients with recent acute myocardial infarction: results of one year follow-up. *Br Med J* 1992;304:1015–1019.
65. Singh RB, Ghosh S, Singh R. Effects on serum lipids of adding fruits and vegetables to prudent diet in the Indian experiment of infarct survival (IEIS). *Cardiology* 1992;80:283–293.
66. Gillman MW, Cupples A, Gagnon D, et al. Protective effect of fruits and vegetables on development of stroke in men. *JAMA* 1995;273:1113–1117.
67. Rimm E, Ascherio A, Giovannucci E, et al. Vegetable, fruit and cereal fiber intake and risk of coronary heart disease among men. *JAMA* 1996;275:447–451.
68. Steinmetz KA, Potter JD. Vegetables, fruit, and cancer. I. Epidemiology. *Cancer Causes Control* 1991;2:325–357.
69. Slavin J, Jacobs D, Marquart L. Whole-grain consumption and chronic disease: protective mechanisms. *Nutr Cancer* 1997;27:14–21.
70. American Heart Association. *Heart and Stroke Facts: 1995 Statistical Supplement.* Dallas, TX: American Heart Association; 1995.
71. Renaud S, de Lorgeril M. Wine, alcohol, platelets, and the French paradox for coronary disease. *Lancet* 1992;339:1523–1526.
72. Willett WC, Sacks F, Trichopoulos A, et al. Mediterranean diet pyramid: a cultural model for healthy eating. *Am J Clin Nutr* 1995;61:1402S–1406S.
73. Willett W. Diet and health: what should we eat? *Science* 1994;264:532–536.
74. Potter JD, Slattery ML, Bostick RM, et al. Colon cancer: a review of the epidemiology. *Epidemiol Rev* 1993;15:499–545.
75. Renaud S, de Lorgeril M, Delaye J, et al. Cretan Mediterranean diet for prevention of coronary disease. *Am J Clin Nutr* 1995;61(suppl):1360–1367.
76. Ulbricht TL, Southgate DAT. Coronary heart disease: seven dietary factors. *Lancet* 1991;338:985–992.
77. Fraser GE. Diet and coronary heart disease: beyond dietary fats and low-density-lipoprotein cholesterol. *Am J Clin Nutr* 1994;59(suppl):1117–1123.
78. Anderson TW. Vitamin E in angina pectoris. *Can Med Assoc J* 1974;110:406–410.
79. Jha P, Flather M, Lonn E, et al. The antioxidant vitamins and cardiovascular disease. *Ann Intern Med* 1995;123:860–872.
80. Steinberg D. Modified forms of low-density lipoprotein and atherosclerosis. *J Intern Med* 1993;233:227–232.
81. Ross R. The pathogenesis of atherosclerosis. In: *Heart Disease.* 4th ed. 1992;1106–1124.
82. O'Keefe JH Jr, Lavie CJ Jr, McCallister BD. Insights into the pathogenesis and prevention of coronary artery disease. *Mayo Clin Proc* 1995;70:69–79.
83. Steinberg D, et al. Antioxidants in the prevention of human atherosclerosis: summary proceedings of a National Heart, Lung, and Blood Institute Workshop. *Circulation* 1992;85:2337–2347.
84. Kohlmeier L, Hastings SB. Epidemiologic evidence of a role of carotenoids in cardiovascular disease prevention. *Am J Clin Nutr* 1995;62(suppl):1370–1376.
85. Sies H, Stahl W. Vitamins E and C, β-carotene, and other carotenoids as antioxidants. *Am J Clin Nutr* 1995;62(suppl):1315–1321.
86. Clifton PM. Antioxidant vitamins and coronary heart disease risk. *Curr Opin Lipid* 1995;6:20–24.

87. Bordia A, Verma SK. Effects of Vitamin C on blood lipids, fibrinolytic activity and platelet aggregation in coronary artery disease patients. *Clin Cardiol* 1985;255:552–554.
88. Halliwell B, Gutteridge JMC, Cross CE. Free radicals, antioxidants, and human disease: where are we now? *J Lab Clin Med* 1992;119:498–620.
89. Formica JV, Regelson W. Review of the biology of quercetin and related biovlavonoids. *Food Chem Toxicol* 1995;33:1061–1080.
90. Handelman G, Packer L, Cross C. Destruction of tocopherols, carotenoids and retinol in human plasma by cigarette smoke. *Am J Clin Nutr* 1996;63:559–565.
91. Beard C, Barnard J, Robbins D, et al. Effects of diet and exercise on qualitative and quantitative measures of LDL and its susceptibility to oxidation. *Arterioscler Vasc Biol* 1996;16:201–207.
92. Kardinaal AF, Kok FJ, Ringstad J, et al. Antioxidants in adipose tissue and risk of myocardial infarction: the EURAMIC study. *Lancet* 1993;342:1379–1384.
93. Kushi L, Folsom A, Prineas R, et al. Dietary antioxidant vitamins and death from coronary heart disease in post menopausal women. *N Engl J Med* 1996;334:1156–1162.
94. Losonczy KG, Harris TB, Havlik RJ. Vitamin E and Vitamin C supplement use and risk of all cause and coronary heart disease mortality in older persons: the Established Populations for Epidemiologic Studies of the Elderly. *Am J Clin Nutr* 1996;64:190–196.
95. Rimm E, Stampfer MJ, Ascherio A, et al. Vitamin E consumption and risk of coronary disease in men. *N Engl J Med* 1993;328:1450–1456.
96. Stampfer MJ, Hennekens CH, Manson JE, et al. Vitamin E consumption and the risk of coronary disease in women. *N Engl J Med* 1993;328:1444–1449.
97. Stampfer MJ, Rimm EB. Epidemiologic evidence for Vitamin E in prevention of cardiovascular disease. *Am J Clin Nutr* 1995;62(suppl):1365–1369.
98. Knekt P, Reunanen A, Jarvinen R, et al. Antioxidant vitamin intake and coronary mortality in a longitudinal population study. *Am J Epidemiol* 1994;139:1180–1189.
99. Pandey DK, Shekelle R, Selwyn BJ, et al. Dietary Vitamin C and β-carotene and risk of death in middle-aged men: the Western Electric Study. *Am J Epidemiol* 1995;5:255–260.
100. Gaziano JM, Manson JE, Branch LG, et al. A prospective study of consumption of carotenoids in fruits and vegetables and decreased cardiovascular mortality in the elderly. *Ann Epidemiol* 1995;5:255–260.
101. DeMaio SJ, King SB, Lembo NJ, et al. Vitamin E supplementation, plasma lipids and incidence of restenosis after percutaneous transluminal angioplasty (PTCA). *J Am Coll Nutr* 1992;11:131–138.
102. Blot WJ, Li J, Taylor PR, et al. Nutrition intervention trials in Linxian, China: supplementation with specific vitamin/mineral combinations, cancer incidence, and disease-specific mortality in the general population. *J Natl Cancer Inst* 1993;85:1483–1492.
103. The α-Tocopherol β-Carotene Research Group. The effect of Vitamin E and β-carotene on the incidence of lung cancer and other cancers in male smokers. *N Engl J Med* 1994;330:1029–1035.
104. Rapola JM, Virtamo J, Haukka JK, et al. Effect of Vitamin E and β-carotene on the incidence of angina pectoris: a randomized, double-blind, controlled trial. *JAMA* 1996;9:693–698.
105. Omenn GS, Goodman GE, Thornquist MD, et al. Effects of a combination of β-carotene and Vitamin A on lung cancer and cardiovascular disease. *N Engl J Med* 1996;334:1150–1155.

106. Hennekens C, Buring J, Manson J, et al. Lack of effect of long-term supplementation with β-carotene on the incidence of malignant neoplasms and cardiovascular disease. *N Engl J Med* 1996;334:1145–1149.
107. Stephens N, Parsons A, Schonfield P, et al. Randomised controlled trial of Vitamin E in patients with coronary disease: Cambridge Heart Antioxidant Study (CHAOS). *Lancet* 1996;347:781–786.
108. Livingston P, Jones C. Treatment of intermittent claudication with Vitamin E. *Lancet* 1958;2:602–604.
109. Williams HTG, Fenna D, MacBeth RA. α-tocopherol in the treatment of intermittent claudication. *Surg Gynecol Obstet* 1971;132:662–666.
110. Haeger K. Long-time treatment of intermittent claudication with Vitamin E. *Am J Clin Nutr* 1974;27:1179–1181.
111. Manson JE, Gaziano JM, Spelsberg A, et al. A secondary prevention trial of antioxidant vitamins and cardiovascular disease in women. *Ann Epidemiol* 1995;5:261–269.
112. Hertog M, Hollman J. Potential health effects of the dietary flavonoids. *Eur J Clin Nutr* 1996;50:63–71.
113. Safe SH. Environmental and dietary estrogens and human health: is there a problem? *Environ Health Perspect* 1995;103:346–351.
114. Middleton JE, Kandaswami C. Effects of flavonoids on immune and inflammatory cell functions. *Biochem Pharmacol* 1992;43:1167–1179.
115. Hertog MGL, Hollman PCH, Katan MB, et al. Intake of potentially anticarcinogenic flavonoids and their determinants in adults in the Netherlands. *Nutr Cancer* 1993;20:21–29.
116. Hertog MG, Feskens EJM, Hollman PCH, et al. Dietary antioxidant flavonoids and risk of coronary heart disease: the Zutphen Study. *Lancet* 1993; 342:1007–1011.
117. Hertog MGL, Hollman PCH, Katan MB. Content of potentially anticarcinogenic flavonoids of 28 vegetables and 9 fruits commonly consumed in the Netherlands. *J Agric Food Chem* 1992;40:2379–2383.
118. Keli S, Hertog M, Feskens E, et al. Dietary flavonoids, antioxidant vitamins and the incidence of stroke: the Zutphen Study. *Arch Intern Med* 1996; 156:637–642.
119. Brandi ML. Flavonoids: biochemical effects and therapeutic applications. *Bone Mineral* 1992;19(suppl):3–14.
120. Anderson J, Smith B, Gustafson N. Health benefits and practical aspects of high-fiber diets. *Am J Clin Nutr* 1994;59(suppl):1242–1247.
121. Truswell AS. Dietary fibre and blood lipids. *Curr Opin Lipid* 1995;6:14–19.
122. Slavin JL. Dietary fiber: classification, chemical analyses, and food source. *J Am Diet Assoc* 1987;87:1164–1171.
123. Marlett JA. Content and composition of dietary fiber in 117 frequently consumed foods. *J Am Diet Assoc* 1992;92:175–186.
124. Ripsin C, Keenan J, Jacobs D, et al. Oat products and lipid-lowering: a meta-analysis. *JAMA* 1992;267:3317–3325.
125. Slavin JL, Jacobs DR, Marquart L. Whole grain consumption and chronic disease: protective mechanisms. *Nutr Cancer* 1997;27:14–21.
126. Kushi LH, Lew RA, Stare FJ. Diet and 20-year mortality from coronary heart disease: the Ireland-Boston Diet-Heart Study. *N Engl J Med* 1984;312:811–818.
127. Messina M, Messina V. Increasing use of soyfoods and their potential role in cancer prevention. *J Am Diet Assoc* 1991;91:836–840.
128. Fraser GE, eds. *Preventive Cardiology.* New York, NY: Oxford University Press; 1986.

129. Anderson J, Johnstone B, Cook-Newell M. Meta-analysis of the effects of soy protein intake on serum lipids. *N Engl J Med* 1995;333:276–282.

130. Knopp RH, Zhu X, Bonet B. Effects of estrogens on lipoprotein metabolism and cardiovascular disease in women. *Atherosclerosis* 1994;110(suppl):83–91.

131. Granfone A, Campos H, McNamara JR. Effects of estrogen replacement on plasma lipoproteins and apolipoproteins in postmenopausal, dyslipidemic women. *Metabolism* 1992;41:1193–1198.

132. Van Itallie TB. Health implications of overweight and obesity in the United States. *Ann Intern Med* 1985;103:983–988.

133. Kumanyika SK. Special issues regarding obesity in minority populations. *Ann Intern Med* 1993;119:650–654.

134. National Institutes of Health Consensus Development Conference. *Health Implications of Obesity*. Bethesda, MD: National Institutes of Health; 1985.

135. Hubert HB, Feinleib M, McNamara PM, et al. Obesity as an independent risk factor for cardiovascular disease: a 26-year follow-up of participants in the Framingham Heart Study. *Circulation* 1983;67:968–977.

136. Manson JE, Colditz GA, Stampfer MJ, et al. A prospective study of obesity and risk of coronary heart disease in women. *N Engl J Med* 1990;322:882–889.

137. Barrett-Connor EL. Obesity, atherosclerosis, and coronary artery disease. *Ann Intern Med* 1985;103:1010–1019.

138. Higgins M, Kannel W, Garrison R, et al. Hazards of obesity—the Framingham experience. *Acta Med Scand* 1988;723(suppl):23–36.

139. Bild DE, Jacobs DR, Liu K, et al. Seven-year trends in plasma low-density-lipoprotein-cholesterol in young adults: the CARDIA Study. *Ann Epidemiol* 1996;6:235–245.

140. Colditz GA, Wilett WC, Stampfer MJ. Weight as a risk factor for clinical diabetes in women. *Am J Epidemiol* 1990;132:501–513.

141. Ashley FW, Kannel WB. Relationship to weight change in atherogenic traits: the Framingham Study. *J Chron Dis* 1974;27:103–114.

142. Denke MA, Sempos CT, Grundy SM. Excess body weight: an underrecognized contributor to high blood cholesterol levels in white American men. *Arch Intern Med* 1993;153:1093–1103.

143. Messerli FH. Obesity in hypertension: how innocent a bystander? *Am J Med* 1984;77:1077–1082.

144. Messerli FH, Nunez BD, Ventura HO, et al. Overweight and sudden death: increased ventricular ectopy in cardiopathy of obesity. *Arch Intern Med* 1987;147:1725–1728.

145. Prineas RJ, Grimm R, Grandits G, et al. The effect of dietary sodium and body weight on echocardiographic measures of left ventricular mass among treated hypertensive men and women: four-year change in the TOMHS Study. *Nieren Hochdruckkrankheiten* 1994;23(suppl):14–21.

146. Folsom AR, Wu KK, Davis CE, et al. Population correlates of plasma fibrinogen and factor VII$_c$, putative cardiovascular risk factors. *Atherosclerosis* 1991;91:191–205.

147. Iso H, Folsom AR, Wu KK, et al. Hemostatic variables in Japanese and Caucasian men: plasma fibrinogen, factor VII$_c$, factor VIII$_c$, and von Willebrand factor and their relations to cardiovascular disease risk factors. *Am J Epidemiol* 1989;130:925–934.

148. Folsom AR, Conlan MG, Davis CE, et al. Relations between hemostasis variables and cardiovascular risk factors in middle-aged adults. *Ann Epidemiol* 1992;2:481–494.

149. Williamson DF, Kahn HS, Byers T. The 10-y incidence of obesity and major weight gain in black and white US women aged 30–55 y. *Am J Clin Nutr* 1991;53(suppl):1515–1518.
150. Wing RR, Matthews KA, Kuller LH, et al. Weight gain at the time of menopause. *Arch Intern Med* 1991;151:97–102.
151. Keppel KG, Taffle SM. Pregnancy-related weight gain and retention: implications of the 1990 Institute of Medicine Guidelines. *Am J Public Health* 1983;83:1100–1103.
152. Van Itallie TB. The perils of obesity in middle-aged women. *N Engl J Med* 1990;322:928–929.
153. Smith DE, Lewis CE, Caveny JL, et al. Longitudinal changes in adiposity associated with pregnancy. The CARDIA Study. Coronary artery risk development in young adults study. *JAMA* 1994;271:1747–1751.
154. Berns MAM, de Vries JHM, Katan MB. Increase in body fatness as a major determinant of changes in serum total cholesterol and high density lipoprotein cholesterol in young men over a 10-year period. *Am J Epidemiol* 1989;130:1109–1122.
155. Despres J, Lupien PJ, Tremblay A, et al. Regional distribution of body fat, plasma lipoproteins, and cardiovascular disease. *Arteriosclerosis* 1990;10: 497–511.
156. Folsom AR, Kaye SA, Sellers TA, et al. Body fat distribution and 5-year risk of death in older women. *JAMA* 1993;269:483–487.
157. Hartz A, Grubb B, Van Nort JJ, et al. The association of waist hip ratio and angiographically determined coronary artery disease. *Int J Obes* 1990;14:657–665.
158. Willett WC, Manson JA, Stampfer MJ, et al. Weight, weight change, and coronary heart disease in women: risk with the "normal" weight range. *JAMA* 1995;273:461–465.
159. Lee IM, Manson JE, Hennekens CH, et al. Body weight and mortality: a 27-year follow-up of middle-aged men. *JAMA* 1993;270:2823–2828.
160. Seidell JC, Bakc KC, Deurenberg P, et al. Overweight and chronic illness—a retrospective cohort study, with a follow-up of 6–17 years, in men and women of initially 20–50 years of age. *J Chron Dis* 1986;39:585–593.
161. Lew EA, Garfinkel L. Variations in mortality by weight among 750 000 men and women. *J Chron Dis* 1979;32:563–576.
162. Seidell JC, de Groot LCP, van Sonsbeek JLA, et al. Associations of moderate and severe overweight with self-reported illness and medical care in Dutch adults. *Am J Public Health* 1986;76:264–269.
163. Joint National Committee on Detection Evaluation and Treatment of High Blood Pressure. The fifth report of the Joint National Committee on Detection, Evaluation, and Treatment of High Blood Pressure (JNC V). *Arch Intern Med* 1993;153:154–183.
164. Working Group on Primary Prevention of Hypertension. Report of the National High Blood Pressure Education Program Working Group on Primary Prevention of Hypertension. *Arch Intern Med* 1993;153:186–208.
165. Cutler JA. Randomized clinical trials of weight reduction in nonhypertensive persons. *Ann Epidemiol* 1991;1:363–370.
166. Stamler R, Stamler J, Gosch FC, et al. Primary prevention of hypertension by nutritional-hygienic means: final report of a randomized, controlled trial. *JAMA* 1989;262:1801–1807.
167. Stamler R, Stamler J, Grimm R, et al. Nutritional therapy for high blood pressure: final report of a four-year randomized controlled trial—the Hypertension Control Program. *JAMA* 1987;257:1484–1491.

168. Hypertension Prevention Trial Research Group. The Hypertension Prevention Trial: three-year effects of dietary changes on blood pressure. *Arch Intern Med* 1990;150:153–162.
169. Grimm RH, Grandits GA, Elmer PJ. The Treatment of Mild Hypertension Study: final results of quality of life measures with diet and drug treatment of mild hypertension. *Arch Intern Med* 1997;157:638–648.
170. Wassertheil-Smoller S, Blaufox MD, Oberman A, et al. Effect of antihypertensives on sexual function and quality of life: the TAIM Study. *Ann Intern Med* 1991;114:613–620.
171. Wadden TA. Treatment of obesity by moderate and severe caloric restriction: results of clinical research trials. *Ann Intern Med* 1993;119:688–693.
172. Wing RR. Weight cycling in humans: a review of the literature. *Ann Behav Med* 1992;14:113–119.
173. Van Dale D, Saris WH. Repetitive weight loss and regain: effects on weight reduction, resting metabolic rate, and lipolytic activity before and after exercise and/or diet treatment. *Am J Clin Nutr* 1989;49:409–416.
174. Blackburn GL, Wilson GT, Kanders BS. Weight cycling: the experience of human dieters. *Am J Clin Nutr* 1989;49:1105–1109.
175. Jeffrey RW, Wing RR, French SA. Weight cycling and cardiovascular risk factors in obese men and women. *Am J Clin Nutr* 1992;55:641–644.
176. Lee IM, Paffenbarger RS. Change in body weight and longevity. *JAMA* 1992;268:2045–2049.
177. National Task Force on Prevention of Obesity. Weight cycling. *JAMA* 1994;272:1196–1202.
178. Stunkard A. Current views on obesity. *Am J Med* 1996;100:230–236.
179. Jeffrey RW, French SA, Schmid TL. Attribution for dietary failures: problems reported by participants in the Hypertension Prevention Trial. *Health Psychol* 1990;9:315–329.
180. Brownell KD, Jeffrey RW. Improving long term weight loss: pushing the limits of treatment. *Behav Ther* 1987;18:353–374.
181. Nicolosi R, Becker D, Elmer PJ, et al. Special report: American Heart Association Guidelines for Weight Management Programs for Healthy Adults. *Heart Dis Stroke* 1994;3:221–228.
182. National Task Force on the Prevention and Treatment of Obesity. Very low calorie diets. *JAMA* 1993;270:967–974.
183. The Trials of Hypertension Prevention Collaborative Research Group. The effects of nonpharmacologic interventions on blood pressure of persons with high normal levels: results of the Trials of Hypertension Prevention, Phase I. *JAMA* 1992;267:1213–1220.
184. Jeffery RW. Behavioral treatment of obesity. *Ann Behav Med* 1987;9:20–24.
185. Pavlou KN, Krey S, Steffee WP. Exercise as an adjunct to weight loss and maintenance in moderately obese subjects. *Am J Clin Nutr* 1989;49:1115–1123.
186. Bouchard C, Depres JP, Tremblay A. Exercise and obesity. *Obes Res* 1993;1:133–147.
187. Dishman RK, Buckworth J. Increasing physical activity: a quantative synthesis. *Medi Sci Sports Exerc* 1996;28:706–719.
188. Hill JO, Drougas H, Peters JC. Obesity treatment: can diet composition play a role? *Ann Intern Med* 1993;119:694–697.
189. Lissner L, Heitmann BL. Dietary fat and obesity: evidence from epidemiology. *Eur J Clin Nutr* 1995;49:79–90.
190. Safer DJ. Diet, behavior modification, and exercise: a review of obesity treatments from a long-term perspective. *South Med J* 1991;84:1470–1474.

191. Blackburn GL. Comparison of medically supervised and unsupervised approaches to weight loss and control. *Ann Intern Med* 1993;119:714–718.
192. Barrett S, Herbert V, eds. *The Vitamin Pushers: How the "Health Food" Industry Is Selling America a Bill of Goods.* Amherst, NY: Prometheus Books; 1994.
193. Abernethy JD. The need to treat mild hypertension. Misinterpretation of results from the Australian trial. *JAMA* 1986;256:3134–3137.
194. National High Blood Pressure Education Program (NHBPEP) and National Cholesterol Education Program (NCEP). *Working Group Report on Management of Patients With Hypertension and High Blood Cholesterol.* Bethesda, MD: National Institutes of Health; 1990.
195. Cutler JA, Follmann D, Allender PS. Randomized trials of sodium reduction: an overview. *Am J Clin Nutr* 1997;65(suppl):643–651.
196. Kumanyaku SK, Obarzanek E, Stevens VJ, et al. Weight-loss experience of black and white participants in NHLBI-sponsored clinical trials. *Am J Clin Nutr* 1991;53(suppl):161–168.
197. Neaton J, Grimm R, Prineas R, et al. Treatment of Mild Hypertension Study (TOMHS): final results. *JAMA* 1993;270:713–724.
198. Whelton PK, Applegate WB, Ettinger WH, et al. Efficacy of weight loss and reduced sodium intake in the Trial of Nonpharmacologic Interventions in the Elderly (TONE). *Circulation* 1996;94:I-178.
199. Blackburn H, Prineas R. Diet and hypertension: anthropology, epidemiology, and public health implications. *Prog Biochem Pharmacol* 1983;19:31–79.
200. Sacks FM, Obarzanek E, Windhauser MM, et al. Rationale and design of the Dietary Approaches to Stop Hypertension Trial (DASH): a multicenter controlled-feeding study of dietary patterns to lower blood pressure. *Ann Epidemiol* 1995;5:108–118.
201. National Academy of Sciences, eds. *Recommended Dietary Allowances.* Washington, DC: National Academy Press; 1989.
202. Appel LJ, Moore TJ, Obarzanek E, et al. A clinical trial of the effects of dietary patterns on blood pressure. *N Engl J Med* 1997;336:1117–1124.

Chapter 6

Special Issues in the Management of Dyslipidemias

Peter H. Jones, MD
and Antonio M. Gotto, Jr, MD, PhD

The relation of elevated low-density lipoprotein cholesterol (LDL-C) to increased risk for coronary heart disease (CHD) is well known. Many clinical trials demonstrated reductions in clinical CHD event rates, including in CHD death, with lipid-regulating therapy.[1] Reductions in total mortality rate were shown as well, both in patients with a history of myocardial infarction (MI) or angina pectoris[2] and in patients without previous MI.[3] In addition, numerous angiographically monitored clinical trials of lipid regulating with diet, single- and combination-drug therapy, and/or surgery in patients with CHD showed less coronary lesion progression, less new lesion formation, and, in some patients, evidence of lesion regression with intervention.[4]

Other dyslipidemias also increase CHD risk. For example, in both the primary-prevention Helsinki Heart Study[5] and the observational Prospective Cardiovascular Münster study,[6] subjects with an elevated triglyceride concentration and an elevated LDL-C/high-density lipoprotein cholesterol (HDL-C) ratio were at the highest risk for CHD events. For many dyslipidemias, clear clinical trial evidence of benefit from treatment is lacking, despite an observed high risk for atherosclerotic vascular disease development. This chapter reviews some of these special issues, in-

From Robinson K, (ed): *Preventive Cardiology*. Armonk, NY: Futura Publishing Company, Inc. © 1998.

cluding isolated low concentrations of HDL-C, severe hypertriglyceridemia, dyslipidemias in cardiac and renal transplantation, dyslipidemias in renal disease, the use of apolipoproteins and lipoproteins to refine treatment decisions, and combination-drug therapy.

Isolated Low High-Density Lipoprotein Cholesterol

A reduced plasma level of HDL-C is a strong, independent predictor of CHD risk in observational studies.[7,8] Available epidemiological evidence suggests that, for every 1-mg/dL decrease in HDL-C, the risk for CHD is increased 2% to 3%.[8] In 321 men aged <60 (mean, 50 years) who had angiographically documented CHD, the most common lipid abnormality, occurring in 36% of the subjects, was low HDL-C,[9] defined as concentrations in the lowest 10th percentile of Lipid Research Clinic values for age and sex. In comparison, low HDL-C was present in only 9% of the 901 control subjects (selected from the Framingham Offspring Study) who did not have clinical manifestations of CHD, cerebrovascular disease, or peripheral vascular disease and who were not taking lipid-regulating drugs. Isolated low HDL-C was found in 19% of the case subjects compared with 4% of the control subjects.[9] For purposes of the present discussion, isolated low HDL-C is defined as HDL-C <35 mg/dL with total cholesterol <200 mg/dL and triglyceride <200 mg/dL in a fasting blood sample.

Nascent HDL particles, produced by the liver and intestine, are discoidal, lipid-poor particles containing phospholipid, cholesterol, and apolipoproteins. Through the action of lecithin:cholesterol acyltransferase, acquired free cholesterol is esterified in the core, and the disk is transformed into spherical HDL_3. HDL_3 acquires additional free cholesterol from cells and additional cholesterol, phospholipid, and apolipoproteins from the redundant surface layer of hydrolyzed triglyceride-rich lipoproteins—chylomicrons and very-low-density lipoproteins (VLDL)—which results in the formation of larger, fully mature HDL_2. Most of the variation in HDL-C concentrations among individuals is attributable to variation in HDL_2 cholesterol concentration.

The observed lower risk for CHD in patients with normal or elevated concentrations of HDL-C is not completely understood. Postulated beneficial actions of HDL that have antiatherosclerotic potential include reverse cholesterol transport (the posited mechanism whereby cholesterol is returned from the periphery to the liver for excretion),[10] increased endothelial repair,[11] prostacyclin stabilization,[12] and inhibition of LDL oxidation.[13] Low HDL-C may increase CHD risk by compromising these protective activities.

Previous clinical trials of lipid-regulating intervention focused on LDL-C reduction; although HDL-C was frequently increased as well, HDL-C was not the target of intervention. However, two trials currently in progress are designed to monitor the effect of increasing HDL-C on clinical CHD events. The HDL Intervention Trial (HIT) is a Veterans Affairs cooperative study of approximately 2500 men aged ≤73 years with known CHD as documented by history of MI, coronary artery revascularization, angiographic evidence of coronary atherosclerosis, or angina with evidence of ischemia.[14] The lipid entry criteria are HDL-C ≤40 mg/dL, LDL-C ≤140 mg/dL, and triglyceride ≤300 mg/dL. Subjects are randomized to receive the fibric-acid derivative gemfibrozil 1200 mg/day or placebo; projected average follow-up is 6 years. The Bezafibrate Infarction Prevention (BIP) study is being conducted in approximately 3000 men and women aged 45–74 with known CHD as documented by MI 6 months to 5 years before randomization or by clinically evident angina.[15] Lipid entry criteria are HDL-C ≤45 mg/dL, total cholesterol 180–250 mg/dL, LDL-C ≤180 mg/dL (≤160 mg/dL in patients aged <50), and triglyceride ≤300 mg/dL. Subjects are randomized to receive the fibric-acid derivative bezafibrate 400 mg/day or placebo for an average of 6 years. Both HIT and BIP have a primary end point of CHD mortality plus nonfatal MI, and both trials are expected to end in 1998.

Treatment

Despite the absence of clinical trial evidence, the observed high risk for CHD in patients with isolated low HDL-C warrants a detection and treatment strategy. The National Cholesterol Education Program (NCEP)[16] recommends that HDL-C be measured in addition to total cholesterol at least every 5 years in all individuals aged 20 or older. In individuals found to have isolated low HDL-C, the primary management should be the reduction of other CHD risk factors. Deleterious lifestyle habits associated with a low HDL-C concentration, such as obesity, cigarette smoking, and a sedentary lifestyle, should be identified and corrected. In particular, regular aerobic exercise can have a substantial effect on increasing HDL-C. Also, drugs such as anabolic steroids, progestational agents, and certain β-blockers can reduce HDL-C and should be discontinued if possible. In high-risk patients without CHD in whom the above mentioned nonpharmacologic treatments do not increase HDL-C sufficiently and in patients with CHD, pharmacologic treatment should be strongly considered. The NCEP guidelines recommend selecting a lipid-regulating drug that not only reduces LDL-C but also increases HDL-C (Table 1).

The drug most likely to improve both LDL-C and HDL-C concentrations is nicotinic acid, which has the capacity to reduce LDL-C by 10% to

Table 1
Lipid-Regulating Drug Mechanisms and Effects

Lipid-Regulating Agents	Mechanisms	Effects on Lipids
Bile-acid sequestrants Cholestyramine Colestipol	Decrease intrahepatic cholesterol by nonspecific binding of bile acids Increased activity of LDL receptors	LDL-C decreases 15% to 30% HDL-C increases 3% to 5% TG usually not affected; may increase
Nicotinic acid	Decreased production of VLDL Decreased mobilization of free fatty acids from peripheral adipocytes	LDL-C decreases 10% to 25% HDL-C increases 15% to 35% TG decreases 20% to 50%
HMG-CoA reductase inhibitors Atorvastatin Cerivastatin Fluvastatin Lovastatin Pravastatin Simvastatin	Decrease in cholesterol synthesis caused by partial inhibition of HMG-CoA reductase	LDL-C decrease 20% to 60% HDL-C increases 5% to 15% TG decreases 10% to 40%
Fibric-acid derivatives Bezafibrate Ciprofibrate Clofibrate Fenofibrate Gemfibrozil	Increases activity of lipoprotein lipase Decreased release of free fatty acids from peripheral adipose tissue	LDL-C decreases 10% to 15% with high LDL-C; may increase with high TG HDL-C increases 10% to 15% TG decreases 20% to 50%

HDL-C = high-density lipoprotein cholesterol; LDL = low-density lipoprotein; LDL-C = low-density lipoprotein cholesterol; TG = triglyceride; VLDL = very-low-density lipoprotein.
Reproduced with permission from Reference 86.

25% and to increase HDL-C by 15% to 35% at dosages of 1500–3000 mg/ day. Studies of the efficacy of nicotinic acid in patients with isolated low HDL-C showed that either immediate-release or sustained-release preparations increase HDL-C by 30% and reduce LDL-C by 20%.[17] Nicotinic acid has the additional advantage of being the least expensive pharmacologic lipid-regulating agent. However, compliance with high-dose nicotinic acid regimens may be limited by cutaneous flushing and pruritus, and potential biochemical side effects such as elevated transaminase, uric acid, and glucose concentrations may restrict its universal use. Sustained-release nicotinic acid is generally not recommended because of increased prevalence of hepatic toxicity with these preparations.[18] In patients with diabetes mellitus (DM) or a predisposition to diabetes or gout, nicotinic acid should only be used with caution and careful clinical monitoring.

Fibric-acid derivatives (fibrates) were also shown to increase HDL-C concentrations, particularly in patients with baseline hypertriglyceridemia. The fibric-acid derivatives currently approved in the United States are gemfibrozil, clofibrate, which is little used, and fenofibrate, which is not currently marketed. Other fibrates approved for use in other countries are bezafibrate and ciprofibrate. Although gemfibrozil is better tolerated and has fewer biochemical side effects than nicotinic acid, it is less efficacious than nicotinic acid in increasing HDL-C in subjects with isolated low HDL-C. In general, gemfibrozil 1200 mg/day increases HDL-C by 10% to 15% and decreases LDL-C by 10% to 15%; however, LDL-C may increase in patients with hypertriglyceridemia.

An alternative treatment strategy for patients with CHD and isolated low HDL-C is to focus entirely on aggressive reduction of LDL-C. The 3-hydroxy-3-methylglutaryl coenzyme A (HMG-CoA) reductase inhibitors (statins), because of their proven safety and efficacy in lowering LDL-C, are ideal candidates as alternatives to nicotinic acid treatment. Atorvastatin 10–80 mg/day, cerivastatin 0.3 mg/day, fluvastatin 20–80 mg/day, lovastatin 10–80 mg/day, pravastatin 10–40 mg/day, or simvastatin 5–40 mg/day decreases LDL-C from 20% to 60% and increases HDL-C by 5% to 15%, depending on which agent is used. In a comparison of gemfibrozil and lovastatin in patients with isolated low HDL-C, both drugs produced similar, small increases in HDL-C, but lovastatin resulted in a much greater reduction in LDL-C.[19]

Severe Hypertriglyceridemia

Severely elevated plasma triglyceride (>1000 mg/dL) represents an infrequent yet clinically important dyslipidemia that can be frustratingly difficult to treat. Most cases of severe hypertriglyceridemia are primary, familial disorders, but secondary conditions such as DM, obesity, alcohol use, nephrotic syndrome, oral estrogen use, pregnancy, and hypothyroidism may contribute significantly to the dyslipidemia. Acute pancreatitis is the most important short-term consequence of severe hypertriglyceridemia and is associated with serious complications such as hypocalcemia, hypotension, retroperitoneal hemorrhage, pseudocyst formation, and occasionally death. For this reason, the NCEP recommends immediate hygienic and, if necessary, pharmacologic treatment for patients with severe hypertriglyceridemia.[16] Although the role of triglyceride-rich lipoproteins in atherogenesis remains controversial, prevention of CHD is not the principal intent of intervention in these cases.

Chylomicrons and VLDL are the initial particles in the transport of exogenous and endogenous lipids, respectively. These lipoproteins are hydrolyzed through the activity of lipoprotein lipase, which is activated by apolipoprotein (apo) C-II on the lipoprotein surface. The resulting remnant particles, chylomicron remnants and intermediate-density lipoprotein (IDL), are believed to increase CHD risk, but the precursor particles are not.

Severe hypertriglyceridemia is usually caused by an elevation of both chylomicrons and VLDL in the fasting state, phenotype V hyperlipidemia. Most cases of type V hyperlipidemia occur in adults. The principal metabolic abnormality in type V hyperlipidemia is thought to be marked overproduction of VLDL, resulting in the competition of these particles with chylomicrons for lipoprotein lipase catabolism and, thus, a decrease in the postprandial clearance of chylomicrons. Typically, patients have plasma triglyceride concentrations in the 1000- to 3000-mg/dL range. Total cholesterol may also be increased, with the cholesterol/triglyceride ratio ranging from 0.2 to 0.5 mg/dL. However, LDL-C and HDL-C concentrations are usually subnormal. The triglyceride-rich lipoproteins in patients with the type V pattern are heterogeneous, with all sizes and densities of VLDL and chylomicrons present. In some members of affected kindreds, hypertriglyceridemia may be caused predominantly by increased VLDL—phenotype IV hyperlipidemia—suggesting some variability in the genetic expression. Uncommonly in type IV hyperlipidemia, fasting triglyceride concentrations exceed 1000 mg/dL. In type IV and in type V, early CHD is seen in some families but not others.

Type V hyperlipidemia may be associated with a variety of other metabolic disturbances such as low HDL-C, hyperuricemia and gout, hypertension, and noninsulin-dependent DM (NIDDM). This clustering of metabolic abnormalities is termed syndrome X and is associated with insulin resistance.[20] Although many patients with type V hyperlipidemia are insulin resistant, it is not clear that insulin resistance is the primary genetic defect responsible for the hypertriglyceridemia.

Rarely, a fasting elevation of chylomicrons alone may occur, referred to as type I hyperlipidemia. Familial chylomicronemia typically manifests in childhood, principally as episodes of abdominal pain and overt pancreatitis. The genetic causes of chylomicronemia are lipoprotein lipase deficiency and apo C-II deficiency, both of which result in defective chylomicron clearance. Familial chylomicronemia was been associated with increased CHD risk.

Treatment

Nonpharmacologic treatment options for severe hypertriglyceridemia include alcohol cessation, weight loss, low-fat diet, increased physical activity, discontinuation of estrogen, and, for hypothyroidism, thyroid replacement. Very–low-fat diets with calorie and carbohydrate restriction are helpful for patients with the type V pattern and are the only effective treatment for patients with type I hyperlipidemia. (Intake of medium-chain triglycerides may assist in the dietary treatment of type I hyperlipidemia.) Restriction of dietary fat only, with increased consumption of carbohydrate to balance calories, may result in minimal benefit on plasma triglyceride concentration because VLDL synthesis may be enhanced. In obese patients, weight loss can improve insulin sensitivity, which will substantially lower triglyceride levels.

Many cases of severe hypertriglyceridemia occurring with poorly controlled diabetes result from a combination of an underlying familial dyslipidemia and the stimulation of hepatic VLDL production and reduced lipoprotein lipase activity secondary to hyperinsulinemia and insulin resistance. Weight loss and exercise are the traditional treatment modalities to improve insulin sensitivity in patients with NIDDM and can simultaneously reduce plasma glucose and triglyceride concentrations. Oral hypoglycemics and/or exogenous insulin have variable effects on triglyceride concentration. The biguanide metformin can reduce triglyceride concentration by up to 50% and was shown to be effective in obese patients with NIDDM when used alone or in combination with the sulfonylurea glyburide; however, triglyceride concentrations were not severely elevated at baseline in these patients.[21]

According to the NCEP guidelines,[16] pharmacologic treatment for severe hypertriglyceridemia should be considered if the above mentioned therapies fail to reduce triglyceride to below 1000 mg/dL. The goal of therapy in these patients is triglyceride <200 mg/dL, although achievement of triglyceride <500 mg/dL may be considered a success. As noted above, drug therapy is usually not helpful in type I hyperlipidemia.

Nicotinic acid is the first choice for drug treatment in patients with hypertriglyceridemia. If tolerated in dosages of at least 1500 mg/day, nicotinic acid can produce dramatic reductions in triglyceride—generally 20% to 50%—that are thought to be mediated through the inhibition of lipolysis in adipose tissues and a decrease in hepatic VLDL synthesis.[22] One disadvantage of nicotinic acid therapy is its negative effect on glucose tolerance[23]; this agent can unmask the latent diabetes so frequently present in subjects with type V hyperlipidemia or worsen glucose control in patients with known diabetes. This effect of nicotinic acid, however, should not deter the clinician from using the agent in high-risk patients who have recurrent bouts of pancreatitis secondary to uncontrolled hypertriglyceridemia. Also, nicotinic acid can increase serum uric acid concentration,[24] which may already be elevated and is associated with gout in these patients. Use of allopurinol may permit continuation of a successful nicotinic acid regimen in such patients.

Gemfibrozil is known to reduce plasma triglyceride concentration, primarily by enhancing lipoprotein lipase activity.[25] In general, gemfibrozil at a dosage of 1200 mg/day decreases triglyceride by 20% to 50%. Gemfibrozil may be useful in combination with nicotinic acid in patients who have an inadequate response to either agent alone.

The n-3 fatty acids eicosapentaenoic acid and docosahexaenoic acid, found in high concentrations in fish oils, were shown to reduce hepatic VLDL production and increase clearance of VLDL particles from the circulation, thereby lowering plasma triglyceride concentration.[26] Studies of supplemental fish oil intake, primarily conducted in subjects with fasting triglyceride concentrations <1000 mg/dL, demonstrated up to a 30% reduction in triglyceride.[27] Although the benefit of n-3 fatty acids in severe hypertriglyceridemia was not established, fish oil at a dosage of at least 6 g/day may be useful as an adjunct to nicotinic acid, gemfibrozil, or both in refractory hypertriglyceridemia.

Steroid hormones with androgenic activity were shown to reduce triglyceride concentration in patients with type V hyperlipidemia. The progestational agent norethindrone acetate at a dosage of 5 mg/day reduced triglyceride in women with type V hyperlipidemia by an average of 50%.[28] This treatment may be considered as monotherapy in hysterectomized women who are intolerant of or unresponsive to nicotinic acid and/or gemfibrozil, or as adjunctive therapy to these medications in refractory cases.

Dyslipidemias in Cardiac and Renal Transplantation

Lipid abnormalities after cardiac and renal transplantation are very common, occurring in as many as 65% of recipients during the first year after transplantation.[29] Posttransplantation dyslipidemia is characterized by elevated total cholesterol, LDL-C, and triglyceride concentrations. Typically, the total cholesterol and LDL-C concentrations increase progressively during the first 6 months after transplantation, reaching a maximum at 6–12 months. Although a variable decline follows during the next 1–2 years, the recipient's cholesterol usually persists above pretransplant values; in most cases, total cholesterol concentration remains >200 mg/dL. Triglyceride follows a similar pattern, with a progressive increase during the first 12 months after transplantation; however, triglyceride tends to decline to acceptable concentrations thereafter. HDL-C concentration is usually normal or even high and tends to increase slowly during the first 12 months after transplantation.

The factors responsible for posttransplant dyslipidemia are multiple and appear to relate to the type and dosage of immunosuppressive therapy, amount of weight gain, glucose concentration, and presence of genetic lipid disorders.[28] The immunosuppressive agents cyclosporine and corticosteroids may be important causes of posttransplant dyslipidemia, particularly in the first 6 months. Cyclosporine can increase LDL-C, and corticosteroids can increase both cholesterol and triglyceride as well as impair glucose tolerance. The use of alternate-day steroids[30] or corticosteroid-free maintenance immunosuppression[31] was shown to minimize or ameliorate posttransplant lipid abnormalities.

Cardiac Transplantation

Accelerated CHD is the leading cause of morbidity and mortality in cardiac transplant recipients who survive more than 1 year after transplantation.[32] The risk factors for the development of transplant arteriopathy are multiple and include both immune and nonimmune mechanisms. Experimental animal models demonstrate a strong relation between hypercholesterolemia and transplant coronary atherosclerosis.[33]

Treatment

Early reports of treatment of transplant dyslipidemia using maximum-dosage lovastatin demonstrated excellent LDL-C reductions, but there were high rates of myositis[34] and rhabdomyolysis.[35] Subsequent studies suggested that increased inhibition of HMG-CoA reductase, secondary to an interaction between reductase inhibitors and cyclosporine, is most likely responsible for the myopathy.[36] In several single-center reports, using lower doses of HMG-CoA reductase inhibitors markedly reduced the myositis risk in cyclosporine-treated cardiac transplant patients.[37–39]

In a prospective, nonblinded study, 97 cardiac transplant recipients were randomized to receive either pravastatin 20–40 mg/day beginning 1–2 weeks after transplantation or no lipid-regulating treatment.[37] All patients received cyclosporine, prednisone, azathioprine, and dietary counseling. During a 12-month follow-up, patients treated with pravastatin had significant reductions in incidence of transplant arteriopathy, hemodynamically significant rejection, and mortality compared with the group that did not receive pravastatin. In a subgroup of 20 consecutive patients, natural-killer-cell cytotoxicity was significantly lower in the pravastatin group than in the control group.

Larger prospective studies are necessary to answer fully concerns about myositis risk and clinical benefit of treating posttransplant dyslipidemia with HMG-CoA reductase inhibitors. However, the available data support the use of these agents at their recommended starting dosages with appropriate caution in cardiac transplant patients. Careful monitoring of plasma cyclosporine concentration to avoid toxicity; avoidance of concomitant use of medications such as antifungal agents, gemfibrozil, and macrolide antibiotics, which can alter cyclosporine and/or HMG-

CoA reductase inhibitor metabolism; and periodic measurement of creatine kinase levels are recommended when HMG-CoA reductase inhibitors are administered in transplant recipients.

The appropriateness of other lipid-regulating drugs in cardiac transplant patients was not extensively evaluated. Gemfibrozil is not as effective as HMG-CoA reductase inhibitors in lowering LDL-C and is not recommended as monotherapy in transplant patients. Nicotinic acid is a reasonable alternative as monotherapy, but compliance is a limiting factor. The bile-acid resins cholestyramine and colestipol are effective in reducing LDL-C; however, the concern about altered absorption of concomitantly administered medications, particularly cyclosporine, makes them less desirable as first-line therapy.

Renal Transplantation

Renal transplant recipients were reported to have a marked increase in atherosclerotic risk, and persistent cholesterol elevations are among several factors that predict atherosclerotic complications in these patients.[40] As in cardiac transplant patients, immunosuppressive drug regimens can contribute to the development of posttransplant dyslipidemia in renal transplant recipients.[41] Although no studies demonstrating the benefit of lowering LDL-C on subsequent CHD events in renal transplant recipients were reported, the clear clinical benefit with aggressive LDL-C reduction in nontransplant patients warrants a prudent treatment strategy.

Treatment

Because of their excellent tolerability and efficacy in lowering LDL-C, the HMG-CoA reductase inhibitors are first-line treatment in renal transplant patients. The same precautions described for cardiac transplant patients are required in renal transplant patients because of the concomitant use of cyclosporine. Several studies of HMG-CoA reductase inhibitor treatment in renal transplant recipients showed that lower dosages result in LDL-C reductions of approximately 40% without evidence of clinically significant myositis or rhabdomyolysis.[42,43]

Dyslipidemia in Renal Disease

Nephrotic Syndrome

One of the more clinically significant causes of secondary dyslipidemia is nephrotic syndrome. The defining clinical manifestations of this disease include albuminuria, hypoalbuminemia, peripheral edema, and severe hypercholesterolemia. The increase in cholesterol is predominantly in the LDL fraction, and LDL-C concentration exceeds 200 mg/dL in many severe cases of nephrosis. An increase in triglyceride concentration may also be seen but usually develops later in the course of the disease, particularly when serum creatinine concentration rises.

The mechanisms responsible for nephrotic hypercholesterolemia most likely involve hepatic overproduction of both cholesterol and apo B-containing lipoproteins (VLDL and LDL).[44] The enhanced cholesterol and lipoprotein production is probably related to the severity of hypoalbuminemia induced by the albuminuria.[45] The liver may respond to the low serum albumin and low oncotic pressure with a general increase in the synthesis of albumin and other proteins such as apoproteins. An increase in hepatic cholesterol synthesis down-regulates hepatic LDL receptor expression, thereby reducing the removal of LDL from the circulation. This combination of enhanced lipoprotein synthesis and reduced receptor-mediated catabolism results in severe elevations of LDL-C.[46]

The hypertriglyceridemia that can develop in nephrotic patients is thought to result from the overproduction of VLDL combined with defective lipolysis of VLDL.[47] This defective lipolysis may be related to one or more sources such as qualitative lipoprotein lipase deficiency, reduced hepatic triglyceride lipase activity, and urinary loss of lipoprotein lipase activators such as apo C-II.[43] High-dose steroid therapy, which is frequently used to induce remission of nephrosis, may cause substantial triglyceride elevation by further stimulating VLDL synthesis.

HDL-C concentrations in nephrotic patients are variable; low,[48] normal,[49] and elevated[50] concentrations were observed. Low HDL-C may result from loss of HDL particles in the urine; at least one study, however, failed to detect any immunoreactive intact apo A-I in the urine of nephrotic subjects.[44]

The consequences of severe hypercholesterolemia, such as CHD and other vascular disease, are not well documented in nephrosis. The relation of LDL-C elevation to CHD risk in the general population reflects many years of exposure to high LDL-C, but adults with nephrosis-induced hypercholesterolemia typically did not have this length of exposure. However, the severity of LDL-C elevation seen in many nephrotic patients may partially offset the time factor. Therefore, aggressive lipid-regulating treatment may be warranted in nephrotic patients whose disease is not likely to remit or be corrected by transplantation in the near future. Also, treatment of the dyslipidemia accompanying nephrosis may slow the progression of glomerulosclerosis.[51]

Treatment

Treatment for nephrotic dyslipidemia should include a low-fat diet, although this therapy alone will not usually normalize LDL-C concentration. Calorie restriction, weight loss, and alcohol cessation may lower triglyceride concentration. In most cases, drug treatment is necessary and should be directed at lowering LDL-C.

The bile-acid resins were shown to reduce LDL-C by approximately 20% to 30% in nephrotic patients but did not satisfactorily control the markedly elevated LDL-C.[52,53] Because bile-acid resins can increase triglyceride concentration, they are not an ideal choice as monotherapy in nephrotic patients with combined elevations in LDL and VLDL.

Nicotinic acid is an attractive treatment for nephrotic dyslipidemia because its mechanism of action is the inhibition of hepatic lipoprotein synthesis. Unfortunately, there are no systematic studies of its efficacy and tolerability in nephrotic syndrome. Theoretically, nicotinic acid would be most useful for treatment of patients who manifest combined dyslipidemia rather than an increase in LDL-C alone.

The HMG-CoA reductase inhibitors were shown to maintain their efficacy in nephrotic syndrome, reducing LDL-C by approximately 30% to 45%.[54-56] In the studies reported, which were fairly short in duration, the HMG-CoA reductase inhibitors were free of clinically significant side effects.

Combination-drug therapy may be warranted for some nephrotic patients whose LDL-C is not adequately controlled with an HMG-CoA reductase inhibitor alone or who have combined hyperlipidemia. LDL-C reduction can be augmented by adding a resin at a low dosage, such as 4–12 g/day of cholestyramine, to an HMG-CoA reductase inhibitor. For combined hyperlipidemia, nicotinic acid and an HMG-CoA reductase inhibitor should produce excellent responses in LDL-C and triglyceride concentrations. However, this combination was not adequately studied for either safety or efficacy in nephrotic patients and should be used with caution; as discussed at the end of this chapter, this combination carries a possible increased risk for myopathy or liver dysfunction in nonnephrotic patients.

Chronic Renal Disease

The dyslipidemia of chronic renal disease, seen in as many as 30% of patients with renal failure,[43] consists of elevated triglyceride and low HDL-C concentrations. Triglyceride concentration is usually 200–800 mg/dL but may exceed this range if there are accompanying factors such as poorly controlled DM, medications such as steroids and β-blockers, and rapid weight gain. Nearly one-fourth of all adults with chronic renal failure in the United States have diabetes, and the presence of abnormal glucose tolerance and insulin resistance may contribute significantly to the hypertriglyceridemia of uremia.

The metabolic cause of uremic hypertriglyceridemia, which primarily represents increased VLDL, appears to be defective lipolysis of triglyceride-rich lipoproteins, resulting from a deficiency in lipoprotein lipase, hepatic triglyceride lipase, or both.[43] The reduced HDL-C concentration is probably the result of the delayed clearance of triglyceride-rich lipoproteins. Treatment of uremia with either hemodialysis or chronic ambulatory peritoneal dialysis not only fails to correct hypertriglyceridemia but may make it worse; high glucose concentrations in dialysate may serve as a substrate for enhanced hepatic VLDL production, especially in patients with impaired glucose tolerance.[57]

Atherosclerotic vascular events, predominantly CHD related, are common in patients with chronic renal failure who are treated by dialysis.[58] It is not clear to what extent elevated triglyceride and low HDL-C concentrations contribute to this accelerated atherosclerosis. Many uremic patients have concomitant CHD risk factors, such as hypertension and diabetes. Whether treatment directed at lowering triglyceride and increasing HDL-C will reduce CHD risk in uremic patients is not known.

Treatment

Diet, exercise, and attainment of a reasonable body weight are the initial therapy for hypertriglyceridemia in patients with chronic renal failure. Improved glucose control in diabetic patients, discontinuation of β-blockers if possible, discontinuation of oral estrogens, and alcohol cessation are also important steps that can lower plasma triglyceride. If fasting triglyceride remains >500 mg/dL after implementation of these hygienic measures, pharmacologic therapy should be strongly considered to reduce the risk for acute pancreatitis. Gemfibrozil has a mechanism of action—enhanced lipoprotein lipase activity—that should correct the postulated metabolic defect in uremia. Gemfibrozil was shown to be effective in reducing triglyceride and increasing HDL-C in uremic patients.[59] However, the excretion of this medication is dependent on renal function, and myositis was reported when fibric-acid derivatives were used in patients with renal failure.[60] Fibrates are also highly protein bound and are not removed by dialysis. Therefore, it is recommended that the dose of gemfibrozil be reduced to 600–900 mg/day if creatinine clearance is 20–50 mL/minute and that the risk to benefit ratio of using gemfibrozil in patients whose creatinine clearance is <20 mL/minute be weighed carefully. There are no controlled studies of nicotinic acid therapy in uremic patients, and the agent's mechanism of action—reduced hepatic VLDL production—would not address the defective lipolysis underlying uremic hypertriglyceridemia. However, because excretion of nicotinic acid is not predominantly through the kidney, a trial of this agent in dialysis-dependent patients may be worthwhile.

Clinical Utility of Apolipoprotein and Lipoprotein (a) Measurement

Because many patients with premature CHD have neither severely elevated LDL-C nor very low HDL-C, other lipid markers may provide better discrimination in predicting CHD risk.

A Apolipoproteins

Apo A-I and apo A-II are the major apolipoproteins of HDL. It is generally thought that the differences in HDL-C concentration between individuals are due to differences in the production or catabolic rates of apo A-I. For example, the reduction in HDL-C caused by a low-fat diet is caused by a decrease in apo A-I transport rate.[61] Nevertheless, epidemiological studies do not support total apo A-I concentration as a better inverse marker for CHD risk than HDL-C. The concentration of HDL particles that contain apo A-I but not apo A-II (termed Lp A-I) was reported to be a better inverse predictor of premature CHD risk than the concentration of HDL particles that contain both apo A-I and apo A-II (Lp A-I/A-II).[62] Lp A-I but not Lp A-I/A-II was also shown to increase cellular cholesterol efflux in vitro.[63] However, the clinical significance of these HDL subspecies requires further study, and the assay for these particles is not readily available for clinical use.

Apolipoprotein B-100

Apo B-100 is produced by the liver and incorporated into VLDL. The single apo B-100 protein in each VLDL particle remains with the lipoprotein as it is converted to LDL by the consecutive delipidating activity of lipoprotein lipase and hepatic triglyceride lipase. Therefore, a measure of apo B is the quantitative guide to the number of VLDL and LDL particles in plasma. This one-to-one ratio of apo B to LDL particles is constant, even if the cholesterol content of LDL varies. For example, individuals with a preponderance of small, dense, cholesterol-poor LDL particles, termed LDL subclass pattern B or LDL phenotype B,[64] usually have an LDL-C concentration that is deceptively normal, with an elevated apo B concentration that reflects an increased number of small, dense LDL particles. This pattern is characteristic of familial combined hyperlipidemia and hyperapobetalipoproteinemia. These dyslipidemias have a dominant mode of inheritance and are associated with increased CHD risk.

Apo B-100 concentration was found in some studies to be a stronger predictor of CHD than LDL-C concentration.[65] Therefore an elevated apo B concentration—apo B >125 mg/dL—may help identify patients at risk who have a relatively normal lipid profile (ie, major lipids) but who may have a strong family history of premature CHD. Also, elevated apo B in a patient with elevated plasma triglyceride and low HDL-C may indicate the presence of familial combined hyperlipidemia, and consequently an increased risk for CHD, rather than familial hypertriglyceridemia, which carries a lower risk for CHD (increased risk in some families but not others).

Treatment Decisions

Determination of apo B concentration should not be part of routine screening lipid profiles. However, measurement of apo B may be helpful in guiding treatment decisions in two clinical situations. In patients with CHD whose LDL-C concentration remains 100–130 mg/dL despite diet, elevated apo B is probably sufficient reason to initiate pharmacologic therapy directed at lowering concentrations of apo B-containing lipoproteins, using medications such as statins, nicotinic acid, and resins. In addition, for primary prevention in patients with a strong family history of premature CHD and either LDL-C of 130–160 mg/dL or a combination of elevated triglyceride and low HDL-C, elevated apo B may indicate the need for pharmacologic lipid-lowering therapy. It should be remembered that apo B assays are not governed by universal standardization and reference methods at this time and therefore are subject to substantial variability among laboratories.

Apolipoprotein E

Apo E plays an important role in the metabolism of lipoproteins, particularly chylomicrons, VLDL, and IDL. It is the ligand for chylomicron remnant uptake by the liver and for IDL uptake by the hepatic LDL receptor. In humans, three major isoforms—apo E_2, apo E_3, and apo E_4— are codominantly inherited. These isoforms differ by the presence of arginine or cysteine at residues 112 and 158. The most common allele is $\epsilon3$, which has a relative frequency of approximately 0.80[66]; as a result, most individuals inherit the $\epsilon3/\epsilon3$ genotype.

Many observational studies evaluated the effect of apo E polymorphism on plasma lipid concentrations and on risk for CHD.[67] Although individuals in populations with apo E_4 have elevated total cholesterol and LDL-C concentrations, these individuals were not consistently shown to have increased risk for CHD.

Type III hyperlipidemia, or familial dysbetalipoproteinemia, arises from an apo E-linked metabolic defect yielding the E_2/E_2 phenotype. Apo E_2 reduces affinity for binding to the remnant receptor and the B/E receptor (LDL receptor), and type III hyperlipidemia is characterized by delayed clearance and resulting accumulation of IDL particles. Typically, fasting triglyceride is 400–800 mg/dL (but may be much higher) and total cholesterol is 300–600 mg/dL in type III, and palmar or tuberoeruptive xanthomas may occur. However, although about 1 in 100 individuals in the United States is homozygous for apo E_2, type III hyperlipidemia occurs in only about 1 in 5000. Other metabolic factors—such as DM, obesity, or hypothyroidism—are usually required for full expression. Because type III hyperlipidemia is associated with premature CHD, peripheral vascular disease, and stroke, aggressive lipid-lowering intervention is warranted.

Treatment Decisions

For routine clinical evaluation and treatment of patients at risk for CHD, the data do not support measurement of total apo E. For patients with combined hyperlipidemia resulting from an elevated concentration of IDL particles, determination of apo E isoforms can be useful to confirm type III hyperlipidemia. Patients with type III hyperlipidemia should be treated with diet and, if overweight, weight loss; appropriate pharmacologic agents are fibrates and, in patients without diabetes or insulin resistance, nicotinic acid. Apo E isoforms should also be determined in first-degree relatives of patients with type III hyperlipidemia. Isoelectric focusing to determine apo E phenotype is available at specialty lipid centers. The $\epsilon4$ allele was suggested as a risk factor for Alzheimer's disease, but a recent consensus statement recommends that apo E isoform determinations not be used for clinical diagnostics or predictive testing for Alzheimer's disease.[68]

Lipoprotein (a)

Lipoprotein (a) [Lp(a)] is identical to LDL except for the addition of a unique apolipoprotein, apo(a), joined to apo B by a disulfide bond.[69] Apo(a) has structural homology to plasminogen[70] and was shown to inhibit the generation of plasmin, thereby reducing fibrinolytic activity.[71] Lp(a) was identified in human atherosclerotic lesions.[72] Therefore, this lipid particle may contribute to CHD events through either direct atherogenicity or enhanced thrombogenesis or possibly through both mechanisms.

Lp(a) concentration is genetically determined and was established as an independent risk factor for CHD.[68] In general, an Lp(a) concentration >30 mg/dL is considered elevated. Some clinical trial evidence suggests that elevated Lp(a) is most predictive of CHD when LDL-C is also elevated[73] and that the adverse effects of both are removed when LDL-C alone is lowered.[74] No prospective primary- or secondary-prevention trials attempted to reduce CHD events through manipulation of Lp(a) concentration alone. Therefore the clinical utility of Lp(a) measurements as part of a screening lipid profile is unknown, and routine Lp(a) measurements for the purpose of attempting to treat elevated concentrations are not recommended. Lp(a) measurements are not yet standardized and can vary among laboratories.

Treatment Decisions

Lp(a) measurements may be useful in making treatment decisions in certain clinical scenarios. In patients with CHD and LDL-C that remains 100–130 mg/dL despite lifestyle modifications (including diet), documentation of elevated Lp(a) suggests that pharmacologic therapy, probably with a statin, should be used to lower LDL-C to below 100 mg/dL. In patients without CHD but with LDL-C that remains 130–160 mg/dL with diet and with a strong family history of CHD, an elevated Lp(a) concentration suggests the need for instituting pharmacologic therapy with nicotinic acid or a statin, with the primary goal of lowering LDL-C to below 130 mg/dL. Statins and resins did not prove effective in reducing Lp(a), but high-dosage nicotinic acid (4 g/day) was shown to lower Lp(a) by approximately 40%.[75] Lp(a) concentration can also be lowered by neomycin, certain steroids (eg, stanozolol), and n-3 fatty acids.[76,77]

Combination-Drug Therapy

Two or more lipid-lowering drugs may be used in combination to treat severe, usually primary, dyslipidemia (Table 2). Patients with familial hypercholesterolemia obtained successful lipid lowering with various combinations of bile-acid resins, nicotinic acid, HMG-CoA reductase inhibitors, and probucol.[78,79] In one study, the combination of a resin and a statin in addition to diet decreased LDL-C by approximately 50% from baseline, and the addition of nicotinic acid as a third pharmacologic agent reduced LDL-C by approximately 65% from baseline.[75] The clinical safety of nicotinic acid or a statin is not altered by the addition of a resin, since resins are nonabsorbable.

Combination-drug therapy with a statin and either nicotinic acid[80] or a fibric-acid derivative[81,82] was reported in patients with familial combined hyperlipidemia or type III hyperlipidemia. The combination of a statin and nicotinic acid may increase risk for myopathy or liver dysfunction, and the combination of a statin and a fibrate increases risk for myopathy and must be used with caution. Despite several reports of clinically significant myositis and a few reports of rhabdomyolysis with statin-fibrate combination therapy,[83] in more recent reports this combination did not cause severe creatine kinase elevations or rhabdomyolysis.[84,85] The combined clinical study experience with the sta-

Table 2
Drug Selection: National Cholesterol Education Program Adult Treatment Panel II

Hyperlipidemia	Single Drug	Combination Drug
Elevated LDL cholesterol and triglyceride <200 mg/dL	Bile-acid sequestrant HMG-CoA reductase inhibitor Nicotinic acid	Bile-acid sequestrant + HMG-CoA reductase inhibitor Bile-acid sequestrant + nicotinic acid HMG-CoA reductase inhibitor + nicotinic acid*
Elevated LDL cholesterol and triglyceride 200–400 mg/dL	Nicotinic acid HMG-CoA reductase inhibitor Gemfibrozil	Nicotinic acid + HMG-CoA reductase inhibitor* HMG-CoA reductase inhibitor + gemfibrozil† Nicotinic acid + bile-acid sequestrant Nicotinic acid + gemfibrozil

HMG-CoA = 3-hydroxy-3-methylglutaryl coenzyme A; LDL = low-density lipoprotein.
* Possible increased risk for myopathy or liver dysfunction.
† Increased risk for myopathy; must be used with caution.
Reproduced with permission from Reference 87.

tins does not suggest that any particular statin is safer to use in combination with gemfibrozil. Because the risk for severe myositis appears to be much lower than previously thought, careful treatment of patients with CHD and mixed dyslipidemia with these drug combinations can retain a favorable risk to benefit ratio. Patients should be instructed to report any unexplained muscle pain or soreness to allow for prompt determination of creatine kinase concentrations and, if indicated, discontinuation of the medications. Myositis should resolve within several weeks after discontinuation of the drugs. The decision of whether to rechallenge the patient with a lower statin dose or with another type of statin in addition to gemfibrozil depends on the severity of CHD risk and dyslipidemia and on the judgment of the clinician.

References

1. Levine GN, Keaney JF Jr, Vita JA. Cholesterol reduction in cardiovascular disease: clinical benefits and possible mechanisms. *N Engl J Med* 1995;332: 512–521.
2. Scandinavian Simvastatin Survival Study Group. Randomised trial of cholesterol lowering in 4444 patients with coronary heart disease: the Scandinavian Simvastatin Survival Study (4S). *Lancet* 1994;344:1383–1389.

3. Shepherd J, Cobbe SM, Ford I, et al. Prevention of coronary heart disease with pravastatin in men with hypercholesterolemia. *N Engl J Med* 1995;333: 1301–1307.
4. Gotto AM Jr. Lipid lowering, regression, and coronary events: a review of the Interdisciplinary Council on Lipids and Cardiovascular Risk Intervention, Seventh Council Meeting. *Circulation* 1995;92:646–656.
5. Manninen V, Tenkanen L, Koskinen P, et al. Joint effects of serum triglyceride and LDL cholesterol and HDL cholesterol concentrations on coronary heart disease risk in the Helsinki Heart Study: implications for treatment. *Circulation* 1992;85:37–45.
6. Assmann G, Schulte H. Role of triglycerides in coronary artery disease: lessons from the Prospective Cardiovascular Münster study. *Am J Cardiol* 1992; 70:10H–13H.
7. Gordon T, Castelli WP, Hjortland MC, et al. High density lipoprotein as a protective factor against coronary heart disease. The Framingham Study. *Am J Med* 1977;62:707–714.
8. Gordon DJ, Probstfield JL, Garrison RJ, et al. High-density lipoprotein cholesterol and cardiovascular disease: four prospective American studies. *Circulation* 1989;79:8–15.
9. Genest J Jr, McNamara JR, Ordovas JM, et al. Lipoprotein cholesterol, apolipoprotein A-I and B and lipoprotein (a) abnormalities in men with premature coronary artery disease. *J Am Coll Cardiol* 1992;19:792–802.
10. Barter P. High-density lipoproteins and reverse cholesterol transport. *Curr Opin Lipidol* 1993;4:210–217.
11. Kuhn FE, Mohler ER, Satler LF, et al. Effects of high-density lipoprotein on acetylcholine-induced coronary vasoreactivity. *Am J Cardiol* 1991;68:1425–1430.
12. Aoyama T, Yui Y, Morishita H, et al. Prostacyclin stabilization by high density lipoprotein is decreased in acute myocardial infarction and unstable angina pectoris. *Circulation* 1990;81:1784–1791.
13. Mackness MI, Abbott C, Arrol S, et al. The role of high-density lipoprotein and lipid-soluble antioxidant vitamins in inhibiting low-density lipoprotein oxidation. *Biochem J* 1993;294:829–834.
14. Rubins HB, Robins SJ, Iwane MK, et al. Rationale and design of the Department of Veterans Affairs High-Density Lipoprotein Cholesterol Intervention Trial (HIT) for secondary prevention of coronary artery disease in men with low high-density lipoprotein cholesterol and desirable low-density lipoprotein cholesterol. *Am J Cardiol* 1993;71:45–52.
15. Goldbourt U, Behar S, Reicher-Reiss H, et al. Rationale and design of a secondary prevention trial of increasing serum high-density lipoprotein cholesterol and reducing triglycerides in patients with clinically manifest atherosclerotic heart disease (the Bezafibrate Infarction Prevention trial). *Am J Cardiol* 1993;71:909–915.
16. National Cholesterol Education Program. Second report of the Expert Panel on Detection, Evaluation, and Treatment of High Blood Cholesterol in Adults (Adult Treatment Panel II). *Circulation* 1994;89:1329–1445.
17. Lavie CJ, Mailander L, Milani RV. Marked benefit with sustained-release niacin therapy in patients with "isolated" very low levels of high-density lipoprotein cholesterol and coronary artery disease. *Am J Cardiol* 1992;69:1083–1085.
18. Rader JI, Calvert RJ, Hathcock JN. Hepatic toxicity of unmodified and time-release preparations of niacin. *Am J Med* 1992;92:77–81.

19. Vega GL, Grundy SM. Comparison of lovastatin and gemfibrozil in normolipidemic patients with hypoalphalipoproteinemia. *JAMA* 1989;262:3148–3153.
20. Reaven GM. Role of insulin resistance in human disease (syndrome X): an expanded definition. *Annu Rev Med* 1993;44:121–131.
21. DeFronzo RA, Goodman AM. Efficacy of metformin in patients with non-insulin-dependent diabetes mellitus. *N Engl J Med* 1995;333:541–549.
22. Drood JM, Zimetbaum PJ, Frishman WH. Nicotinic acid for the treatment of hyperlipoproteinemia. *J Clin Pharmacol* 1991;31:641–650.
23. Kreisberg RA. Niacin: a therapeutic dilemma. "One man's drink is another's poison." *Am J Med* 1994;97:313–316.
24. Coronary Drug Project Research Group. Clofibrate and niacin in coronary heart di~ease. *JAMA* 1975;231:360–381.
25. Zimetbaum P, Frishman WH, Kahn S. Effects of gemfibrozil and other fibric acid derivatives on blood lipids and lipoproteins. *J Clin Pharmacol* 1991; 31:25–37.
26. Leaf A, Weber PC. Cardiovascular effects of n-3 fatty acids. *N Engl J Med* 1988;318:549–557.
27. Harris WS. Dietary fish oil and blood lipids. *Curr Opin Lipidol* 1996;7:3–7.
28. Glueck CJ, Levy RI, Fredrickson DS. Norethindrone acetate, postheparin lipolytic activity, and plasma triglycerides in familial types I, III, IV, and V hyperlipoproteinemia: studies in 26 patients and 5 normal persons. *Ann Intern Med* 1971;75:345–352.
29. Kubo SH, Peters JR, Knutson KR, et al. Factors influencing the development of hypercholesterolemia after cardiac transplantation. *Am J Cardiol* 1992; 70:520–526.
30. Curtis JJ, Galla JH, Woodford SY, et al. Effect of alternate-day prednisone on plasma lipids in renal transplant recipients. *Kidney Int* 1982;22:42–47.
31. Renlund DG, Bristow MR, Crandall BG, et al. Hypercholesterolemia after heart transplantation: amelioration by corticosteroid-free maintenance immunosuppression. *J Heart Transplant* 1989;8:214–219.
32. Cooper DKC, Lanza RP, Boyd ST, et al. Factors influencing survival following heart transplantation. *Heart Transplant* 1983;3:86–91.
33. Tanaka H, Sukhova GK, Libby P. Interaction of the allogeneic state and hypercholesterolemia in arterial lesion formation in experimental cardiac allografts. *Arterioscler Thromb* 1994;14:734–745.
34. Norman DJ, Illingworth DR, Munson J, et al. Myolysis and acute renal failure in a heart-transplant recipient receiving lovastatin. Letter. *N Engl J Med* 1988;318:46–47.
35. East C, Alivizatos PA, Grundy SM, et al. Rhabdomyolysis in patients receiving lovastatin after cardiac transplantation. Letter. *N Engl J Med* 1988;318:47–48.
36. Regazzi MB, Iacona I, Campana C. Clinical efficacy and pharmacokinetics of HMG-CoA reductase inhibitors in heart transplant patients treated with cyclosporin A. *Transplant Proc* 1994;26:2644–2645.
37. Ballantyne CM, Radovancevic B, Farmer JA, et al. Hyperlipidemia after heart transplantation: report of a 6-year experience, with treatment recommendations. *J Am Coll Cardiol* 1992;19:1315–1321.
38. Kobashigawa JA, Katznelson S, Laks H, et al. Effect of pravastatin on outcomes after cardiac transplantation. *N Engl J Med* 1995;333:621–627.
39. Vanhaecke J, Van Cleemput J, Van Lierde J, et al. Safety and efficacy of low dose simvastatin in cardiac transplant recipients treated with cyclosporine. *Transplantation* 1994;58:42–45.
40. Kasiske BL. Risk factors for accelerated atherosclerosis in renal transplant recipients. *Am J Med* 1988;84:985–992.

41. Vathsala A, Weinberg RB, Schoenberg L, et al. Lipid abnormalities in cyclo-sporine-prednisone-treated renal transplant recipients. *Transplantation* 1989; 48:37–43.
42. Kandus A, Kovac D, Koselj M, et al. Lovastatin treatment of hyperlipidemia in kidney transplant recipients on cyclosporine immunosuppression. *Transplant Proc* 1994;26:2642–2643.
43. Yoshimura N, Ohmori Y, Tsuji T, et al. Effect of pravastatin on renal transplant recipients treated with cyclosporine—4-year follow-up. *Transplant Proc* 1994; 26:2632–2633.
44. Grundy SM. Management of hyperlipidemia of kidney disease. *Kidney Int* 1990;37:847–853.
45. Joven J, Villabona C, Vilella E, et al. Abnormalities of lipoprotein metabolism in patients with the nephrotic syndrome. *N Engl J Med* 1990;323:579–584.
46. Hutchison FN. Proteinuria, hyperlipidemia, and the kidney. *Miner Electrolyte Metab* 1993;19:127–136.
47. Wheeler DC, Bernard DB. Lipid abnormalities in the nephrotic syndrome: causes, consequences, and treatment. *Am J Kidney Dis* 1994;23:331–346.
48. Alexander JH, Schapel GJ, Edwards KD. Increased incidence of coronary heart disease associated with combined elevation of serum triglyceride and choles-terol concentrations in the nephrotic syndrome in man. *Med J Aust* 1974; 2:119–122.
49. Appel GB, Blum CB, Chien S, et al. The hyperlipidemia of the nephrotic syn-drome: relation to plasma albumin concentration, oncotic pressure, and vis-cosity. *N Engl J Med* 1985;312:1544–1548.
50. Ohta T, Matsuda I. Lipid and apolipoprotein levels in patients with nephrotic syndrome. *Clin Chim Acta* 1981;117:133–143.
51. Kees-Folts D, Diamond JR. Relationship between hyperlipidemia, lipid me-diators, and progressive glomerulosclerosis in the nephrotic syndrome. *Am J Nephrol* 1993;13:365–375.
52. Rabelink AJ, Hene RJ, Erkelens DW, et al. Effects of simvastatin and chole-styramine on lipoprotein profile in hyperlipidaemia of nephrotic syndrome. *Lancet* 1988;2:1335–1338.
53. Valeri A, Gelfand J, Blum C, et al. Treatment of the hyperlipidemia of the nephrotic syndrome: a controlled trial. *Am J Kidney Dis* 1986;8:388–396.
54. Golper TA, Illingworth DR, Morris CD, et al. Lovastatin in the treatment of multifactorial hyperlipidemia associated with proteinuria. *Am J Kidney Dis* 1989;13:312–320.
55. Kasiske BL, Velosa JA, Halstenson CE, et al. The effects of lovastatin in hy-perlipidemic patients with the nephrotic syndrome. *Am J Kidney Dis* 1990; 15:8–15.
56. Thomas ME, Harris KPG, Ramaswamy C, et al. Simvastatin therapy for hy-percholesterolemic patients with nephrotic syndrome or significant protein-uria. *Kidney Int* 1993;44:1124–1129.
57. Ramirez G, Bercaw BL, Butcher DE, et al. The role of glucose in hemodialysis: the effects of glucose-free dialysate. *Am J Kidney Dis* 1986;7:413–420.
58. Lindner A, Charra B, Sherrard DJ, et al. Accelerated atherosclerosis in pro-longed maintenance hemodialysis. *N Engl J Med* 1974;290:697–701.
59. Pasternack A, Vanttinen T, Solakivi T, et al. Normalization of lipoprotein li-pase and hepatic lipase by gemfibrozil results in correction of lipoprotein ab-normalities in chronic renal failure. *Clin Nephrol* 1987;27:163–168.
60. Pierides AM, Alvarez-Ude F, Kerr DN. Clofibrate-induced muscle damage in patients with chronic renal failure. *Lancet* 1975;2:1279–1282.

61. Brinton EA, Eisenberg S, Breslow JL. A low-fat diet decreases high density lipoprotein (HDL) cholesterol levels by decreasing HDL apolipoprotein transport rates. *J Clin Invest* 1990;85:144–151.
62. Puchois P, Kandoussi A, Fievet P, et al. Apolipoprotein A-I containing lipoproteins in coronary artery disease. *Atherosclerosis* 1987;68:35–40.
63. Fruchart JC, Ailhaud G. Apolipoprotein A-containing lipoprotein particles: physiological role, quantification, and clinical significance. *Clin Chem* 1992; 38:793–797.
64. Austin MA, Breslow JL, Hennekens CH, et al. Low-density lipoprotein subclass patterns and risk of myocardial infarction. *JAMA* 1988;260:1917–1921.
65. Sniderman A, Shapiro S, Marpole D, et al. Association of coronary atherosclerosis with hyperapobetalipoproteinemia [increased protein but normal cholesterol levels in human plasma low density (b) lipoproteins]. *Proc Natl Acad Sci U S A* 1980;77:604–608.
66. Davignon J, Gregg RE, Sing CF. Apolipoprotein E polymorphism and atherosclerosis. *Arteriosclerosis* 1988;8:1–21.
67. de Knijff P, Havekes LM. Apolipoprotein E as a risk factor for coronary heart disease: a genetic and molecular biology approach. *Curr Opin Lipidol* 1996; 7:59–63.
68. American College of Medical Genetics/American Society of Human Genetics Working Group on Apo E and Alzheimer Disease. Statement on use of apolipoprotein E testing for Alzheimer disease. *JAMA* 1995;274:1627–1629.
69. Loscalzo J. Lipoprotein (a): a unique risk factor for atherothrombotic disease. *Arteriosclerosis* 1990;10:672–679.
70. McLean JW, Tomlinson JE, Kuang W-J, et al. cDNA sequence of human apolipoprotein (a) is homologous to plasminogen. *Nature* 1987;330:132–137.
71. Loscalzo J, Weinfeld M, Fless GM, et al. Lipoprotein (a), fibrin binding, and plasminogen activation. *Arteriosclerosis* 2990;10:240–245.
72. Beisiegel U, Niendorf A, Wolf K, et al. Lipoprotein (a) in the arterial wall. *Eur Heart J* 1990;11(suppl):174–183.
73. Armstrong VW, Cremer P, Eberle E, et al. The association between serum Lp(a) concentration and angiographically assessed coronary atherosclerosis. Dependence on serum LDL levels. *Atherosclerosis* 1986;62:249–257.
74. Maher VMG, Brown BG, Marcovina SM, et al. Effects of lowering elevated LDL cholesterol on the cardiovascular risk of lipoprotein (a). *JAMA* 1995; 274:1771–1774.
75. Carlson LA, Hamsten A, Asplund A. Pronounced lowering of serum levels of lipoprotein Lp(a) in hyperlipidaemic subjects treated with nicotinic acid. *J Intern Med* 1989;226:271–276.
76. Howard GC, Pizzo SV. Lipoprotein (a) and its role in atherothrombotic disease. *Lab Invest* 1993;69:373–386.
77. Soma MR, Osnago-Gadda I, Paoletti R, et al. The lowering of lipoprotein (a) induced by estrogen plus progesterone replacement therapy in postmenopausal women. *Arch Intern Med* 1993;153:1462–1468.
78. Malloy MJ, Kane JP, Kunitake ST, et al. Complementarity of colestipol, niacin, and lovastatin in treatment of severe familial hypercholesterolemia. *Ann Intern Med* 1987;107:616–623.
79. Witztum JL, Simmons D, Steinberg D, et al. Intensive combination drug therapy of familial hypercholesterolemia with lovastatin, probucol, and colestipol hydrochloride. *Circulation* 1989;79:16–28.
80. Davignon J, Roederer G, Montigny M, et al. Comparative efficacy and safety of pravastatin, nicotinic acid and the two combined in patients with hypercholesterolemia. *Am J Cardiol* 1994;73:339–345.

81. Feussner G, Eichinger M, Ziegler R. The influence of simvastatin alone or in combination with gemfibrozil on plasma lipids and lipoproteins in patients with type III hyperlipoproteinemia. *Clin Invest* 1992;70:1027–1035.
82. Yeshurun D, Abukarshin R, Elias N, et al. Treatment of severe, resistant familial combined hyperlipidemia with a bezafibrate-lovastatin combination. *Clin Ther* 1993;15:355–363.
83. Pierce LR, Wysowski DK, Gross TP. Myopathy and rhabdomyolysis associated with lovastatin-gemfibrozil combination therapy. *JAMA* 1990;264:71–75.
84. Glueck CJ, Oakes N, Speirs J, et al. Gemfibrozil-lovastatin therapy for primary hyperlipoproteinemias. *Am J Cardiol* 1992;70:1–9.
85. Wiklund O, Angelin B, Bergman M, et al. Pravastatin and gemfibrozil alone and in combination for the treatment of hypercholesterolemia. *Am J Med* 1993;94:13–20.
86. Farmer JA, Gotto AM Jr. Currently available hypolipidemic drugs and future therapeutic developments. *Baillieres Clin Endocrinol Metab* 1995;9:825–847.
87. National Cholesterol Education Program. Second report of the Expert Panel on Detection, Evaluation, and Treatment of High Blood Cholesterol in Adults (Adult Treatment Panel II). *Circulation* 1994;89:1329–1445.

Chapter 7

Homocysteine

Anjan Gupta, MD,
Donald W. Jacobsen, PhD,
and Killian Robinson, MD

Homocysteine, a sulfur-containing amino acid, was discovered in the 1930s by du Vigneaud[1] in studies on the demethylation of methionine. In homocystinuria, an autosomal recessive inborn error of metabolism first reported by Carson and Neil in 1962,[2] 50- to 100-fold increases above normal in the concentrations of homocysteine are seen in plasma and urine. This disorder was later shown by Mudd and others[3] to be due to a lack of cystathionine β-synthase, an enzyme essential for the metabolism of homocysteine through the transulfuration pathway. In homocystinuria, skeletal, ocular, and neuropsychiatric disorders are typical. Severe premature vascular disease and thromboembolism are also characteristic and are the major causes of death in these patients.[4] Subsequently, McCully[5] suggested that the excessively high concentrations of homocysteine might be directly responsible for the vascular lesions. These observations led to many investigations of the relation between milder increases in plasma homocysteine concentrations and vascular disease.

Different Forms of Homocysteine in Plasma

There are two main fractions of homocysteine in human plasma (see Figure 1). Some 80% is covalently associated with albumin and other

From Robinson K, (ed): *Preventive Cardiology.* Armonk, NY: Futura Publishing Company, Inc. © 1998.

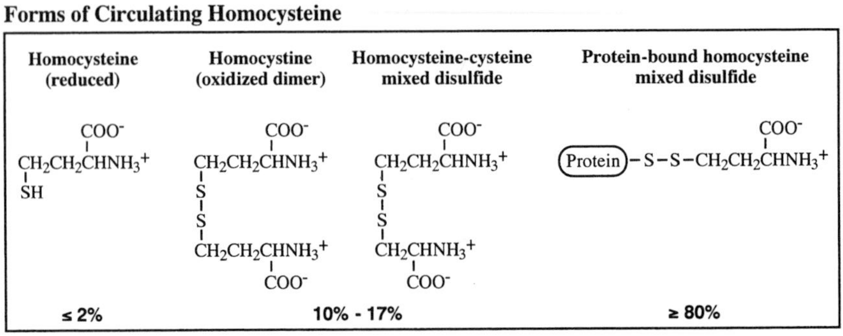

Forms of Circulating Homocysteine

Homocysteine (reduced)	Homocystine (oxidized dimer)	Homocysteine-cysteine mixed disulfide	Protein-bound homocysteine mixed disulfide
$\begin{array}{c} COO^- \\ \| \\ CH_2CH_2CHNH_3{}^+ \\ \| \\ SH \end{array}$	$\begin{array}{c} COO^- \\ \| \\ CH_2CH_2CHNH_3{}^+ \\ \| \\ S \\ \| \\ S \\ \| \\ CH_2CH_2CHNH_3{}^+ \\ \| \\ COO^- \end{array}$	$\begin{array}{c} COO^- \\ \| \\ CH_2CH_2CHNH_3{}^+ \\ \| \\ S \\ \| \\ S \\ \| \\ CH_2CHNH_3{}^+ \\ \| \\ COO^- \end{array}$	$\text{(Protein)} - S - S - CH_2CH_2CHNH_3{}^+ \quad \overset{COO^-}{\|}$
≤ 2%	10% - 17%		≥ 80%

Figure 1. *The main fractions of homocysteine in human plasma.*

plasma proteins by a disulfide bridge to form the "protein-bound fractions." The remaining unbound fraction is referred to as free homocysteine and exists mostly as homocystine and homocysteine-cysteine mixed disulfide. Protein-bound homocysteine, homocystine, and the mixed disulfide with cysteine are referred to as oxidized forms of homocysteine. Free homocysteine itself with its reactive sulfhydryl group is present at very low concentrations. The sum of all these free and protein-bound homocysteine species is referred to as total homocysteine.[4] Usually, total fasting plasma homocysteine values lie in the range of 5–15 μmol/L. The prevalence of high concentrations in the general population is uncertain due to definitions of normality. The normal range is often based on arbitrary cut points such as the 95th percentile for "healthy controls," but many patients with atherosclerosis have levels in this range, which may therefore be too high.

Homocysteine Metabolism

Homocysteine is an intermediate formed during metabolism of the essential amino acid methionine (see Figure 2). The average daily methionine intake is about 2 g/day.[6] Although this amino acid plays an important role in protein synthesis, most of the dietary methionine is converted to S-adenosylmethionine (SAM), a reaction catalyzed by methionine adenosyltransferase and then to S-adenosylhomocysteine. Hydrolysis of the latter leads to adenosine and homocysteine. Homocysteine may then be metabolized either by transsulfuration or transmethylation, depending on the availability of methionine. In the presence of excess methionine, homocysteine enters the transsulfuration pathway.[7] Under normal conditions, about 50% of homocysteine is metabolized in this way. Entry into this pathway is regulated by cystathionine β-synthase, which requires pyridoxal 5'-phosphate (vitamin B$_6$) as cofactor.

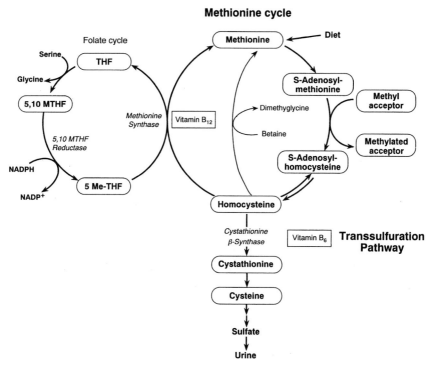

Figure 2. *The metabolic pathways for the metabolism of homocysteine. THF, tetrahydrofolate; MTHF, methylenetetrahydrofolate; Me-THF, methyltetrahydrofolate.*

Under most conditions, this reaction is irreversible in vivo, and the homocysteine moiety is thus committed to the transsulfuration pathway.[7] Cystathionase, another enzyme requiring pyridoxal 5'-phosphate, catalyzes the conversion of cystathionine to cysteine, which is subsequently converted to glutathione, taurine, and other metabolites.[7] Most cells in the body remethylate homocysteine back to methionine using 5-methyl-tetrahydrofolate-homocysteine methyltransferase (methionine synthase).[8] 5-Methyltetrahydrofolate (derived from folic acid) and cobalamin (vitamin B_{12}) are necessary as cosubstrate and cofactor, respectively, for this reaction. Homocysteine can also be remethylated to methionine in liver and kidney in a reaction that utilizes betaine as a substrate and the enzyme betaine-homocysteine methyltransferase.

Regulation of the Metabolic Pathway

Regulation of this metabolic pathway is dependent on the presence of adequate levels of enzymes or their inherent kinetic properties as affected by both the concentrations of substrate and the products of the metabolic reaction. Dietary factors including protein content or methionine, hormone administration, and aging can affect levels of the enzymes of methionine metabolism.[7] Methionine supplementation usually leads to a decreased activity of the enzyme methionine synthase and increased activity of the transsulfuration enzymes.[8] SAM serves as a primary allosteric effector of homocysteine metabolism, regulating the flow of this amino acid between the transsulfuration (positive effector) and remethylation (negative effector) pathways, depending upon the availability of methionine.[7] Increased concentrations of SAM reflect methionine excess and favor transsulfuration by stimulating cystathionine β-synthase. SAM also inhibits methylenetetrahydrofolate reductase (MTHF), reducing methyltetrahydrofolate availability and methionine biosynthesis.[7]

Factors Influencing Homocysteine Metabolism

Because several enzymes, cofactors, and cosubstrates are essential for the metabolism of homocysteine, both genetic and environmental factors play important roles in this process.

Age and Gender

Homocysteine levels increase progressively with age in both sexes[9,10] and, in general, men have higher fasting and postmethionine-load homocysteine concentrations compared to women[9,11,12] (see Figure 3). Some studies demonstrated higher fasting homocysteine concentrations after menopause, and postmenopausal women may attain the level found in men.[4,9,11] The age and sex differences in homocysteine concentrations may be secondary to differences in sex hormones, changes in enzyme or cofactor levels,[13] protein and vitamin intake,[14,15] or renal function.[9]

Genetic Factors

The important role of several enzymes in homocysteine metabolism is reflected by significant correlations between homocysteine concentrations in identical twins and other siblings. Levels also correlate strongly between plasma samples from the same individual that were stored for >14 years, suggesting that environmental influences also remain constant. Absent or reduced enzyme activity may all be associated with elevated homocysteine levels.[14]

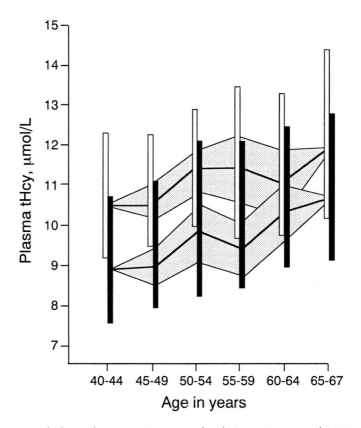

Figure 3. *Total plasma homocysteine (tHcy) levels in 7591 men and 8585 women according to different age groups. The solid lines are median values, and the shaded area indicates the 95% confidence intervals; vertical bars showing the 25th- to 75th-percentile intervals and are open for men and closed for women. (Reproduced with permission from Nygård et al. JAMA 1995;274:1526–1533, copyright 1995, American Medical Association.)*

Cystathionine β-Synthase Deficiency

The first of these abnormalities to be described was deficiency of cystathionine β-synthase, an autosomal recessive disease originally described in a survey of mentally retarded children in Ireland.[2] The condition is rare with a prevalence in the United States of about 1 in 400 000 births[16] and worldwide of 1 in 200 000. Characteristically, lens dislocations (90% to 100%), mental retardation (40% to 60%), seizures, disproportionate growth, and osteoporosis are seen. There is a high prevalence of thromboembolic episodes, with a 50% risk of such an event by age 30.[16] This risk was attributed to the extremely high circulating plasma homocysteine concentrations that may be seen in untreated patients.[14] Enzyme activity is low in various tissues from homozygous patients.[16]

MTHFR Deficiency

MTHFR catalyzes the conversion of 5,10-methylenetetrahydrofolate to 5-methyltetrahydrofolate. Severe hyperhomocysteinemia due to deficiency of this enzyme was reported to cause neurological abnormalities, mental retardation, arteriosclerosis, and thrombosis.[17] This condition is associated with high plasma homocysteine levels, reduced or low methionine concentrations in plasma, low plasma folate levels, and very low MTHFR activity in both fibroblasts and lymphocytes.[18-23] More recently, a thermolabile variant of MTHFR was described.[24] This is caused by a common 677 C to T mutation of the MTHFR gene and is detectable by genotyping or by *in vitro* enzyme activity analysis in peripheral leukocytes.[25] Originally, thermolabile enzyme activity was found in 17% of 212 patients with coronary artery disease but only in 5% of 202 controls. Both patients and controls with the variant enzyme had high homocysteine concentrations. Homozygotes for the thermolabile MTHFR deficiency have a specific activity of about 50% of normal and a residual activity of <30% after heat inactivation, compared with 50% residual activity in control subjects.[24]

Recent genotyping studies revealed the complex nature of the prevalence and significance of thermolabile MTHFR. Jacques et al[26] measured MTHFR activities and folate levels in 365 subjects. Among those who were homozygous for C677T, fasting homocysteine concentrations were 24% higher than in those with normal genotypes but only in the lower range of plasma folate levels. There was no statistical difference in homocysteine levels between genotypes among those with plasma folate concentrations >15 nmol/L. Harmon et al[27] detected the homozygous thermolabile MTHFR genotype in 11.5% of 625 men. Thermolabile MTHFR had a prevalence of 48.4% in the top 5% of homocysteine values, a 35.5% prevalence in the top 10%, and a 23.4% prevalence in the top 20%. Thermolabile MTHFR is therefore common in those with the highest homocysteine levels. Serum folate was lowest in those who were homozygous for C677T. In a screened population of 18 043 subjects aged between 40 and 67 years, Guttormsen et al[28] detected homocysteine values of 40 μmol/L or greater in 67 individuals (0.4%). Homozygosity for thermolabile MTHFR occurred in >70% of this subset compared with 10% of controls, and folate levels were lower. This large population study shows that hyperhomocysteinemia in the range of four to five times normal is uncommon in the general population. When it occurs, it is likely to represent low plasma folate levels combined with the thermolabile MTHFR mutation.

Other Enzyme Disorders

Inherited disorders of cobalamin metabolism may also affect the cobalamin-dependent enzyme methionine synthase, leading to increased homocysteine concentrations.[4]

Nutritional Factors

Deficiencies of folate, vitamin B_{12}, and vitamin B_6 usually cause elevation in homocysteine concentrations, and there is negative correlation with all these vitamins, even in subjects with normal vitamin levels.[4,14] The usually weak correlations may, however, belie the importance of these vitamins as, at lower plasma vitamin levels, homocysteine levels rise more steeply. Riboflavin is cofactor for MTHFR, and deficiency might produce high homocysteine concentrations. In 37 patients studied at this institution with high homocysteine concentrations and normal folate, vitamin B_{12}, and vitamin B_6 levels, the concentrations of riboflavin were no different than in those of controls (unpublished data).

Renal Failure

Homocysteine correlates positively with creatinine, and levels therefore rise in patients with chronic renal failure.[4] In 1977, Cohen et al[29] reported increased homocysteine concentrations in these patients. The concentrations of other amino acids, including cysteine, were also increased, and later similar findings were also noted by Wilcken and Gupta.[30] Furthermore, cysteine-homocysteine-mixed disulfide, cystine, and creatinine levels were all significantly reduced by hemodialysis. Protein-bound homocysteine levels also rise in renal failure, and both pre- and postdialysis protein-bound homocysteine concentrations are higher than in controls.[31] Increased total homocysteine is seen in the early stages of chronic renal failure and rise progressively with the worsening of this disorder.[32,33] Homocysteine concentrations also rise in patients with chronic renal failure on chronic ambulatory peritoneal dialysis.[34–36]

Pathophysiology of Increased Homocysteine Concentrations in Renal Failure

The mechanisms for the high circulating plasma concentrations of sulfur-containing amino acids, including homocysteine, in patients with renal failure are poorly understood but appear to be principally related to impaired homocysteine metabolism.[37] Other proposed mechanisms include reduced glomerular filtration[38,39] and deranged tubular reabsorption,[33,39] although these are unlikely to play a major role. In addition, serine is also essential for normal homocysteine metabolism by both transsulfuration and remethylation pathways,[7] and levels are commonly low in renal failure. Low levels of folate, vitamin B_{12}, and vitamin B_6 are associated with high homocysteine concentrations.[4,14] Inhibition of their normal function may also be a contributing factor. Indeed, despite normal or even high levels of folate, hyperhomocysteinemia persists in end-stage renal failure.[34,36] The relation of these findings to the risk of atherosclerosis in these patients is discussed later.

Diabetes Mellitus

Diabetes does not influence plasma homocysteine concentrations. In a study of patients with type I diabetes mellitus, Hultberg et al demonstrated that, in patients with an increased albumin/creatinine clearance ratio, the increased homocysteine concentrations were probably related to underlying diabetic nephropathy.[40] Diabetics with macroangiopathy have higher homocysteine concentrations than diabetics without.[41]

Hypothyroidism

For unclear reasons, homocysteine levels rise in hypothyroidism and fall in hyperthyroidism.[42] This might partially explain the increased atherosclerotic risk of hypothyroid patients.

Psoriasis

Severe psoriasis is associated with elevated homocysteine concentrations, perhaps related to increased cell turnover,[43] and may predispose these patients to increased incidence of vascular disease.[44] This may be accompanied by lower folate levels.[45]

Cancer

High homocysteine levels are seen with acute leukemia and fall after treatment with cytotoxic drugs. This might be secondary to altered methionine metabolism due to rapid turnover of malignant cells,[46] although patients with solid tumors have normal homocysteine concentrations.[47]

Drugs Affecting Folate, Vitamin B_{12}, and Vitamin B_6 Metabolism

Plasma homocysteine levels can be influenced by various pharmacologic agents, including methotrexate, phenytoin, carbamazepine, nitrous oxide (NO), estrogen-containing oral contraceptives, and penicillamine.[4] Methotrexate can induce a transient increase in plasma homocysteine concentration by depleting 5-methyltetrahydrofolate.[45,48–50] Anticonvulsants such as phenytoin and carbamazepine also increase plasma homocysteine concentration by interfering with folate metabolism.[47] NO inactivates vitamin B_{12}-dependent methionine synthase, thus increasing homocysteine concentrations.[47] Azaribine, a drug formerly used in treatment of psoriasis, causes increased homocysteine concentration by acting as a vitamin B_6 antagonist.[51] The drug was withdrawn because of its association with increased thromboembolism. In one study, treatment of postmenopausal women with estradiol and dydrogesterone produced a 10.9% decrease in fasting homocysteine levels. This reduction was greatest for women with high baseline concentrations, but no change was seen in those with low baseline levels.[52] Although Wong and Kang observed marked reduction in plasma homocysteine concentrations in some women taking oral contraceptive pills, others had high homocysteine levels.[53] Contraceptives may induce a vitamin B_6 deficiency and could therefore increase homocysteine concentrations in susceptible individuals by this mechanism. Diuretics[54] and the lipid-lowering agent colestipol in combination with niacin were also associated with increased homocysteine levels.[55] The increased homocysteine levels observed may be due to interference with folate absorption by the bile acid-binding resin. Niacin may increase homocysteine levels by stimulating the production of S-adenosylhomocysteine after undergoing methylation.[14] Penicillamine, a copper chelating agent used in the treatment of Wilson's disease, lowers plasma homocysteine concentrations possibly by forming a mixed disulfide.[47]

Determination of Homocysteine in Plasma

In vitro, after blood is drawn, homocysteine becomes rapidly bound to plasma proteins, even when samples are frozen immediately.[14] Thus, even though free homocysteine is variable, total homocysteine remains constant. If samples are left to stand without removal of the cellular elements, total plasma homocysteine may rise due to export from erythrocytes.[56] Mixed disulfide, homocystine, or protein-bound homocysteine concentrations were assayed in the past, but techniques for determination of total homocysteine developed by Refsum et al[57] and Jacobsen et al[58] are now standard. Most often, fasting samples are used for determination of plasma homocysteine, although postprandial samples may give similar results.[14] Samples of blood should be placed on ice immediately upon drawing, and plasma should be removed from cellular components within a few hours.

Methionine Loading Test

In some individuals, the fasting concentrations of homocysteine may fall within limits that are currently defined as normal, but levels may become abnormal following ingestion of a methionine load. This test, first described by Brenton et al[59] for the detection of heterozygotes for homocystinuria,[59] reflects the capacity for normal transsulfuration and therefore reflects the status of cystathionine β-synthase and of vitamin B_6. Oral ingestion of methionine leads to a rapid peak in its plasma concentration within 1 hour. The increase in methionine is associated with increases in the concentrations of free, protein-bound, and total homocysteine (see Figure 4). Total homocysteine concentration reaches a maximum in 6–8 hours and has a half-life of about 12–24 hours.[60] Abnormalities in homocysteine metabolism, including the carrier state for cystathionine β-synthase deficiency and deficiency of vitamin B_6, may be latent in the fasting state but may be exposed by a methionine load. Methionine is administered at doses of 0.1 g/kg of body weight, and plasma homocysteine concentra-

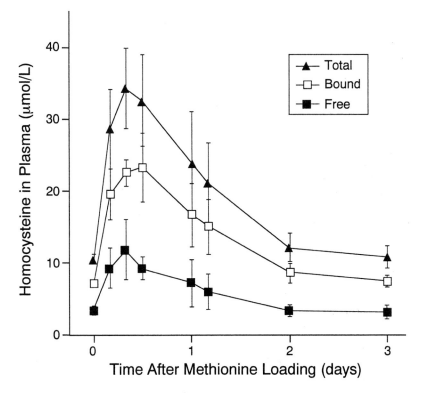

Figure 4. *Oral ingestion of methionine leads to a rapid peak in plasma concentration within 1 hour (not shown) and is accompanied by a rise in the free, protein-bound, and total homocysteine concentrations in plasma after methionine loading. (Reproduced with permission from Ueland et al., Arteriosclerotic Cardiovascular Disease, Hemostasis, and Endothelial Function. 1992: 183–236, courtesy of Marcel Dekker, Inc.)*

tions may be measured at 2, 4, 6, or 8 hours later. Abnormalities of the test have arbitrary definitions. Postload homocysteine concentrations, or increases above preload values, exceeding the 95th percentile or the mean plus two standard deviations for control subjects are often considered abnormal. Recent studies of homocysteine in vascular disease utilized fasting total plasma homocysteine concentrations[61-65] with conclusions similar to those seen in earlier studies utilizing the methionine loading test.[66-68]

Pathology of Vascular Disease Seen in Patients with High Homocysteine Concentrations

The severe vascular changes seen in patients with cystathionine β-synthase deficiency are similar to changes observed in patients with homozygous methionine synthase deficiency and MTHFR deficiency.[18] The lesions are usually focal and involve the large, medium-sized, and small arteries in many organs. The typical features of atherosclerosis seen in patients with homocystinuria compared with conventional atherosclerosis are summarized in Table 1. Focal intimal and medial fibrosis narrows the arterial lumen and is often associated with fraying and discontinuity of internal elastic membranes. There is focal proliferation of perivascular connective tissue with increase in fibroblasts, small collagen bundles, and

Table 1
Summary of Pathological Changes

	Classic Atherosclerosis	Homocystinuria Atherosclerosis
Intima	Intimal thickening and increase in formation of collagen fibrils and new elastic fibers and proliferation of smooth muscle cells	Intimal fibrosis; intimal hyperplasia; fibrous intimal plaque formation from focal splitting, fraying, and disruption of intimal elastic membrane; proliferation of intimal loose fibrous connective tissue
Media	Formation of fibrous cap consisting of layer of smooth muscle cells surrounded by macrophages and lymphocytes; beneath cell-rich region lies area of necrosis containing cholesterol crystals and foam cells	Fragmentation and disruption of elastic lamellae; prominent deposits of interstitial material staining positively for collagen; arteries surrounded by increased perivascular loose connective tissue consisting of collagen bundles and fibroblasts

Reproduced with permission from References 21, 69, and 70.

small elastic fibers, similar to findings in animals.[69] In a study of patients who died from homocystinuria, Gibson et al demonstrated the presence of multiple thromboses in intracranial venous sinuses, inferior vena cava, and peripheral veins. Fibrous endophlebitis of the renal vein was also seen.[70] Both arterial and venous thromboses are common and can cause serious complications including optic atrophy, seizures, and focal neurological signs due to cerebral thrombosis. Cor pulmonale due to recurrent pulmonary thromboembolism and secondary hypertension due to renal infarcts may also occur.[4]

Role of Homocysteine in Pathophysiology of Vascular Disease

Experimental and clinical studies demonstrated that high homocysteine concentrations are associated with atherosclerotic and thromboembolic events. Although the precise mechanism(s) is unclear, the balance of evidence favors an adverse effect of homocysteine on endothelial cells perhaps by increasing oxidant stress.

Effect on Endothelium

Hydrogen Peroxide: In Vitro

In vitro studies examined the direct cytotoxic effect of homocysteine on cultured endothelial cells.[71–73] D,L-Homocysteine produced dose-dependent endothelial cell damage preventable by catalase, suggesting that hydrogen peroxide may have been responsible.[71] Cultured bovine aortic endothelial cells exposed to homocysteine underwent lysis that was also inhibited by catalase,[73] consistent with these findings. The direct toxic effects may be followed by the loss of normal protective mechanisms. For example, the protective effect of endothelium-dependent relaxing factor against adverse effects of homocysteine on the blood vessel wall may be lost with endothelial damage.[74] Homocysteine has a growth-promoting effect on smooth muscle cells at relatively high levels,[75] but it also causes a decrease in endothelial cell DNA synthesis at low concentrations.[75a]

An intracellular accumulation of homocysteine could occur in the presence of relative deficiency of intraendothelial cystathionine β-synthase and account for endothelial damage from within.[76] In one study, the transsulfuration pathway was inoperative in endothelial cells and vascular tissues, which may explain the risk of vascular complications associated with hyperhomocysteinemia.[77]

Hydrogen Peroxide: In Vivo

The in vitro findings are consistent with early studies that showed patchy desquamation of aortic endothelium following infusion of homocysteine in baboons.[78] In one investigation, a decrease in platelet survival time was noted, and it was suggested that arterial damage might result from homocysteine-mediated endothelial injury, possibly with secondary atherogenic effects from platelet consumption. The extent of endothelial damage rose with increasing homocysteine concentrations, and antiplatelet agents were able to reverse some of these effects.[79] The conflicting results of other animal studies[80–87] suggest species-dependent responses or variations due to the use of different forms and concentrations of homocysteine. More recently, in a study of minipigs, feeding of a methionine-rich caseinate-based diet induced hyperhomocysteinemia, which reproduced the metabolic and histopathological findings in homocystinuric patients.[88] Diet-induced moderate hyperhomocyst(e)inemia is also associated with vascular dysfunction in cynomolgus monkeys.[89] Vasomotor responses were assessed in vivo by quantitative angiography and Doppler measurement of blood-flow velocity. In response to activation of platelets by intraarterial infusion of collagen, blood flow to the leg decreased in monkeys fed modified diet, compared with monkeys fed normal diet. Responses of resistance vessels to the endothelium-dependent vasodilators acetylcholine and adenosine diphosphate (ADP) were markedly impaired in the hyperhomocyst(e)inemic animals, suggesting that increased vasoconstriction in response to collagen may be caused by decreased vasodilator responsiveness to platelet-generated ADP. Thrombomodulin anticoagulant activity in aorta also decreased. Similar findings were reported in humans.[90]

Effect on Platelets

Older studies reported inconsistent abnormalities of platelet morphology, survival, and adhesiveness in patients with cystathionine β-synthase deficiency.[14]

Prostaglandins

High concentrations of hydrogen peroxide inhibit synthesis of prostacyclin[91] at the arterial wall. Because prostacyclin is a potent inhibitor of platelets, reduced synthesis could predispose to thrombosis. Enhanced platelet activity was also suggested by Quere et al,[92] who demonstrated inhibition of cyclooxygenase activity by homocysteine in human endothelial cells. Abnormal ADP-induced platelet aggregation in response to high circulating homocysteine was also demonstrated.[16] Graeber et al showed that in vitro D,L-homocysteine alters arachidonic acid metabolism of normal platelets so that 12-hydroxy-5,8,10 heptatrienoic acid and thromboxane A_2 are increased compared to controls.[93] Altered arachidonic acid metabolism induced by homocysteine that results in the accumulation of platelet aggregators provides a possible mechanism for thrombosis. These findings of altered platelet metabolism or function are consistent with in vivo studies in which high homocysteine concentrations are associated with thrombosis or vascular damage and also with the observation of high thromboxane A_2 concentrations in patients with homocystinuria.

Effect on Coagulation

In addition to effects on endothelium and platelets, other studies also showed effects of homocysteine on constituents of the clotting cascade. In a number of studies, serum antithrombin III activity was reduced in seven homocystinuric patients when compared with age- and sex-matched controls.[94–96] Using cultured porcine aortic endothelial cells, Nishinaga et al[97] demonstrated that homocysteine, cysteine, or 2-mercaptoethanol inhibited antithrombin III binding to the cell surface. This effect was blocked by catalase, suggesting that hydrogen peroxide generated from sulfhydryl oxidation was involved in the mechanism. Homocysteine also activated factor V in a dose-dependent manner and increased prothombin activation of factor Xa in cultured bovine aortic endothelial cells.[98] Homocysteine also inhibited protein C activation in cultured human umbilical veins and bovine aortic endothelial cells,[99] although mRNA levels of thrombomodulin in cultured human umbilical vein endothelial cells were actually stimulated.[100] However, the passage of thrombomodulin through the secretory pathway was blocked, resulting in inhibition of cell surface expression. Secretion of plasminogen activator inhibitor I was not affected by homocysteine.[100] Homocysteine induced thrombomodulin mRNA synthesis in cultured human umbilical vein endothelial cells[101] and directly inhibited the cofactor activity of cell surface thrombomodulin.[101] Synthesis of tissue factor mRNA was stimulated by homocysteine, which increased the cellular activity of tissue factor in cultured human umbilical vein endothelial cells.[102] Homocysteine disrupted the processing and secretion of von Willebrand factor in cultured human umbilical vein endothelial cells.[103] Homocysteine but not other sulfhydryl compounds blocked the binding of tissue-plasminogen activator to cultured human umbilical vein endothelial cells.[104] Reduced levels of factor V[105] and factor VII[16,96] were also reported.

In summary, disparate effects of homocysteine were reported on the clotting process. The role of these abnormalities in the genesis of clinically manifest atherosclerosis is unclear, although some may occur as a consequence of disrupted endothelial cell function. Some observations may also be difficult to interpret physiologically, since in many of these studies doses of thiols far in excess of those circulating under normal circumstances were used. Some of these actions may also be nonspecific effects of thiols in general.

Effect on Cholesterol and Other Lipid Subfractions

Low-Density Lipoprotein

A high serum level of low-density lipoprotein cholesterol (LDL-C) is an established risk factor for CAD.[106] When oxidized, LDL-C is taken up by scavenger receptors located on endothelial cells and macrophages in the blood vessels. Modification of the LDL-C particle by reactive oxygen species may depend on the presence of thiols.[14] This was supported by demonstration of cell-independent oxidation of LDL-C in the presence of thiols, including homocysteine.[107,108] Incubation with homocysteine was also associated with oxidation of LDL-C, which was concentration dependent.[109] However, indices of lipid peroxidation are no different in patients with homocystinuria and controls.[110] Oral administration of homocysteine thiolactone may lead to increases in plasma homocysteine concentrations and triglyceride levels in rats, possibly by inhibition of fatty-acid oxidation.[111] Increased binding of lipoprotein (a) with fibrin was also seen in the presence of homocysteine, suggesting a possible biochemical relation among sulfhydryl compounds, thrombosis, and atherogenesis.[112]

Clinical Studies on Homocysteine and Atherosclerosis

Homocysteine and Coronary Artery Disease

The association between CAD and more modest elevations of homocysteine than those seen in homocystinuria was first reported by Wilcken and Wilcken[66] from Australia. In this study, using the methionine loading test, higher postload homocysteine was demonstrated in 25 patients under age 50 with angiographically proven CAD compared to 22 healthy controls. Since then, numerous case-control studies had similar findings,[4,14] and several prospective nested case-control studies (see Table 2) also support the hypothesis that a high plasma homocysteine is an independent predictor for the subsequent development of CAD and stroke[113,114] (see Figure 5). The various studies suggest a gradient of risk with rising homocysteine concentrations,[113,114,117] irrespective of age and gender[117] (see Figure 6). Curiously, high levels may not be a risk factor in the Chinese,[118] and African blacks may have more efficient methionine metabolism, perhaps for dietary reasons, which may protect against coronary disease.[119] The exact prevalence of high concentrations in patients with coronary disease is unclear and depends on the definition of hyperhomocysteinemia. In one study, when levels at the 80th percentile for

Table 2
Prospective Studies of Risk of Atherosclerotic Vascular Disease Associated with High Homocysteine Concentrations

Author	Year	Number of Patients	Population	Risk of Vascular Disease
Stampfer et al[116]	1992	14 916	US male physicians	RR of 3.4 for AMI
Eritsland et al[165]	1194	610	CABG patients	None
Alfthan et al[115]	1993	7 424	Finnish	None
Arnesen et al[114]	1995	21 826	Norway	RR of 1.32 for CHD
Perry et al[113]	1995	5 661	United Kingdom	RR of 2.8 for stroke
Chasan-Taber et al[166]	1996	14 916	US male physicians	RR of 2.0 for AMI

controls were used, the prevalence of high concentrations was as high as 45% in men, 56% in women, and 58% in the elderly.[117] Longer follow-up will help with the more precise identification of the levels of homocysteine that predispose to vascular disease and hence with definition of normal concentrations.

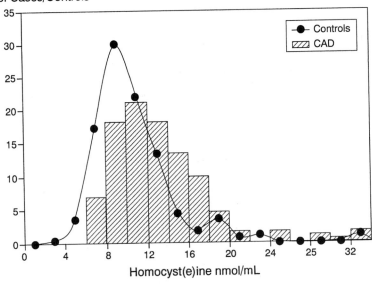

Figure 5. *Homocyst(e)ine level distribution in 255 control subjects and 170 patients with coronary artery disease (CAD). (Reproduced with permission from Genest et al., J Am Coll Cardiol 1990; 2(5): 1114–1119.)*

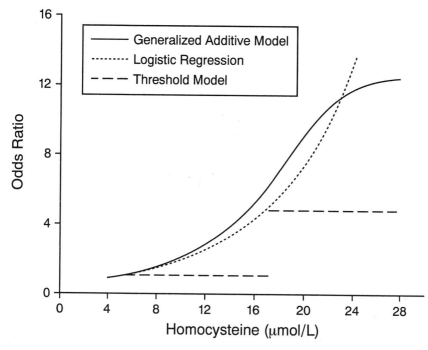

Figure 6. *Plot of odds ratio for CAD using three different models. The simple thresh-old model uses a cutoff point at 14 µmol/L to yield an odds ratio of 4.8 in those with levels greater than this value. When logistic regression or generalized additive models are used, increased odds ratios for CAD are seen at plasma homocysteine concentrations below 14 µmol/L and within a normal range. (Reproduced with permission from Robinson et al., Circulation 1995;92:2825–2830.)*

Mechanisms for the high homocysteine concentrations in these patients are unclear. Homocysteine concentrations correlate negatively with folate, vitamin B_6, and vitamin B_{12}, pointing to inadequate nutrient intake in these patients.[4] Pancharuniti et al[120] in 1994 reported an increasing odds ratio for CAD per quartile increase in homocysteine concentrations independent of all other traditional risk factors. A low vitamin B_6 level is commonly seen in patients with vascular disease and may also contribute to increased vascular risk either by increasing homocysteine levels or by other mechanisms.[10,117]

Decreased activity of enzymes responsible for the metabolism of homocysteine could also play a role (see Table 3). In one study the thermolabile form of MTHFR, which is associated with impaired homocysteine metabolism, was found in 17% of cardiac patients compared with 5% of controls and was associated with higher homocysteine concentrations.[24] Engbersen et al observed the thermolabile variant of this enzyme in 11 of 39 premature vascular disease patients with mild hyperhomocys-

Table 3

Association of Mutation of 5,10-Methylenetetrahydrofolate Reductase and Atherosclerotic Vascular Disease

Author	Country	Number of Subjects	Mutation Present	Association with Atherosclerosis Present
Kang et al[24]	United States	212	17% of cardiac patients	Yes
Engbersen et al[121]	The Netherlands	68	28% of hyperhomocysteinemic patients with vascular disease	Yes
Adams et al[167]	United Kingdom	310	10% of patients with MI	No
Kluijtmans et al[168]	The Netherlands/Canada	60	15% of cardiovascular patients	Yes
Izumi et al[169]	Japan	250	25% of patients with ischemic heart disease	Yes
Wilcken et al[170]	Australia	565	11% of patients with CAD	No

teinemia after methionine loading.[121] No thermolabile MTHFR was observed among 28 patients with premature vascular disease with normal homocysteine levels. In another study by Frosst et al,[25] it was observed that homozygotes for the mutation had about 30%, and heterozygotes about 65%, of normal enzyme activity. It was also found in the same study that individuals who were homozygous for the mutation had significantly elevated homocysteine concentrations. These findings were later confirmed by van der Put et al, who showed that the mutation was not only associated with thermolability of the enzyme and increased plasma homocysteine but also with increased red blood cell folate, although the plasma folate tended to be in the low-normal range.[122] Among patients with low folate concentrations, those with the homozygous mutant genotype may have higher total fasting homocysteine levels than those with the normal genotype, suggesting a higher folate requirement.[26] However, not all studies supported these observations linking MTHFR abnormalities to hyperhomocysteinemia. There are several other recent studies that address the relations among the thermolabile MTHFR mutation, hyperhomocysteinemia, folate status, and risk of CAD.[123–127] Schmitz et al[123] studied MTHFR polymorphism, homocysteine, and folate intake in 190 patients with a myocardial infarction (MI) compared to 188 controls. The C677T genotype was absent in 37.8%, heterozygous in 47.8%, and homozygous in 14.4% of controls and was similar to cases. The relative risk of MI was similar in homozygotes. Total homocysteine values were normal and were similar among the genotypes. According to this study, the thermolabile MTHFR defect is relatively common in the general population but is not associated with either hyperhomocysteinemia or reduced folate levels and is not more prevalent in those with an acute MI. A second study[124] of 555 whites with angiographically established CAD was also negative. Ma et al[125] studied the relation among MTHFR polymorphisms, homocysteine, and folate levels in 293 physicians with CAD and compared the finding with 290 control subjects. The genotype frequencies were 41% heterozygous and 12% homozygous for the C677T mutation. Similar to Schmitz et al,[123] the relative risk of MI was similar among the three genotypes, although those who were homozygous had higher homocysteine values. The difference was especially notable among men with folate levels in the lowest quartile of normal. Homozygous thermolabile MTHFR was, therefore, associated with higher homocysteine and lower folate levels but not with increased risk of MI. Christensen et al reported similar findings in a French Canadian population.[126] Recently, Gallagher et al[127] studied 111 patients with clinical evidence of CAD and 105 controls. The prevalence of homozygous C677T was 17% in patients and 7% in controls. Homozygosity for C677T was significantly more frequent in patients than in controls but heterozygosity was not. The CAD group had higher fasting homocysteine levels, and this was related to homozygosity

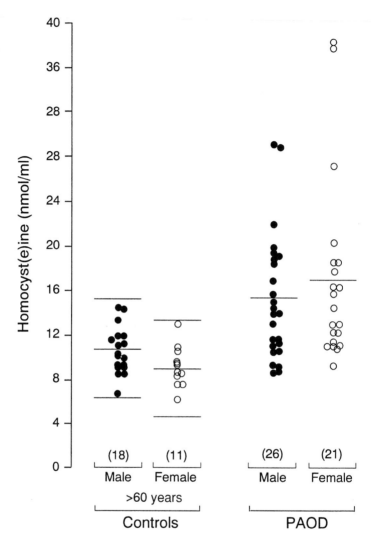

Figure 7. *Plot of plasma homocyst(e)ine concentrations in older control subjects and in patients with peripheral arterial occlusive disease (PAOD); number of subjects is indicated between parentheses. Values are expressed in nanomoles per millilters of homocysteine. Horizontal lines indicate mean 2 SD. In PAOD patients, only means are indicated. (Reproduced with permission from Malinow et al., Circulation 1989; 79(6): 1180–1184.)*

for C677T. Kang et al[24] provide likely explanations for the varied clinical observations regarding thermolabile MTHFR and prevalent coronary disease. The moderate genetic defects such as homozygosity for C677T are insufficient within themselves to cause hyperhomocysteinemia. Nongenetic factors such as nutrition may amplify or mask the phenotypic expression of these genetic defects.

Reduced cystathionine β-synthase activity is associated with high homocysteine concentrations. Although earlier studies emphasized the possible importance of this,[67,68,128] the mutation commonly associated with cystathionine β-synthase deficiency is rare. The gene for methionine synthase was also recently cloned, but its role in hyperhomocysteinemia and vascular disease remains as yet unknown.[129] Many patients with vascular disease may also have coexisting renal disease, which may be an important contributing factor.[13]

In summary, in spite of a small number of studies (see Table 2) to the contrary, most investigations confirm that a high plasma homocysteine is a risk factor for CAD and also for peripheral vascular disease and cerebrovascular disease[4,14] (see Figure 7). Underlying causes and relations with vitamins are probably multifactorial but represent a complex interaction between genetic and nutritional influences.

Other Thiols and Atherosclerosis

High homocysteine concentrations are commonly seen in atherosclerosis patients with stroke, coronary disease, and peripheral vascular disease.[4,14] Higher levels of cysteine[11,130] and cystine[14] were also reported in patients with stroke. In one study, slightly greater cysteine levels were seen in patients with coronary disease than in controls, although this did not achieve statistical significance.[131] These observations are of importance because some of the deleterious effects of homocysteine may also be observed with other thiols. For example, mercaptoethanol, like homocysteine, also induced endothelial damage, suggesting that this property may be common to sulfhydryl-containing compounds in general.[71] Methionine may alter platelet function,[16] and both cysteine and methionine may alter factor V activation.[98] In one study, a decrease in protein C activation with cysteine and methionine was seen.[132] Homocysteine was noted to have a relatively specific effect on reduction of tissue plasminogen activator binding sites in one study in which similar effects were not seen with methionine, cysteine, cystine, or glutathione.[104] A reduction in PGI$_2$ by the addition of homocysteine and other thiols was observed in two studies.[92,133] Recently, Tsai et al reported a growth-promoting effect of homocysteine on smooth muscle cells and a decrease in endothelial cell DNA synthesis in vitro but had no other thiol as a positive control.[75] In minipigs fed a methionine-rich diet, both high homocysteine and methionine concentrations were seen after 4 months, and two of the 16 animals developed thromboemboli.[88] Further investigations are required to clarify the specificity of the adverse effects of homocysteine.

Hyperhomocysteinemia and Other Risk Factors for Atherosclerosis

Several studies have demonstrated a positive correlation between homocysteine and total or LDL-C levels.[13,24,114] In the Norwegian Hordaland Study, in which more than 12 000 community subjects were studied, homocysteine rose with the concentrations of both cholesterol and triglycerides[9] and also correlated with the number of cigarettes smoked and with blood pressure (BP). An inverse relation was seen between homocysteine levels and physical exercise. The higher levels in smokers may be related to an effect on pyridoxal levels.[134] The clustering of these risk factors was also evident in a recent study by Glueck et al in patients with hyperlipidemia.[135] Positive correlations were observed between homocysteine and hypertension, serum triglycerides, and smoking. Negative correlations were observed between homocysteine and high-density lipoprotein cholesterol (HDL-C). Hyperlipidemic patients were at greatest risk for an atherosclerotic event in the presence of high homocysteine concentrations and low concentrations of HDL-C. In a recent multicenter European case-control investigation of approximately 1600 patients, correlations among homocysteine, total cholesterol, systolic and diastolic BPs, and cigarette consumption were studied.[10] Significant interactions of homocysteine with other risk factors were demonstrated. Interactions were also seen among smoking, hypertension, and hyperhomocysteinemia. These studies are consistent with in vitro investigations showing significant interactions between homocysteine and LDL-C.

Homocysteine and Venous Thrombosis

Venous thrombosis is the most frequent atherothrombotic complication of homocystinuria. Several studies have documented high homocysteine concentrations in patients with venous thrombosis without homocystinuria.[136–142] The major studies are shown in Table 4. The evidence favors an association between high homocysteine concentrations and deep venous thrombosis and pulmonary emboli. The role of high homocysteine concentrations, if any, in the pathogenesis for primary arterial thrombosis remains unclear. Further work is needed to define the mechanisms of high homocysteine concentrations in these patients. Recently, a mutation in the gene coding for factor V (factor V Leiden) was discovered and is responsible for resistance to activated protein C. The combination of this genetic abnormality and high homocysteine concentrations has been shown to substantially increase the risk of thrombosis in patients with homocystinuria.[143] The role of this combination in the pathogenesis of venous thrombosis is unknown.

Table 4
Association between Hyperhomocysteinemia and Venous
and Arterial Thromboembolism

Author	Year	Number of Patients	Arterial Thrombosis	Association Present
Brattström et al[142]	1991	42	No	No
Bienvenu et al[139]	1993	50	Yes	Yes
Falcon et al[137]	1994	80	No	Yes
den Heijer et al[138]	1995	185	No	Yes
Fermo et al[171]	1995	85	Yes	Yes
Kottke-Marchant et al[136]	1997	60	Yes	Yes
Amundsen et al[172]	1995	35	No	No
den Heijer et al[173]	1996	269	No	Yes

In all studies, venous thrombosis was included.

Hyperhomocysteinemia and Vascular Disease in Renal Failure

Since the observation of Wilcken et al that homocysteine rises in renal failure,[30] assessment of this amino acid as a risk factor for atherosclerosis and thrombosis in these patients was undertaken in a number of studies. These showed significant associations between higher homocysteine concentrations and vascular complications.[34,36,144,145] In one study, higher concentrations were associated with an independent increase in the risk of atherosclerotic and thrombotic complications, with an odds ratio for vascular events of 2.9 for the upper two quintiles of plasma homocysteine values compared with the lower three.[34] High homocysteine concentrations are commonly seen in patients with end-stage renal disease on hemodialysis and on peritoneal dialysis.[29–36] Overall, hyperhomocysteinemia may be seen in over 80% of patients with end-stage renal disease. In our studies, the most important predictors of hyperhomocysteinemia were lower folate and vitamin B_{12} levels, high serum creatinine concentrations, and the length of time on dialysis.

Homocysteine in Patients Undergoing Organ Transplantation

After initial complications of infection and rejection, cardiovascular complications are the leading cause of death in patients undergoing organ transplantation. The causes are multifactorial and may include the worsening of traditional risk factors following the transplant procedure possibly due to immunosuppression. Attention has been fo-

Table 5

Hyperhomocysteinemia in Organ Transplantation and Risk of
Atherosclerotic and Thromboembolic Vascular Complications

Author	Year	Organ Transplanted	Number of Patients	Mean tHCY (μmol/L)	Association with Vascular Complication Present
Wilcken et al[146]	1981	Kidney	27	6.0 ± 3.2	No
Ambrosi et al[149]	1994	Heart	27	15.4 ± 7	No
Massy et al[147]	1994	Kidney	42	14.5 ± 5.9	Yes
Berger et al[150]	1995	Heart	44	21.2 ± 12.7	No
Arnadottir et al[148]	1996	Kidney	120	19 ± 6.9	Yes
Gupta et al[151]	1996	Heart	189	19.1 ± 13	Yes

cused on homocysteine as a possible risk factor for vascular disease in
these populations (see Table 5).

Renal Transplantation

Wilcken et al, in 1981, explored the effects of renal transplantation on
the metabolism of sulfur-containing amino acids, including homocysteine
and cysteine.[146] Concentrations of both these were increased compared to
controls and correlated with serum creatinine. When folic acid, vitamin
B_{12}, and vitamin B_6 were administered, levels of the amino acids decreased. Other studies have been reported with similar conclusions.[147,148]
In one, patients on cyclosporine had levels higher than others, suggesting
interference with folate-assisted remethylation. This may also explain the
increased homocysteine concentrations seen in recipients of other organs.[149,150] Homocysteine concentrations were significantly increased in
renal transplant patients with a history of atherosclerotic complications
compared to those without.[147]

Cardiac Transplantation

In 1994, Ambrosi et al[149] demonstrated high homocysteine concentrations in over 50% of patients who underwent cardiac transplantation. Folic
acid and vitamin B_{12} levels were no different than those of controls. The
authors suggested cyclosporine-induced renal insufficiency as a possible
mechanism. No correlation was found between hyperhomocysteinemia
and angiographic evidence of atherosclerosis of the grafted coronary vessels. The size of the study was, however, probably too small to establish
this correlation. Berger et al demonstrated similar findings in over 50% of

patients undergoing cardiac transplantation.[150] Concentrations of folic acid and vitamin B_{12} decreased 20% and 49%, respectively, within 3 months after transplantation. Mean glomerular filtration rate also fell by 25%. In a recent case-control study, higher homocysteine concentrations were seen in 180 cardiac transplant patients compared to controls.[151] Concentrations of folate and pyridoxal 5'-phosphate were lower in the transplant patients. Hyperhomocysteinemia was seen more often in patients with vascular complications compared to those without. In multivariate analysis folate and increasing age were predictive of high homocysteine concentrations. The mechanism of high homocysteine concentrations in these patients is likely to be multifactorial and to be related both to derangements in B vitamins and renal function, which commonly occur in these patients. The role of the antifolate actions of immunosuppressive drugs and of these metabolic derangements in the development of cardiac transplant vasculopathy or conventional atherosclerotic complications in these patients remains to be elucidated.

Therapeutic Implications

Homocysteine concentrations may be reduced by a variety of techniques. Dietary methionine restriction will reduce homocysteine production and, presumably, will also encourage recycling of homocysteine in order to conserve methionine. This technique is widely used in patients with homocystinuria but may also be effective in patients with vascular disease.[152]

The cornerstone of therapy to reduce plasma homocysteine is folic acid, which encourages remethylation of homocysteine to methionine.[4,14] In normal subjects, maximum effects are seen in a few weeks, although patients with folate deficiency may respond even more rapidly. Doses of folic acid as low as 400 μg orally are effective in reducing homocysteine levels,[154] although higher doses were used in some studies.[131] Determinants of response to folate include baseline vitamin status, including that of vitamin B_{12}, pretreatment homocysteine values, the presence of the C677T mutation in MTHFR, as well as abnormal renal and possibly low thyroid function. The use of other drugs such as niacin, colestipol, antifolate drugs, or methylxanthanes may also influence the response.

The presence of the C677T mutation in the MTHFR gene may also play a role. For example, in the Hordaland study, 67 of 18 043 subjects, (0.4%) had homocysteine levels ≥40 mmol/L.[28] These patients also had lower folate and cobalamin levels, and 73.1% were homozygous for the mutation in the MTHFR gene compared to 10.2% of controls. In 21 of 37 subjects treated with low-dose (0.2 mg per day) folic acid, homocysteine was normalized within 7 months. In most of the remaining subjects, a normal homocysteine level was obtained with 5 mg per day.[28] In the

NHLBI Family Heart Study,[155] among individuals with lower plasma folate concentrations (<15.4 nmol/L), those homozygous for thermolabile MTHFR had total fasting homocysteine levels that were 24% greater than individuals with the normal genotype. A difference between genotypes was not seen among individuals with higher folate levels, suggesting that the thermolabile MTHFR may increase folate requirement for regulation of plasma homocysteine concentrations.

The high homocysteine concentrations seen in patients with end-stage renal disease on chronic hemodialysis and peritoneal dialysis also respond to folic acid. Normal values may not be obtained, however, even with doses as high as 15 mg per day. The reasons for this are unclear but may be related to the loss of functioning renal tissue that may have a role in the metabolism of homocysteine.[37] In some patients with end-stage renal disease, however, homocysteine levels may be within the upper-normal range (see Figure 8) and may be seen in association with high-circulating folate concentrations,[34] suggesting a possible role for even higher doses of folic acid.

The efficacy of folic acid may be blunted by the use of other medications. For example, in patients who underwent organ transplantation, high homocysteine levels may be reduced by folic acid, although, in one study of patients who underwent renal transplantation, higher levels were seen in patients on cyclosporine, suggesting interference of folate-dependent remethylation.[148]

Several studies also addressed the treatment of high homocysteine concentrations following a methionine load. In these circumstances, vitamin B_6 may be useful adjunctive treatment to folic acid. Because hyperhomocysteinemia is a risk factor for atherosclerosis, folic acid is now undergoing extensive investigation in patients with vascular disorders. In 1983, Wilcken et al[156] administered folic acid to two identical twins with premature CAD. These findings were reproduced in many other studies.[4,129,131,157–161] In a placebo-controlled study of patients with CAD, homocysteine concentrations were reduced by folic acid supplements in doses as low as 400 μg per day with no added benefit seen with larger doses.[162] The effects of such a reduction on the long-term prognosis in these patients needs further study. Fortification of the food supply with folic acid mandated by the Food and Drug Administration will soon begin. The addition of 140 μg per 100 g of cereal-grain product may lower elevated homocysteine concentrations[15] and may also decrease the risk of heart disease.[15]

There are various other potential agents that may be of use in lowering homocysteine concentrations. These include choline and betaine,[128] which have already been successfully used in patients with vascular disease. Serine may be of theoretical use, as it is required both for transsulfuration and remethylation of homocysteine, but, in one study of patients

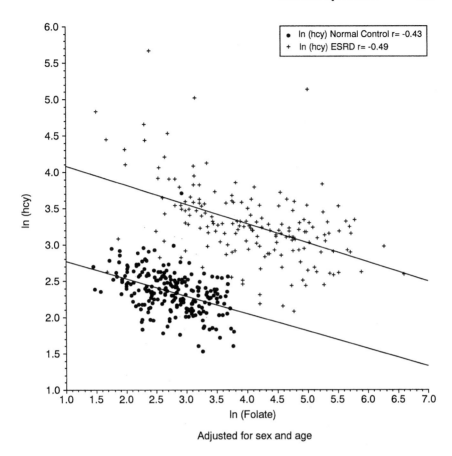

Figure 8. *Concentrations of folate and homocysteine (hcy) in patients with end-stage renal disease (ESRD) and normal subjects. (Reproduced with permission from Robinson et al., Circulation 1996;94:2743–2748.)*

with renal failure, it failed to lower homocysteine levels. Other preparations that may lower plasma homocysteine levels include N-acetylcysteine[163] and estrogen.[164]

Conclusion

A high homocysteine concentration is frequently seen in patients with vascular disease and, in many case-control and prospective studies, is an independent risk factor for atherosclerosis. The underlying cause for this elevation is complex and probably multifactorial. The mechanism, if any, by which homocysteine causes vascular damage is obscure but may relate to an increased oxidant stress on endothelial cells. Treatment of high homocysteine concentrations is possible using folic acid either alone or in combination with other B vitamins. The doses necessary to lower homocysteine levels still remain unclear.[168] Other non–vitamin-based treatment options are also possible. Any effects of lowering homocysteine levels on prognosis, either in patients with established cardiovascular disorders or in those at risk, remain unknown and are currently being evaluated by appropriate clinical trials.[169,170] Such treatment may have substantial benefits on mortality from vascular disorders.[15,171]

References

1. du Vigneaud V, Ressler C, Rachele JR. The biological synthesis of labile methyl groups. *Science* 1950;112:267–271.
2. Carson NAJ, Neill DW. Metabolic abnormalities detected in a survey of mentally backward individuals in Northern Ireland. *Arch Dis Child* 1962; 37:505–513.
3. Mudd SH, Finkelstein JD, Irreverre F, et al. Homocystinuria: an enzymatic defect. *Science* 1964;143:1443–1445.
4. Mayer EM, Jacobsen DW, Robinson K. Homocysteine and coronary atherosclerosis. *J Am Coll Cardiol* 1996;27:517–527.
5. McCully KS. Vascular pathology of homocysteinemia: implications for the pathogenesis of arteriosclerosis. *Am J Pathol* 1969;56:111–128.
6. Subcommittee on the Tenth Edition of the RDAs. *Recommended Dietary Allowances.* 10th ed. Washington, DC: Food and Nutrition Board, Commission on Life Sciences, National Research Council; 1989.
7. Finkelstein JD. Methionine metabolism in mammals. *J Nutr Biochem* 1990; 1:228–237.
8. Finkelstein JD, Martin JJ. Methionine metabolism in mammals. Adaptation to methionine excess. *J Biol Chem* 1986;261:1582–1587.
9. Nygård O, Vollset SE, Refsum H, et al. Total plasma homocysteine and cardiovascular risk profile. The Hordaland homocysteine study. *JAMA* 1995; 274:1526–1533.
10. Graham IM, Daly LE, Refsum HM, et al. Plasma homocysteine as a risk factor for vascular disease: the European Concerted Action Project. *JAMA* 1997; 277:1775–1781.
11. Andersson A, Brattström L, Israelsson B, et al. Plasma homocysteine before and after methionine loading with regard to age, gender, and menopausal status. *Eur J Clin Invest* 1992;22:79–87.
12. Brattström L, Lindgren A, Israelsson B, et al. Homocysteine and cysteine: determinants of plasma levels in middle-aged and elderly subjects. *J Intern Med* 1994;236:633–641.
13. Wu LL, Wu J, Hunt SC, et al. Plasma homocyst(e)ine as a risk factor for early familial coronary artery disease. *Clin Chem* 1994;40:552–561.
14. Ueland PM, Refsum H, Brattström L. Plasma homocysteine and cardiovascular disease. In: Francis RB Jr, ed. *Atherosclerotic Cardiovascular Disease, Hemostasis, and Endothelial Function.* New York, NY: Marcel Dekker; 1992:183–236.
15. Boushey CJ, Beresford SA, Omenn GS, Motulsky AG. A quantitative assessment of plasma homocysteine as a risk factor for vascular disease. Probable benefits of increasing folic acid intakes. *JAMA* 1995;274:1049–1057.

16. Mudd SH, Levy HL, Skovby F. Disorders of transsulfuration. In: Scriver CR, Beaudet AL, Sly WS, et al, eds. *The Metabolic and Molecular Basis of Inherited Disease.* 7th ed. New York, NY: McGraw-Hill 1995:1279–1327.

17. Rosenblatt DS. Inherited disorders of folate transport and metabolism. In: Scriver CR, Beaudet AL, Sly WS, et al, eds. *The Metabolic and Molecular Basis of Inherited Disease.* 7th ed. New York, NY: McGraw-Hill 1995:3111–3149.

18. Baumgartner R, Wick H, Ohnacker H, et al. Vascular lesions in two patients with congenital homocystinuria due to different defects of remethylation. *J Inher Metab Dis* 1980;3:101–103.

19. Haan EA, Rogers JG, Lewis GP, et al. 5,10-Methylenetetrahydrofolate reductase deficiency. Clinical and biochemical features of a further case. *J Inher Metab Dis* 1985;8:53–57.

20. Holme E, Kjellman B, Ronge E. Betaine for treatment of homocystinuria caused by methylenetetrahydrofolate reductase deficiency. *Arch Dis Child* 1989;64:1061–1064.

21. Kanwar YS, Manaligod JR, Wong PWK. Morphologic studies in a patient with homocystinuria due to 5,10-methylenetetrahydrofolate reductase deficiency. *Pediatr Res* 1976;10:598–609.

22. Wong PWK, Justice P, Hruby M, et al. Folic acid nonresponsive homocystinuria due to methylenetetrahydrofolate reductase deficiency. *Pediatrics* 1977; 59:749–756.

23. Erbe RW. Inborn errors of folate metabolism. In: Blakely RL, Whitehead VM, eds. *Folates and Pterins. Nutritional, Pharmacological and Physiological Aspects.* New York, NY: John Wiley & Sons 1986:413–465.

24. Kang S-S, Wong PWK, Susmano A, et al. Thermolabile methylenetetrahydrofolate reductase: an inherited risk factor for coronary artery disease. *Am J Hum Genet* 1991;48:536–545.

25. Frosst P, Blom HJ, Milos R, et al. A candidate genetic risk factor for vascular disease: a common mutation in methylenetetrahydrofolate reductase. *Nat Genet* 1995;10:111–113.

26. Jacques PF, Bostom AG, Williams RR, et al. Relation between folate status, a common mutation in methylenetetrahydrofolate reductase, and plasma homocysteine concentrations. *Circulation* 1996;93:7–9.

27. Harmon DL, Woodside JV, Yarnell JW, et al. The common 'thermolabile' variant of methylene tetrahydrofolate reductase is a major determinant of mild hyperhomocysteinaemia. *QJM* 1996;89:571–577.

28. Guttormsen AB, Ueland PM, Nesthus I, et al. Determinants and vitamin responsiveness of intermediate hyperhomocysteinemia ($>$ or $=$ 40 micromol/liter). The Hordaland homocysteine study. *J Clin Invest* 1996;98:2174–2183.

29. Cohen BD, Patel H, Kornhauser RS. Alternate reasons for atherogenesis in uremia. *Proc Dialysis Transplant Forum* 1977;7:178–180.

30. Wilcken DEL, Gupta VJ. Sulfur containing amino acids in chronic renal failure with particular reference to homocystine and cysteine-homocysteine mixed disulfide. *Eur J Clin Invest* 1979;9:301–307.

31. Kang S-S, Wong PWK, Bidani A, et al. Plasma protein-bound homocyst(e)ine in patients requiring chronic hemodialysis. *Clin Sci* 1983;65:335–336.

32. Soria C, Chadefaux B, Coude M, et al. Concentrations of total homocysteine in plasma in chronic renal failure. *Clin Chem* 1990;36:2137–2138.

33. Hultberg B, Anderson A, Sterner G. Plasma homocysteine in renal failure. *Clin Nephrol* 1993;40:230–234.

34. Robinson K, Gupta A, Dennis V, et al. Hyperhomocysteinemia confers an independent increased risk of atherosclerosis in end-stage renal disease and is closely linked to plasma folate and pyridoxine concentrations. *Circulation* 1996;94:2743–2748.
35. Chauveau P, Chadefaux B, Coude M, et al. Hyperhomocysteinaemia, a risk factor for atherosclerosis in chronic uremic patients. *Kidney Int* 1993; 43(suppl):72–77.
36. Bostom AG, Shemin D, Lapane KL, et al. Hyperhomocysteinemia and traditional risk factors in end-stage renal disease patients on dialysis: a case-control study. *Atherosclerosis* 1995;114:93–103.
37. Bostom AG, Brosnan JT, Hall B, et al. Net uptake of plasma homocysteine by the rat kidney in vivo. *Atherosclerosis* 1995;116:59–62.
38. Wilcken DEL, Gupta VJ, Reddy SG. Accumulation of sulfur-containing amino acids including cysteine-homocysteine in patients on maintenance hemodialysis. *Clin Sci* 1980;58:427–430.
39. Janssen MJFM, van den Berg M, Stehouwer CDA. Hyperhomocysteinaemia: a role in the accelerated atherogenesis of chronic renal failure? *Neth J Med* 1995;46:244–251.
40. Hultberg B, Agardh E, Anderson A, et al. Increased levels of plasma homocysteine are associated with nephropathy but not severe retinopathy in type I diabetes mellitus. *Scand J Lab Clin Invest* 1991;51:277–282.
41. Araki A, Sako Y, Ito H. Plasma homocysteine concentrations in Japanese patients with noninsulin dependent diabetes mellitus—effect of parenteral methylcobalamin therapy. *Atherosclerosis* 1993;103:149–157.
42. Green R, Chong Y, Jacobsen D, et al. Serum homocysteine is high in hypothyroidism: a possible link with coronary artery disease. *Ir J Med Sci* 1995;164:27.
43. Weinstein GD. Biochemical and pathophysiological rationale for amethopterin in psoriasis. *Ann N Y Acad Sci* 1971;186:1782–1784.
44. McDonald CJ, Calabresi P. Psoriasis and occlusive vascular disease. *Br J Dermatol* 1978;99:469–475.
45. Refsum H, Helland S, Ueland PM. Fasting plasma homocysteine as a sensitive parameter to antifolate effect. A study on psoriasis patients receiving low dose methotrexate treatment. *Clin Pharmacol Ther* 1989;46:510–520.
46. Refsum H, Wesenberg F, Ueland PM. Plasma homocysteine in children with acute lymphoblastic leukemia: changes during a chemotherapeutic regimen including methotrexate. *Cancer Res* 1991;51:828–835.
47. Ueland PM, Refsum H. Plasma homocysteine, a risk factor for vascular disease: plasma levels in health, disease and drug therapy. *J Lab Clin Med* 1989;114:473–501.
48. Brattström L, Ueland PM, Refsum H. Adjuvant therapy for breast cancer. *N Engl J Med* 1988;319:443–444.
49. Refsum H, Ueland PM, Kvinnsland S. Acute and long-term effects of high-dose methotrexate treatment on homocysteine in plasma and urine. *Cancer Res* 1986;46:5385–5391.
50. Broxson EH, Stork LC, Allen RH, et al. Changes in plasma methionine and total homocysteine levels in patients receiving methotrexate infusions. *Cancer Res* 1989;49:5879–5883.
51. Drell W, Welch AD. Azaribine-homocystinemia-thrombosis in historical perspective. *Pharmacol Ther* 1989;41:195–206.
52. Miller LT. Oral contraceptives and vitamin B_6 metabolism. In: Reynolds RD, Leklem JE, eds. *Vitamin B_6: Its Role in Health and Disease*. New York, NY: Alan R Liss 1985:243–255.

53. Wong PWK, Kang S-S. Accelerated atherosclerosis. *Am J Med* 1988;84:1093–1094.
54. Taylor LM Jr, DeFrang RD, Harris EJ Jr, et al. The association of elevated plasma homocyst(e)ine with progression of symptomatic peripheral arterial disease. *J Vasc Surg* 1991;13:128–136.
55. Blankenhorn DH, Malinow R, Mack WJ. Colestipol plus niacin therapy elevates plasma homocyst(e)ine levels. *Coron Artery Dis* 1991;2:357–360.
56. Malinow MR, Axthelm MK, Meredith MJ, et al. Synthesis and transsulfuration of homocysteine in blood. *J Lab Clin Med* 1994;123:421–429.
57. Refsum H, Helland S, Ueland PM. Radioenzymic determination of homocysteine in plasma and urine. *Clin Chem* 1985;31:624–628.
58. Jacobsen DW, Gatautis VJ, Green R, et al. Rapid HPLC determination of total homocysteine and other thiols in serum and plasma: sex differences and correlation with cobalamin and folate concentrations in healthy subjects. *Clin Chem* 1994;40:873–881.
59. Brenton DP, Cusworth DC, Dent CE, et al. Homocystinuria: clinical and dietary studies. *QJM* 1966;35:325–346.
60. Mansoor MA, Svardal AM, Ueland PM. Determination of the in vivo redox status of cysteine, cysteinylglycine, homocysteine, and glutathione in human plasma. *Anal Biochem* 1992;200:218–229.
61. Malinow MR, Kang SS, Taylor LM, et al. Prevalence of hyperhomocyst(e)inemia in patients with peripheral arterial occlusive disease. *Circulation* 1989;79:1180–1188.
62. Israelsson B, Brattström LE, Hultberg BL. Homocysteine and myocardial infarction. *Atherosclerosis* 1988;71:227–233.
63. Genest JJ, McNamara JR, Upson B, et al. Prevalence of familial hyperhomocyst(e)inemia in men with premature coronary artery disease. *Arterioscler Thromb* 1991;11:1129–1136.
64. Ubbink JB, Vermaak WJH, Bennett JM, et al. The prevalence of homocysteinemia and hypercholesterolemia in angiographically defined coronary heart disease. *Klin Wochenschr* 1991;69:527–534.
65. Brattström L, Lindgren A, Israelsson B, et al. Hyperhomocysteinaemia in stroke: prevalence, cause, and relationships to type of stroke and stroke risk factors. *Eur J Clin Invest* 1992;22:214–221.
66. Wilcken DEL, Wilcken B. The pathogenesis of coronary artery disease. A possible role for methionine metabolism. *J Clin Invest* 1976;57:1079–1082.
67. Boers GHJ, Smals AGH, Trijbels FJM, et al. Heterozygosity for homocystinuria in premature peripheral and cerebral occlusive arterial disease. *N Engl J Med* 1985;313:709–715.
68. Clarke R, Daly L, Robinson K, et al. Hyperhomocysteinemia: an independent risk factor for vascular disease. *N Engl J Med* 1991;324:1149–1155.
69. McCully KS, Wilson RB. Homocysteine theory of arteriosclerosis. *Atherosclerosis* 1975;22:215–227.
70. Gibson JB, Carson NAJ, Neill DW. Pathological findings in homocystinuria. *J Clin Pathol* 1964;17:427–437.
71. Wall RT, Harlan JM, Harker LA, et al. Homocysteine-induced endothelial cell injury in vitro: a model for the study of vascular injury. *Thromb Res* 1980;18:113–121.
72. Dudman NPB, Hicks C, Lynch JF, et al. Homocysteine thiolactone disposal by human arterial endothelial cells and serum in vitro. *Arterioscler Thromb* 1991;11:663–670.

73. Starkebaum G, Harlan JM. Endothelial cell injury due to copper-catalyzed hydrogen peroxide generation from homocysteine. *J Clin Invest* 1986; 77:1370–1376.
74. Stamler JS, Osborne JA, Jaraki O, et al. Adverse vascular effects of homocysteine are modulated by endothelium-derived relaxing factor and related oxides of nitrogen. *J Clin Invest* 1993;91:308–318.
75. Tsai J-C, Perrella MA, Yoshizumi M, et al. Promotion of vascular smooth muscle cell growth by homocysteine: a link to atherosclerosis. *Proc Natl Acad Sci U S A* 1994;91:6369–6373.
75a. Wang H, Yoshizumi M, Lai K, et al. Inhibition of growth and p21^{ras} methylation in vascular endothelial cells by homocysteine but not cysteine. *J Biol Chem* 1997;272:25380–25385.
76. de Groot PG. Willems C. Boers GHJ, et al. Endothelial cell dysfunction in homocystinuria. *Eur J Clin Invest* 1983;13:405–410.
77. Jacobsen DW, Savon SR, Stewart RW, et al. Limited capacity for homocysteine catabolism in vascular cells and tissues: a pathophysiologic mechanism for arterial damage in hyperhomocysteinemia? *Circulation* 1995;92(suppl):104. Abstract.
78. Harker LA, Slichter SJ, Scott CR, et al. Homocystinemia. Vascular injury and arterial thrombosis. *N Engl J Med* 1974;291:537–543.
79. Harker LA, Ross R, Slichter SJ, et al. Homocystine-induced arteriosclerosis. The role of endothelial cell injury and platelet response in its genesis. *J Clin Invest* 1976;58:731–741.
80. Reddy GSR, Wilcken DEL. Experimental homocysteinemia in pigs: comparison with studies in sixteen homocystinuric patients. *Metabolism* 1982;31:778–783.
81. Smolin LA, Crenshaw TD, Kurtycz D, et al. Homocyst(e)ine accumulation in pigs fed diets deficient in vitamin B$_6$: relationship to atherosclerosis. *J Nutr* 1983;113:2122–2133.
82. Donahue S, Sturman JA, Gaull G, et al. Arteriosclerosis due to homocyst(e)inemia: failure to reproduce the model in weanling rabbits. *Am J Pathol* 1974;77:167–174.
83. McCully KS, Ragsdale BD. Production of arteriosclerosis by homocysteinemia. *Am J Pathol* 1970;61:1–8.
84. Mushett CW, Emerson GA. Arteriosclerosis in pyridoxine-deficient monkeys and dogs. *Fed Proc* 1956;15:526.
85. Hladovec J. Experimental homocystinemia, endothelial lesions and thrombosis. *Blood Vessels* 1979;16:202–205.
86. Rinehart JF, Greenberg LD. Arteriosclerotic lesions in pyridoxine-deficient monkeys. *Am J Pathol* 1949;25:481–491.
87. Rinehart JF, Greenberg LD. Vitamin B$_6$ deficiency in the rhesus monkey with particular reference to the occurrence of atherosclerosis, dental caries, and hepatic cirrhosis. *Am J Clin Nutr* 1956;4:318–328.
88. Rolland PH, Friggi A, Barlatier A, et al. Hyperhomocysteinemia induced vascular damage in the minipig. Captopril-hydrochlorothiazide combination prevents elastic alterations. *Circulation* 1995;91:1161–1174.
89. Lentz SR, Sobey CG, Piegors DJ, et al. Vascular dysfunction in monkeys with diet-induced hyperhomocyst(e)inemia. *J Clin Invest* 1996;98:24–29.
90. Tawakol A, Omland T, Gerhard M, et al. Hyperhomocyst(e)inemia is associated with impaired endothelium-dependent vasodilatation in humans. *Circulation* 1997;95:1119–1121.
91. Panganamala RV, Karpen CW, Merola AJ. Peroxide mediated effects of homocysteine on arterial prostacyclin synthesis. *Prostaglandins Leukot Med* 1986;22:349–356.

92. Quere I, Habib A, Tobelem G, et al. Inhibition of cyclooxygenase activity in human endothelial cells by homocysteine. *Adv Prostaglandin Thromboxane Leuko Res* 1995;23:397–399.

93. Graeber JE, Slott JH, Ulane RE, et al. Effect of homocysteine and homocystine on platelet and vascular arachidonic acid metabolism. *Pediatr Res* 1982; 16:490–493.

94. Giannini MJ, Coleman M, Innerfield I. Antithrombin activity in homocystinuria. Letter. *Lancet* 1975;1:1094.

95. Maruyama I, Fukuda R, Kazama M, et al. A case of homocystinuria with low antithrombin activity. *Acta Haematol Jpn* 1977;40:267–271.

96. Palareti G, Coccheri S. Lowered antithrombin III activity and other clotting changes in homocystinuria: effects of a pyridoxine-folate regimen. *Haemostasis* 1989;19(suppl):24–28.

97. Nishinaga M, Ozawa T, Shimada K. Homocysteine, a thrombogenic agent, suppresses anticoagualnt heparan sulfate expression in cultured porcine aortic endothelial cells. *J Clin Invest* 1993;92:1381–1386.

98. Rodgers GM, Kane WH. Activation of endogenous factor V by a homocysteine-induced vascular endothelial cell activator. *J Clin Invest* 1986;77:1909–1911.

99. Rodgers GM, Conn MT. Homocysteine, an atherogenic stimulus, reduces protein C activation by arterial and venous endothelial cells. *Blood* 1990; 75:895–901.

100. Lentz SR, Sadler JE. Inhibition of thrombomodulin surface expression and protein C activation by the thrombogenic agent homocysteine. *J Clin Invest* 1991;88:1906–1914.

101. Hayashi T, Honda G, Suzuki K. An atherogenic stimulus homocysteine inhibits cofactor activity of thrombomodulin and enhances thrombomodulin expression in human umbilical vein endothelial cells. *Blood* 1992;79:2936.

102. Fryer RH, Wilson BD, Gubler DB, et al. Homocysteine, a risk factor for premature vascular disease and thrombosis, induces tissue factor activity in endothelial cells. *Arterioscler Thromb* 1993;13:327–333.

103. Lentz SR, Sadler JE. Homocysteine inhibits von Willebrand factor processing and secretion by preventing transport from the endoplasmic reticulum. *Blood* 1993;81:683–689.

104. Hajjar KA. Homocysteine-induced modulation of tissue plasminogen activator binding to its endothelial cell membrane receptor. *J Clin Invest* 1993;91:2873–2879.

105. Hilden M, Brandt NJ, Nilsson IM, et al. Investigation of coagulation and fibrinolysis in homocystinuria. *Acta Med Scand* 1974;195:533–535.

106. Kannel WB, Sytkowski PA. Atherosclerosis risk factors. *Pharmacol Ther* 1987;32:207–235.

107. Loscalzo J. The oxidant stress of hyperhomocyst(e)inemia. *J Clin Invest* 1996;98:5–7.

108. Heinecke JW. Superoxide-mediated oxidation of low density lipoproteins by thiols. In: Cerutti PA, Cerutti JM, Mccord I, et al, eds. *Oxy-Radicals in Molecular Biology and Pathology*. New York, NY: Alan R Liss; 1988:443–457.

109. Hirano K, Ogihara T, Miki M, et al. Homocysteine induces iron catalyzed lipid peroxidation of LDL that is prevented by alpha-tocopherol. *Free Radic Res* 1994;21:267–276.

110. Blom HJ, Kleinveld HA, Borr GH, et al. Lipid peroxidation and susceptibility of LDL to in vitro oxidation in hyperhomocysteinemia. *Eur J Clin Invest* 1995;25:149–154.

111. Frauscher G, Karnaukhova E, Muehl A, et al. Oral administration of homocysteine leads to increased plasma triglycerides and homocysteic acid—additional mechanisms in homocysteine induced endothelial damage? *Life Sci* 1995;57:813–817.
112. Harpel PC, Chang VT, Borth W. Homocysteine and other sulfhydryl compounds enhance the binding of lipoprotein (a) to fibrin: a potential biochemical link between thrombin, atherogenesis and sulfhydryl compound metabolism. *Proc Natl Acad Sci U S A* 1992;89:10193–10197.
113. Perry IJ, Refsum H, Morris RW, et al. Prospective study of serum total homocysteine concentrations and risk of stroke in middle aged British men. *Lancet* 1995;346:1395–1398.
114. Arnesen E, Refsum H, Bonaa KH, et al. Serum total homocysteine and coronary heart disease. *Int J Epidemiol* 1995;24:704–709.
115. Alfthan G, Pekkanen J, Jauhiainen M, et al. Relation of serum homocysteine and lipoprotein (a) concentrations to atherosclerotic disease in a prospective Finnish population based study. *Atherosclerosis* 1994;106:9–19.
116. Stampfer MJ, Malinow MR, Willett WC, et al. A prospective study of plasma homocyst(e)ine and risk of myocardial infarction in US physicians. *JAMA* 1992;268:877–881.
117. Robinson K, Mayer EL, Miller DP, et al. Hyperhomocysteinemia and low pyridoxal phosphate. Common and independent reversible risk factors for coronary artery disease. *Circulation* 1995;92:2825–2830.
118. Lolin YI, Sanderson JE, Cheng SK, et al. Hyperhomocysteinemia and premature coronary artery disease in the Chinese. *Heart* 1996;76:117–122.
119. Ubbink JB, Vermaak WJH, Delport R, et al. Effective homocysteine metabolism may protect South African Blacks against coronary heart disease. *Am J Clin Nutr* 1995;62:802–808.
120. Pancharuniti N, Lewis CA, Sauberlich HE, et al. Plasma homocyst(e)ine, folate, and vitamin B-12 concentrations and risk for early-onset coronary artery disease. *Am J Clin Nutr* 1994;59:940–948.
121. Engbersen AMT, Franken DG, Boers GHJ, et al. Thermolabile 5,10-methylenetetrahydrofolate reductase as a cause of mild hyperhomocysteinemia. *Am J Hum Genet Soc* 1995;56:142–150.
122. van der Put NM, Steegers-Theunissen RPM, Frosst P, et al. Mutated methylene-tetrahydrofolate reductase as a risk factor for spina bifida. *Lancet* 1995;346:1070–1071.
123. Schmitz C, Lindpaintner K, Verhoef P, et al. Genetic polymorphism of methylenetetrahydrofolate reductase and myocardial infarction. A case-control study. *Circulation* 1996;94:1812–1814.
124. van Bockxmeer FM, Mamotte CD, Vasikaran SD, et al. Methylenetetrahydrofolate reductase gene and coronary artery disease. *Circulation* 1997;95:21–23.
125. Ma J, Stampfer MJ, Hennekens CH, et al. Methylenetetrahydrofolate reductase polymorphism, plasma folate, homocysteine, and risk of myocardial infarction in US physicians. *Circulation* 1996;94:2410–2416.
126. Christensen B, Frosst P, Lussier-Cacan S, et al. Correlation of a common mutation in the methylenetetrahydrofolate reductase gene with plasma homocysteine in patients with premature coronary artery disease. *Arterioscl Thromb Vasc Biol* 1997;17:569–573.
127. Gallagher PM, Meleady R, Shields DC, et al. Homocysteine and risk of premature coronary heart disease. Evidence for a common gene mutation. *Circulation* 1996;94:2154–2158.
128. Dudman NPB, Wilcken DEL, Wang J, et al. Disordered methionine/homocysteine metabolism in premature vascular disease. Its occurrence,

cofactor therapy, and enzymology. *Arterioscler Thromb* 1993;13:1253–1260.

129. van der Put NM, van der Molen EF, Kluijtmans LA, et al. Sequence analysis of the region of human methionine synthase: relevance to hyperhomocysteinaemia in neural-tube defects and vascular disease. *Q J Med* 1997;90:511–7.

130. Araki A, Sako Y, Fukushima Y, et al. Plasma sulfhydryl-containing amino acids in patients with cerebral infarction and in hypertensive patients. *Atherosclerosis* 1989;79:139–146.

131. Landgren F, Israelsson B, Lindgren A, et al. Plasma homocysteine in acute myocardial infarction: homocysteine-lowering effect of folic acid. *J Intern Med.* 1995;237:381–388.

132. Hilden M, Brandt NJ, Nilsson IM, et al. Investigation of coagulation and fibrinolysis in homocystinuria. *Acta Med Scand* 1974;195:533–535.

133. Wang J, Dudman NPB, Wilcken DEL. Effects of homocysteine and related compounds on prostacyclin production by cultured human vascular endothelial cells. *Thromb Haemost* 1993;70:1047–1052.

134. Bergmark C, Mansoor MA, Swedenborg J, et al. Hyperhomocysteinemia in patients operated for lower extremity ischaemia below the age of 50—effect of smoking and extent of disease. *Eur J Vasc Surg* 1993;7:391–396.

135. Glueck CJ, Shaw P, Lang J, et al. Evidence that homocysteine is an independent risk factor for atherosclerosis in hyperlipidemic patients. *Am J Cardiol* 1995;75:132–136.

136. Kottke-Marchant K, Green R, Jacobsen DW, et al. High plasma homocysteine: a risk factor for arterial and venous thrombosis in patients with normal hypercoagulation profiles. *Clin Appl Thromb Hemost* 1997;3:239–44.

137. Falcon CR, Cattaneo M, Panzeri D, et al. High prevalence of hyperhomocyst(e)inemia in patients with juvenile venous thrombosis. *Arterioscler Thromb* 1994;14:1080–1083.

138. den Heijer M, Blom HJ, Gerrits WBJ, et al. Is hyperhomocystein(a)emia a risk factor for recurrent venous thrombosis? *Lancet* 1995;345:882–885.

139. Bienvenu T, Ankri A, Chadefaux B, et al. Elevated total plasma homocysteine, a risk factor for thrombosis. Relation to coagulation and fibrinolytic parameters. *Thromb Res* 1993;70:123–129.

140. D'Angelo SV, Fermo I, Paroni R, et al. Total plasma homocyst(e)ine in young patients with venous thromboembolic disease. *Thromb Haemost* 1993;69:295A.

141. David J-L, Schoos RR. Homocysteine and venous thromboembolism. *Thromb Haemost* 1993;69:272A.

142. Brattström L, Tengborn L, Lagerstedt C, et al. Plasma homocysteine in venous thromboembolism. *Haemostasis* 1991;21:51–57.

143. Mandel H, Brewner B, Berant M, et al. Coexistence of hereditary homocystinuria and factor V Leiden—Effect on thrombosis. *N Engl J Med* 1996;334:763–768.

144. Kim SS, Hirore S, Tamura H, et al. Hyperhomocysteinemia as a possible role for atherosclerosis in CAPD patients. *Adv Periton Dial* 1994;10:282–285.

145. Bachmann J, Tepel M, Raidt H, et al. Hyperhomocysteinemia and the risk for vascular disease in hemodialysis patients. *J Am Soc Nephrol* 1995;6:121–125.

146. Wilcken DEL, Gupta VJ, Betts AK. Homocysteine in the plasma of renal transplant recipients: effects of cofactors for methionine metabolism. *Clin Sci* 1981;61:743–749.

147. Massy ZA, Chadefaux-Vekemans B, Chevalier A, et al. Hyperhomocystein-aemia: a significant risk factor for cardiovascular disease in renal transplant recipients. *Nephrol Dial Transplant* 1994;9:1103–1108.
148. Arnadottir M, Hultberg B, Vladov V, et al. Hyperhomocysteinemia in cyclos-porine-treated renal transplant recipients. *Transplantation* 1996;61:509–512.
149. Ambrosi P, Barlatier A, Habib G, et al. Hyperhomocysteinaemia in heart transplant recipients. *Eur Heart J* 1994;15:1191–1195.
150. Berger PB, Jones JD, Olson LJ, et al. Increase in total plasma homocysteine concentration after cardiac transplantation. *Mayo Clin Proc* 1995;70:125–131.
151. Gupta A, Moustapha A, Jacobsen DW, et al. High homocysteine, low folate and low vitamin B_6 concentrations: prevalent risk factors for vascular disease in heart transplant recipients. *Transplantation* 1998;65:544–550.
152. Chait A. Effect of a food plan with increased folate and vitamins B_{12} and B_6 on serum homocyst(e)ine levels in high-CVD risk persons. *Circulation* 1996;94(suppl):264.
153. Ubbink JB, Vermaak WJH, van der Merwe A, et al. Vitamin B-12, vitamin B-6, and folate nutritional status in men with hyperhomocysteinemia. *Am J Clin Nutr* 1993;57:47–53.
154. Tucker KL, Mahnken B, Wilson PWF, et al. Folic acid fortification of the food supply. Potential benefits and risks for elderly population. *JAMA* 1996; 276:1879–1885.
155. Jacques PF, Bostom AG, Williams RR, et al. Relation between folate status, a common mutation in methylenetetrahydrofolate reductase, and plasma ho-mocysteine concentrations. *Circulation* 1996;93:7–9.
156. Wilcken DEL, Reddy SG, Gupta VJ, et al. Homocysteinemia, ischemic heart disease and the carrier state for homocystinuria. *Metabolism* 1983;32: 363–370.
157. Brattström LE, Hardebo JE, Hultberg BL. Moderate homocysteinemia—A possible risk factor for arteriosclerotic cerebrovascular disease. *Stroke* 1984; 15:1012–1016.
158. Franken DG, Boers GHJ, Blom HJ, et al. Treatment of mild hyperhomo-cysteinemia in vascular disease patients. *Arterioscler Thromb* 1994;14: 465–470.
159. Ryan M, Robinson K, Clarke R, et al. Vitamin B_6 and folate reduce ho-mocysteine concentrations in coronary artery disease. *Ir J Med Sci* 1993;162:197A.
160. Saltzman E, Mason JB, Jacques PF, et al. B vitamin supplementation lowers homocysteine levels in heart disease. *Clin Res* 1994;42:172A.
161. Naurath HJ, Joosten E, Reizler R, et al. Effects of vitamin B_{12}, folate, and vitamin B_6 supplements in elderly people with normal serum vitamin con-centrations. *Lancet* 1995;346:85–89.
162. Lobo A, Naso A, Arheart K, et al. Reduction of homocysteine levels in cor-onary disease by low-dose folic acid combined with vitamins B6 and B12: a placebo-controlled study. (submitted for publication).
163. Wiklund O, Fager G, Andersson A, et al. *N*-Acetylcysteine treatment lowers plasma homocysteine but not serum lipoprotein (a) levels. *Atherosclerosis* 1996;119:109–106, 1996.
164. Brattström L, Israelsson B, Olsson A, et al. Plasma homocysteine in women on oral oestrogen-containing contraceptives and in men with oestrogen-treated prostatic carcinoma. *Scand J Clin Lab Invest* 1992;52:283–287.
165. Eritsland J, Arnesen H, Seljeflot I, et al. Influence of serum lipoprotein (a) and homocyst(e)ine levels on graft patency after coronary artery bypass grafting. *Am J Cardiol* 1994;74:1099–1102.

166. Chasan-Taber L, Selhub J, Rosenberg IH, et al. A prospective study of folate and vitamin B_6 and risk of myocardial infarction in US Physicians. *J Am Coll Nutr* 1996;15:136–143.

167. Adams M, Smith PD, Martin D, et al. Genetic analysis of thermolabile methylenetetrahydrofolate reductase as a risk factor for myocardial infarction. *QJM* 1996;89:437–444.

168. Homocysteine Lowering Trialists' Collaboration. Lowering blood homocysteine with folic acid based supplements: meta-analysis of randomised trials. *BMJ* 1998;316:894–8.

169. Howard VJ, Chambless LE, Malinow MR, Lefkowitz D, Toole JF. Results of a homocyst(e)ine lowering pilot study in acute stroke patients. *Stroke* 1997;28:234.

170. Aursnes I. Protocol for a nested case-control study with folic acid in hyperhomocysteinemia (abstract). *Can J Cardiol* 1997;13(suppl B):315B.

171. Rimm EB, Willett WC, Hu FB, et al. Folate and vitamin B6 from diet and supplements in relation to risk of coronary artery disease among women. *JAMA* 1998;297:359.

172. Amundsen T, Ueland PM, Waage A. Plasma homocysteine levels in patients with deep vein thrombosis. *Arterioscler Thromb Vasc Biol* 1995;15:1321–1323.

173. den Heijer M, Koster T, Blom HJ, et al. Hyperhomocysteinemia as a risk factor for deep-vein thrombosis. *N Engl J Med* 1996;334:759–762.

Chapter 8

Prevention of Atherosclerosis in Children and Adolescents

Peter O. Kwiterovich Jr, MD

Introduction

Evidence from different scientific fields consistently indicates that the early lesions of atherosclerosis start in children and adolescents and that the risk factors that promote atherosclerosis and coronary artery disease (CAD) in adults are also operative in youth.[1,2]

Pathological Studies

Postmortem studies from the International Atherosclerosis Study indicated that earliest lesions of atherosclerosis, called fatty streaks, begin in the coronary arteries around age 10 and in the abdominal aorta around age 3; some lesions progress into fibrous plaques, which can lead to the clinical complications of atherosclerosis in adulthood (ie, CAD, cerebro-vascular disease, and peripheral vascular disease).[3] Youth from countries where CAD was a major health problem had more extensive early lesions

This report was supported in part by National Institutes of Health grants DISC HL 37975, NHLBI 31497, 1 R01 HD 32193, 1-P50-HL 47212 (Specialized Center of Research in Arteriosclerosis), HL 40518, and HL 02824 and Pediatric Clinical Research Center RR00052. Dr. Feldman is recipient of an award from the Fulbright Scholar program.

of atherosclerosis than youth from countries where CAD was less prevalent.

In the Pathological Determinants of Atherosclerosis in Youth Study, both the cellular and lipid characteristics of atherosclerotic lesions in adolescents and young adults (aged 15–34 years) were indistinguishable from those found later in life.[2,4] The extent and severity of the lesions in both the aorta and right coronary artery were significantly correlated with elevated postmortem serum levels of low-density lipoprotein cholesterol (LDL-C) and very-low-density lipoprotein cholesterol (VLDL-C) but low levels of high-density lipoprotein cholesterol (HDL-C).[5] Cigarette smoking was strongly associated with lesions in the aorta.

In the prospective Bogalusa Heart Study, Berenson et al[6] reported that, in autopsies from 150 persons aged 6–30 years, the degree of atherosclerosis in the aorta was strongly related to antemortem levels of total cholesterol and LDL-C and the ponderal index (weight/height^3); in the coronary arteries, fatty streaks were significantly related to serum levels of VLDL-C and triglyceride, to systolic and diastolic blood pressure (SBP and DBP, respectively), and to ponderal index.

In the prospective Muscatine Study, Mahoney and coworkers[7] used electron-beam computed tomography as a sensitive, noninvasive method for detecting coronary artery calcification, a marker of the atherosclerotic process. In young adulthood, 31% of men and 10% of women had coronary artery calcification. Increased body mass index (BMI) measured during childhood and young adult life and increased BP and decreased HDL-C levels measured during young adult life were associated with the presence of coronary artery calcification in young adults.

Epidemiological Studies

Children from countries that consumed higher amounts of dietary cholesterol and saturated fatty acids had higher mean plasma cholesterol levels. Adults from those countries with higher fat consumption also had higher plasma cholesterol levels and higher rates of CAD.[8–10]

Genetic Studies

Children and adolescents may be at high risk for premature CAD because they inherited a genetic predisposition to a dyslipidemia. Children who have an atherogenic lipoprotein profile (Table 1) are commonly found in families with a high prevalence of CAD in adult relatives.[11–15] Moreover, in the inherited lipid disorder familial hypercholesterolemia (FH), children heterozygous for a gene in the LDL receptor have an average cholesterol of 300 mg/dL and are highly likely to develop premature CAD by middle age.[16] If a child inherited two mutant genes at the

Table 1
Dyslipoproteinemias in Progeny of Fathers with Premature
Angiographically Documented Coronary Atherosclerosis

Dyslipoproteinemia	Progeny ($n = 173$)		
	n	% of Total	% of Abnormal
High LDL-C	20	12	23
Low HDL-C	29	17	33
High LDL-C, low HDL-C	7	4	8
High triglyceride	13	8	15
High triglyceride, high LDL-C	7	4	8
High triglyceride, low HDL-C	5	3	6
High triglyceride, high LDL-C, low HDL-C	6	3	7
Total abnormal	87	51	100

Reproduced with permission from Reference 11.

LDL receptor (ie, an FH homozygote), the cholesterol level often reaches 1000 mg/dL, planar xanthomas develop by age 5, and atherosclerosis of the coronary arteries and aortic valve is not uncommon by age 10, with a significant number succumbing to CAD by age 20.[16]

Apolipoproteins

In addition to the seven dyslipidemic lipoprotein profiles outlined in Table 1, additional information was obtained in families with premature coronary or cerebral atherosclerosis by measuring the major apolipoproteins (apo's) of LDL and HDL, apo B and apo A-I, respectively. Lipoprotein (a) [Lp(a)], a lipoprotein consisting of one molecule of LDL bound covalently through a disulfide bridge to a molecule of apo(a), a protein homologous to plasminogen, was also studied. The plasma levels of apo B, apo A-I, and Lp(a), along with plasma lipid and lipoprotein levels were measured in children born to a parent either with CAD or with cerebrovascular disease, and compared with control children.[17] Levels of plasma total cholesterol, LDL-C, and apo B found in children born to a parent with CAD were significantly higher than those of controls, but levels of HDL-C and apo A-I were lower. Of interest, children born to a parent with cerebrovascular disease had only significantly higher levels of apo B and lower levels of HDL-C and apo A-I than those of controls. Those children born to a parent with CAD, but not cerebrovascular disease, had significantly higher levels of Lp(a) than those of controls.

In Bogalusa,[18] low values in children for plasma apo A-I levels or for the ratio of apo A-I to apo B, or the ratio of LDL-C to apo B, were all strongly related to parental incidence of myocardial infarction (MI); no such relation was found with respect to lipoprotein cholesterol levels. These findings suggest that measurement of apo's can provide additional useful information, particularly if they indicate the presence of small, dense LDL particles.

Other Cardiovascular Disease Risk Factors in Youth

Obesity, high BP, cigarette smoking, diabetes mellitus (DM), and physical inactivity are often present in youth.[1,2] Thus an approach to the prevention of atherosclerosis early in life includes an assessment of the presence of other cardiovascular disease (CVD) risk factors in addition to an assessment of a high-fat diet and dyslipidemia. Such an approach allows an integrated, comprehensive plan for treatment and follow-up.

Obesity

Obesity in children and adolescents is often defined as a BMI (weight/height^2) above the 95th percentile. Excess body weight relative to height (ie, ponderosity) in childhood can predict future obesity through adolescence into adulthood.[19,20] Genetic factors play an important role in determining obesity. The relative risk of dying from CAD in relatives of a "heavy" group of children from the Muscatine Ponderosity Study was significantly higher than that in relatives of the control children.[19] In a subset of these families, where the heavy children also had an elevated SBP, the risk of death from CAD in their adult relatives was further accentuated.[19] Obesity in youth also keeps "bad company" as it does in adults. Obese children have higher levels of plasma LDL-C, apo B, triglycerides, glucose, and insulin but lower levels of HDL-C and apo A-I than nonobese children.[19-22] Such clustering of adverse cardiovascular risk factors in obese adolescents persists into young adulthood.[20] Thus the presence of obesity in youth should prompt a measurement of a lipoprotein profile. Physical inactivity can contribute to both obesity and an abnormal lipid profile.[23] Treatment of obesity in youth with weight control and exercise can often improve a dyslipidemic profile.

Hypertension

Hypertension in children is often secondary to renal, vascular, endocrine, or neurological disease or due to certain medications. If these secondary causes of high BP are ruled out, the hypertension is considered essential. Elevated BP in children is usually defined as a SBP consistently above the age-specific 95th percentile.[24] In certain families prone to essential hypertension, primary elevated BP levels were assessed in children and adolescents. Children born to hypertensive parents had a number of characteristics that appeared to make them "at risk" to develop high BP; examples include overresponsiveness to a high-salt diet or a high protein load, increased renal vasoconstriction, and decreased secretion of renin and aldosterone.[2] As well, in epidemiological studies, almost one-half of the subjects who developed hypertension as adults had elevated SBP and DBP levels as children.[25]

Cigarette Smoking

Cigarette smoking in children and adolescents is often accompanied by significantly higher levels of VLDL and LDL-C but lower levels of HDL-C.[26] Exposure to cigarette smoke also appears to promote the formation of oxidized LDL, which may facilitate the accumulation of cholesteryl esters in macrophages.

Glucose Intolerance

The presence of dyslipidemias in children with type I insulin-dependent DM is well established.[27] However, it is less well appreciated that, in healthy children without overt diabetes, the plasma levels of insulin and glucose are correlated with other CVD risk factors. For example, in Bogalusa, fasting insulin levels were positively related to measures of obesity, plasma levels of LDL, VLDL-C and triglyceride, SBP, and DBP but negatively related to HDL-C levels.[28] In the same study, fasting glucose levels were positively related to VLDL-C and triglyceride levels, obesity, and SBP and DBP.[28] Furthermore, the increased association of insulin levels with adverse lipoprotein levels persisted from childhood into young adulthood, especially in those with obesity.[29]

Aggregation of CAD Risk Factors

When one considers all of the data on cardiovascular risk factors in children and adolescents,[2] it is clear that these risk factors aggregate. Furthermore, such aggregation of CAD risk factors in children persists into adulthood. In Bogalusa, Myers and coworkers[30] found that 21.8% of children who placed in the top quartile for ponderal index, SBP, and cholesterol were clustered 15 years later as adults, whereas only 1.1% of those with no risk factors in the top quartile were clustered as adults. As well, syndrome X, described by Reaven,[31] most likely has its origins in childhood. Indeed, recent data from Bogalusa indicate the persistence of multiple cardiovascular risk "clustering" from childhood to young adulthood.[32] A syndrome probably related to syndrome X, familial dyslipidemic hypertension, was described in Utah pedigrees by Williams et al.[33] In the Utah families, the dyslipidemia that is expressed in children usually precedes the hypertension by about 10 years.

The Expert Panel on Blood Cholesterol Levels in Children and Adolescents of the National Cholesterol Education Program (NCEP)[1] considered the above data in aggregate and made recommendations for lipid and risk factor management in children.

Population Approach to Lipid and Risk Factor Management

The first recommendation of the panel was that all healthy children above age 2 follow a diet reduced in the total amount of fat, saturated fat, and cholesterol (Table 2). Such a public health approach may decrease the mean cholesterol and LDL levels in children by 5% to 10%.[1]

Infants were excluded from the population recommendations of the NCEP panel because of the need for higher fat intake in the first 6 months of life.

There was a concern that, in growing children and adolescents, a low-fat, low-cholesterol diet be nutritionally adequate and contain sufficient calories and a variety of foods to promote normal growth and development. This includes all the vitamins, minerals, and essential nutrients. The recent findings of the Dietary Intervention Study in Children (DISC) indicate that this is indeed the case.[34] As well, the approach here is substitution of acceptable low-fat foods rather than elimination of specific foods. Examples include a substitution of low-fat cheese for regular or whole-milk cheeses, vegetables and fresh fruits for snacks high in fat or salt, substitution of skim or 1% milk for whole milk, and frozen low-fat yogurt for ice cream.

Table 2
Current Versus Recommended Nutrient Intake
in Healthy Children and Adolescents

	Current	Recommended
Total fat, % of calories	35–36	Average no more than 30
Saturated fatty acids, %	14	<10
Polyunsaturated, %	6	Up to 10
Monounsaturated, %	13–14	10–15
Cholesterol, mg/d	193–296	<300

Reproduced with permission from Reference 1.

Individualized Approach to Lipid and Risk Factor Management in High-Risk Children and Adolescents

The panel next developed an individualized approach to the child or adolescent who was considered to be at an increased risk for premature CAD. The rationale was to focus on the detection of youth who may be more likely to develop premature CAD because of a strong family history of CAD or the presence of significant dyslipidemias or essential hypertension or the aggregation of other risk factors for CAD in their family. Such children and adolescents need to be identified, treated, and followed over a long term.

Recommendations for Screening Children and Adolescents

A screening strategy was proposed by the NCEP expert panel[1] to identify youth most likely to be at an increased risk for developing premature CAD. Four recommendations were made, the first three of which focused on CAD or parental hypercholesterolemia, whereas the last focused on those having multiple risk factors for CAD.

1. Perform a lipoprotein profile on children and adolescents whose parents and grandparents at age 55 years or less underwent coronary arteriography or were found to have coronary atherosclerosis, often leading to coronary artery bypass surgery or balloon angioplasty.
2. Perform a lipoprotein profile on children and adolescents whose parents and grandparents or aunts or uncles at age 55 years or less suffered a previously documented MI, angina pectoris, peripheral vascular disease, cerebrovascular disease, or sudden cardiac death.
3. Screen for hypercholesterolemia in offspring of a parent who was found to have a high blood cholesterol that is 240 mg/dL or higher.
4. When parental or grandparental history is unobtainable, children and adolescents who have two or more other CVD risk factors may be screened at the physician's discretion.

Such screening may be performed any time after age 2.

To interpret the results of the plasma total cholesterol and LDL-C analyses, cut points were recommended as guidelines, which are summarized in Table 3. In addition to a high LDL-C level, youths screened based upon the above recommendations may have a low HDL-C level alone (<35 mg/dL) or an elevated triglyceride level alone (>100 mg/dL 2–9 years, >130 mg/dL, 10–19 years), or some children may have a combination of various abnormal levels (see Table 1).[1,2]

Table 3
Cut Points for Plasma Total and Levels in LDL-C Children and Adolescents
from High-Risk Families

Category	Total Cholesterol	LDL-C
High	≥200	≥130
Borderline high	170–199	110–129
Acceptable	≤170	≤100

Reproduced with permission from Reference 1.

The algorithm for high-risk assessment is summarized in Figure 1. First, all those with a positive family history of premature CAD have a lipoprotein analysis as the initial screen. If one only measures a cholesterol in such youth, a number of dyslipidemic children will be missed. For those youth in whom a parent has a blood cholesterol >240 mg/dL, a blood total cholesterol can be measured (Figure 1). Of course, physicians may choose, at their discretion, to obtain a lipoprotein analysis as the first step.

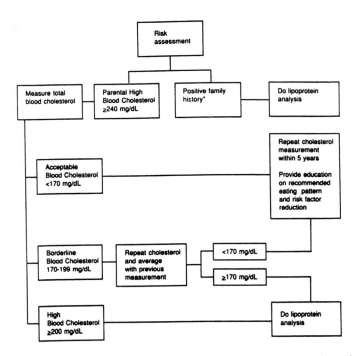

Figure 1. *Algorithm for the assessment of risk for dyslipidemias in youth with parental hypercholesterolemia* (**left**) *or a positive family history of CVD* (**right**). *Reproduced with permission from Reference 1.*

A total cholesterol level <170 mg/dL is considered acceptable, and such a child receives general advice on risk factors and healthy eating patterns; the cholesterol level is screened again in 5 years. If the cholesterol level is borderline, 170–199 mg/dL, the test is repeated and the results averaged. If the average cholesterol is >170 mg/dL, then lipoprotein analysis is performed; if the average is <170 mg/dL, the child is given general risk factor and eating pattern advice and brought back in 5 years (Figure 1). Those children who are found to have a blood cholesterol >200 mg/dL are given a lipoprotein analysis.

Evaluation and Follow-Up

The algorithm developed for evaluation and follow-up of LDL-C levels is found in Figure 2. The average LDL-C value from two lipoprotein profiles (obtained in the fasting state at least 3 weeks apart) is used to determine whether the child receives lipid management. If the average

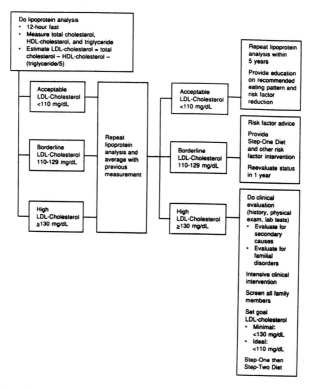

Figure 2. *Algorithm for the evaluation of a high LDL-C level in youth. Reproduced with permission from Reference 1.*

LDL-C is <110 mg/dL, the child receives general risk factor and dietary education and returns in 5 years for a repeat lipoprotein analysis. If the average LDL-C is borderline, 110–129 mg/dL, the child receives more structured dietary intervention and risk factor modification and is brought back in 1 year for a follow-up evaluation. Those youth with an average LDL-C (>130 mg/dL) return for more-detailed clinical and family assessment. This includes a modified physical examination, which includes checking height, weight, BP, corneal arcus, and xanthomas.

Exclusion of Secondary Causes of Dyslipidemia

Secondary causes of dyslipidemia are ruled out systematically by history, physical examination, and blood tests. Common causes of secondary hyperlipidemia include hypothyroidism, the nephrotic syndrome, DM, diseases of the liver, and taking oral contraceptives, prednisone, anabolic steroids (especially by weight lifters), and isotretinoin (Accutane; for acne).[35] In addition, the parents and siblings of such children and adolescents should also have a lipoprotein profile determined.

Genetic Dyslipidemias

Any one of seven general dyslipidemic patterns (Table 1) may be uncovered as a result of using this algorithm for high-risk assessment. Many times the precise genetic etiology of the dyslipidemia will not be elucidated. However, this is not critical to appropriate treatment and follow-up. Three common conditions that may be found in clinics specializing in the evaluation of high-risk children and adolescents include FH, familial combined hyperlipidemia (FCHL), and hyperapobetalipoproteinemia (hyperapo B). Representative values for the plasma lipid, lipoprotein, and apo B levels in pediatric probands with these three conditions are summarized in Table 4.[38]

Familial Hypercholesterolemia

FH is the most commonly recognized and best-understood disorder of lipoprotein metabolism in children.[16,37] FH is an autosomal dominant trait that has a gene dosage effect. In FH heterozygotes (prevalence 1 in 500) the plasma levels of total cholesterol and LDL-C are increased two- to threefold. FH homozygotes (prevalence one in a million) have levels that are elevated up to sixfold.[16,38] FH heterozygote children usually do not have tendon xanthomas or CAD, but about one-half of adult FH heterozygotes develop xanthomas or CAD by middle age.[16] Of interest, Celermajer and coworkers[39] found strong evidence for endothelial cell

Table 4

Plasma Lipid, Lipoprotein, and apo B Levels in Pediatric Probands with FH, FCHL, and Hyperapo B and in Controls

Lipid Disorder	Age	Plasma Concentration (mg/dL)					
		Total Cholesterol	Triglycerides	HDL-C	LDL-C	apo B	LDL-C/apo B Ratio
FH (n = 20)	8.0 ± 4.7	323 ± 44	86 ± 36	44 ± 8	262 ± 45	219 ± 42	1.22 ± 0.22
FCHL (n = 65)	9.3 ± 4.7	220 ± 51	120 ± 91	45 ± 11	149 ± 48	153 ± 39	0.98 ± 0.19
HyperapoB (n = 11)	7.8 ± 4.6	200 ± 20	91 ± 35	52 ± 7	130 ± 16	138 ± 21	0.95 ± 0.10
Control children (n = 110)	8.7 ± 1.8	162 ± 30	70 ± 39	51 ± 10	97 ± 27	85 ± 20	1.15 ± 0.20

Mean ± SD.
Reproduced with permission from Reference 36.

dysfunction in FH heterozygous children, as judged by reduced or absent flow-mediated dilatation. FH homozygote children usually have planar xanthomas by age 5 and coronary atherosclerosis and aortic stenosis by age 10–20.

FH results from a mutation in a cell surface membrane protein, the LDL receptor. The LDL receptor binds and internalizes LDL from plasma. Hobbs et al[40] summarized at least 150 mutations in the human LDL receptor. These insertions, deletions, and missense and nonsense mutations can affect the normal synthesis, transport, clustering (in coated pits), and binding ability of the LDL receptor.[16,40] Although a high Lp(a) level does not invariably accompany FH, when present, it appears to enhance the risk of premature CAD considerably.[41,42]

Familial Defective Apo B$_{100}$

In about one out of 20 families, the presence of high LDL-C levels and xanthomas are not due to FH. There is a defect in the ligand for the LDL receptor, namely, apo B, where glutamine is substituted for arginine at residue 3500.[43] This disorder is called familial defective apo B$_{100}$. The mutant LDL is not bound normally by the LDL receptor, often leading to elevated LDL-C levels. Most patients with familial defective apo B$_{100}$, however, do not have tendon xanthomas, and the LDL-C levels may be normal, moderately, or markedly elevated.[43] It is not necessary in clinical practice to distinguish FH from familial defective apo B$_{100}$, since treatment for these patients is similar.

Familial Combined Hyperlipidemia and Hyperapobetalipoproteinemia

Some youth with elevated LDL-C levels represent FCHL, a disorder first described by Goldstein and coworkers[44] in families of survivors of early MI. In FCHL, three lipoprotein patterns (type IIa, type IIb, or type IV) are expressed in about equal proportion in affected adult relatives.[44] FCHL accounts for at least 10% of survivors of premature CAD. Although the expression of FCHL can be delayed until adulthood, children or adolescents who are ascertained to have a positive family history of premature CAD and/or parental hypercholesterolemia will often have FCHL. For example, Cortner and coworkers[36] found that FCHL was the most prevalent lipid disorder among youth referred to a lipid clinic; FCHL was three times more prevalent than FH (Table 4). Because the LDL-C level in FCHL may actually be normal or borderline high, a subset of patients with FCHL in whom such a lipoprotein pattern is accompanied by high LDL apo B levels (a phenotype called hyperapo B) was identified (Table 4). Thus the measurement of apo B was useful in identifying further children from high-risk families, particularly if these children had hypertriglyceridemia; an elevated apo B level in youth is >110 mg/dL and an elevated triglyceride level is >100 mg/dL in the first decade and >130 mg/dL in the second decade.[45] There is clinical, metabolic, and genetic overlap among FCHL, hyperapo B, syndrome X, familial dyslipidemic hypertension, and LDL subclass pattern B.[46]

Polygenic Hypercholesterolemia

Many children and adolescents with elevated LDL-C levels may have "polygenic hypercholesterolemia."[44] The elevated LDL-C levels will be less marked than those seen in FH or FCHL (Table 4). On average, one-half of the parents and siblings of such children will not have elevated LDL-C levels. Other factors, such as a diet high in saturated fat and cholesterol, obesity, and physical inactivity, may also contribute to polygenic hypercholesterolemia.

Hypertriglyceridemia

When lipoprotein profiles are evaluated in high-risk children and adolescents, a subset will have normal LDL-C levels but elevated plasma triglyceride levels (type IV phenotype). If the LDL-C level is borderline (between 110 and 129 mg/dL) or the LDL apo B levels are elevated (above the 110 mg/dL), FCHL or hyperapo B may be suspected (see previous discussion). However, if the LDL-C and apo B levels are normal, and chylomicrons are absent, then the hypertriglyceridemia may indicate the presence of familial hypertriglyceridemia (FHT).[35] Affected first-degree relatives should also have hypertriglyceridemia with normal LDL-C and apo B levels.[35] Thus the opposite lipoprotein profiles seen in affected members in FCHL families are not found in families with FHT. The HDL-C level is often decreased, secondary to hypertriglyceridemia. FHT is most likely inherited as an autosomal dominant, but delayed penetrance is present (about one in five children born to an affected parent will express FHT).[44] Hyperinsulinism and obesity are often found in children with FHT.[47]

Hypoalphalipoproteinemia

A low HDL-C level (<35 mg/dL) in the presence of normal LDL-C and triglyceride levels (primary hypoalpha) was a common finding in progeny of fathers with premature CAD (Table 1).[11] A number of these hypoalpha children, however, most likely will have borderline high LDL-C levels or elevated LDL apo B levels, indicative of FCHL or hyperapo B.[35] A few of these children will have a primary deficiency of HDL metabolism. If so, other affected members will also have isolated low HDL-C level (hypoalpha) as their major abnormality, indicative of familial hypoalpha.[48] Point mutants in the *APOA-I* gene were found in families with low HDL-C levels.[49] Such families often have enhanced removal of HDL particles that is not accompanied by premature CAD. No abnormal physical findings were reported in children with *APOA-I* point mutations. Several genetic defects were described in the *APOAI/CIII/AIV* gene complex; HDL-C levels are very low, eg, 20–30 mg/dL, and the level of apo AI <10 mg/dL.[49] Some of these patients may have corneal clouding or planar xanthomas. Here, there is a synthetic defect in apo A-I production that is often accompanied by premature CAD.[49]

Dietary Management of Dyslipidemias in Youth

Dietary therapy is the first treatment approach. Two diets were recommended by the NCEP panel[1]: a step-one diet, similar to that suggested for all healthy children, and a step-two diet, which is more restricted in saturated fat and cholesterol (Table 5). The use of a registered dietitian is often essential to achieve long-lasting and significant dietary change. After dietary instruction, the patient returns after 6 weeks, 3 months, and 6 months to see if the goals of therapy, ie, an LDL-C level of <130 mg/dL (minimum) and <110 mg/dL (optimal), were achieved (Figure 3). If the goals are achieved, the child or adolescent is seen about twice a year.

Table 5
Characteristics of Step-One and Step-Two Diets for Children and Adolescents with Dyslipoproteinemia

Nutrient	Recommended Intake	
	Step-One Diet	Step-Two Diet
Total fat, % of calories	Average of no more than 30	Same
Saturated fatty acids, %	<10	<7
Polyunsaturated fatty acids, %	Up to 10	Same
Monounsaturated fatty acids, %	Remaining total fat calories	Same
Cholesterol, mg/d	<300	<200
Carbohydrates, % of calories	About 55	Same
Proteins, % of calories	About 15–20	Same
Calories	To promote normal growth and development and to reach or maintain desirable body weight	Same

Reproduced with permission from Reference 1.

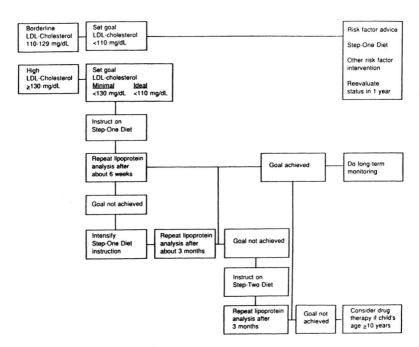

Figure 3. *Algorithm for the treatment of high LDL-C levels in youth. Reproduced with permission from Reference 1.*

Similar dietary management is used for children with hyper triglyceridemia or isolated low HDL-C levels. The addition of dietary oat bran or soybean protein may be acceptable dietary supplements to a low-cholesterol, low-fat diet.[50]

In children with high LDL-C or triglyceride levels or low HDL-C levels, the weight is often too high for the height (ponderosity), or obesity itself is present. Such children will also tend to have higher BP and insulin and glucose levels (see also above). Regular aerobic exercise is an important component, in addition to diet, to help control their weight problem.[51]

Low-fat diets (Table 5) appear safe but only provided that sufficient calories are given.[1,52] Even a balanced vegetarian diet can support normal growth and development.[53] A diet similar to the step-two diet was recently found to be both safe and efficacious in a DISC randomized, controlled clinical trial of moderately hypercholesterolemic adolescents.[34] After 3 years, those in the intervention group had a significantly lower mean LDL-C, but indistinguishable heights, serum ferritin, and Tanner staging compared with those in the usual care group.

Table 6
Guidelines for the Use of Drug Therapy in Children
Aged 10 Years or Older with Primary LDL-C Elevation

Risk Factors for CAD	Postdietary LDL-C Level (mg/dL)
None	≥190
Positive family history for premature CAD	≥160
Two or more other CAD risk factors	

Reproduced with permission from Reference 1.

Drug Management of Dyslipidemias in Youth

The NCEP panel[1] recommendations for the initiation of drug therapy are summarized in Table 6. In the child or adolescent with a positive family history of premature CAD, or with two other CAD risk factors, consider adding an LDL-lowering drug, if after diet the LDL-C level is >160 mg/dL. In a healthy child without such a family history, or other CAD risk factors, the cut point for initiation of drug therapy after diet is a LDL-C of 190 mg/dL (Table 6). These recommendations were made for children older than 10 years, but exceptions may be made based on the judgment of the physician.

Bile Acid Sequestrants

The only drug recommended by the NCEP panel was the use of bile acid sequestrants (Questran, or cholestramine, and Colestipol, or colestid). These drugs were used for reasonably long periods and appear relatively free of side effects. The starting dose in a child is usually one packet or one scoop (4 g) with breakfast and dinner. There was no evidence of fat-soluble vitamin deficiencies, fat malabsorption, steatorrhea, or significant adverse effects on calcium or vitamin D metabolism.[54,55] Whereas serum folate levels often decrease in children on a bile acid sequestrant, erythrocyte folate deficiency was not reported. However, no double-blind, placebo-controlled prospective study of the efficacy and safety of the bile acid binding agents, particularly regarding growth and development, is available. I recommend the addition of a one-a-day, multiple vitamin-mineral supplement containing iron and folic acid to my patients on a bile acid binding resin. This supplement should be taken 1 hour before or 3 hours after the bile acid binding resin.

Inhibitors of Hydroxymethyglutaryl
Coenzyme A Reductase

Inhibitors of hydroxymethyglutaryl coenzyme A (HMGCoA) reductase, the rate-limiting enzyme of cholesterol biosynthesis, were not approved by the Food and Drug Administration for use in persons younger than age 18. However, some children and adolescents may present with a clinical picture that warrants more special consideration of whether to use an HMGCoA reductase inhibitor before age 18. Such clinical characteristics are summarized in Table 7. If a clinician decides to prescribe an HMGCoA reductase inhibitor for such a youth, it is important to explain the rationale for the decision to the patient and his family, review the available efficacy and safety data (see also following text) with them, and to obtain written permission from the family to institute such treatment.

Ducobu and coworkers[56] treated hypercholesterolemic boys and girls, who were presumed FH heterozygotes, with 20 mg/day of simvastatin (Zocor) (in those <10 years of age) or 40 mg/day (in those >10 years of age) for 24–36 months. The LDL-C fell 37.3%, and the HDL-C increased 22.5%.[56] No significant changes were found in growth and development, and no abnormalities were noted in liver function or muscle tests. However, this study was not placebo controlled.

The Lovastatin Adolescent Male Study[57] was a 1-year, double-blind, randomized, multicenter, placebo-controlled trial in FH heterozygotes. The efficacy and safety of lovastatin (Mevacor) was assessed in 132 carefully characterized adolescent males with presumed heterozgous FH. Thirty-seven percent of parents of the participants had premature CAD (59% of fathers, 19% of mothers). The mean baseline plasma levels of total cholesterol and LDL-C (milligrams/deciliter) were (lovastatin group) 325 and 258, respectively, and (placebo group) 320 and 254, respectively. Subjects were seen every 4 weeks. Safety evaluation included Tanner staging (weeks 0, 24, and 48), height, weight, and Quetelet index; tests of liver

---

Table 7
Clinical Characteristics of Children and Adolescents that Warrant Special
Consideration for Treatment with HMGCoA Reductase Inhibitors

Family history of premature CAD in a parent before 35 years of age
Above average levels of plasma total (>300 mg/dL) and LDL-C (>240 mg/dL) for a
    FH heterozygote
Elevated plasma level of Lp(a) (≥30 mg/dL)
Low level of HDL-C (≤35 mg/dL)
Cigarette smoking
Male gender
Poor response to or compliance with bile acid sequestrants

---

function and creatine phosphokinase, hematologies, and coagulation; assessment of thyroid [thyroxine (T4) and thyrotropin (TSH)], adrenal (cortisol, dihydroepiandrosterone, and testosterone), and pituitary (follicle-stimulating hormone and luteinizing hormone) function; and tests of nutrient status (ferritin and vitamins A, D, and E). Those assigned to the lovastatin group were gradually titrated from a dose of 10 mg/day up to a dose 40 mg/day. The percent change versus baseline in the plasma levels of total cholesterol and LDL-C were (lovastatin group) −21% and −26%, respectively, and (placebo) −4% and −5%, respectively. This decrease in LDL-C on lovastatin was similar to that seen in adult patients. There were no significant differences between the lovastatin and placebo groups in the evaluation of growth and development (height, weight, Quetelet index, and testicular volume) and Tanner staging and tests of liver, muscle, and endocrine function.

The Canadian Lovastatin in Children Study Group[58] assessed the efficacy, safety, and tolerance of a shorter-term use of lovastatin in 69 male patients with heterozygous FH in a multicenter, randomized, double-blind trial. After a 4-week placebo period, the patients were allocated to four treatment groups (lovastatin 10, 20, 30, or 40 mg/day) for 8 weeks. Each dose of lovastatin reduced plasma levels of total cholesterol (−17% to −29%) and LDL-C (−21% to −36%). The lovastatin was well tolerated by all the patients, and no serious clinical adverse experience was reported.

Starting Dose of Hydroxymethyglutaryl Coenzyme A Reductase Inhibitors and Follow-Up

In both studies with lovastatin,[57,58] there was a significant response to the lowest dose of lovastatin used (10 mg/day). This is a desirable characteristic for a medication that is to be prescribed long term to optimize the daily dosage and to minimize the occurrence of potential side effects. A gradual increment in a dose of an HMGCoA reductase inhibitor in children or adolescents undergoing such treatment is the optimal approach. For example, the starting dose may be 10 mg/day (for lovastatin or pravastatin), 5 mg/day (for simvastatin), or 20 mg/day (for fluvastatin). Growth and development and liver function need to be monitored. Creatine phosphokinase is measured at baseline and thereafter if the patient develops symptoms suggestive of myositis. As a precautionary note, any female FH heterozygote taking an HMGCoA reductase inhibitor should discontinue the drug before becoming pregnant.

Other Lipid-Lowering Drugs

Experience in the use of other hypolipidemic drugs was limited[54]; nicotinic acid is not routinely recommended for dyslipidemia in children.[1]

Such therapy should be undertaken after consultation at a university lipid clinic. Patients with hypertriglyceridemia, even when it is severe, can usually be managed by dietary therapy alone.[59]

Summary

An extensive body of scientific evidence supports the notion that the harbingers of CAD risk factors start in childhood. As well, several disorders of lipid metabolism that are strongly associated with CAD in affected adults can be detected in youth. A complimentary, dual approach for prevention of CAD seems reasonable: (1) a Mediterranean-like, low-fat diet for all healthy children above age 2, with proper attention to obesity, physical inactivity, and BP levels and prevention of cigarette smoking in adolescence; and (2) the identification and treatment of dyslipidemic children from families at high risk for premature CAD. The management of dyslipidemias and the identification of CAD ideally begin early in life, when the lesions of atherosclerosis are beginning.

Acknowledgments

Pauline Gugliotta provided invaluable help with manuscript preparation.

References

1. National Cholesterol Education Program Report of the Expert Panel on Blood Cholesterol Levels in Children and Adolescents. *Pediatrics* 1992;89:525–584.
2. Kwiterovich PO Jr. Prevention of coronary disease starting in childhood: what risk factors should be identified and treated? *Coron Artery Dis* 1993;4: 611–630.
3. Strong JP, McGill HC Jr. The pediatric aspects of atherosclerosis. *J Atheroscler Res* 1969;9:251–265.
4. Wissler RW. Update on the pathogenesis of atherosclerosis. *Am J Med* 1991;91(suppl):3–9.
5. PDAY Research Group. Relationship of atherosclerosis in young men to serum lipoprotein cholesterol concentrations and smoking. A preliminary report from the Pathobiologcal Determinants of Atherosclerosis in Youth (PDAY) Research Group. *JAMA* 1990;264:3018–3024.
6. Berenson GS, Wattigney WA, Tracy RE, et al. Atherosclerosis of the aorta and coronary arteries and cardiovascular risk factors in persons aged 6 to 30 years and studied at necropsy (the Bogalusa Heart Study). *Am J Cardiol* 1992; 70:851–858.
7. Mahoney LT, Burns TL, Stanford W, et al. Coronary risk factors measured in childhood and young adult life are associated with coronary artery calcification in young adults: the Muscatine Study. *J Am Coll Cardiol* 1996;27: 277–284.

8. Knuiman JT, Hermus RJJ, Hautvast JGAJ. Serum total and high density lipoprotein (HDL) cholesterol concentrations in rural and urban boys from 16 countries. *Atherosclerosis* 1980;36:529–537.
9. Knuiman JT, Westenbrink S, Van der Heyden L. Determinants of total and high density lipoprotein cholesterol in boys from Finland, the Netherlands, Italy, the Philippines and Ghana with special reference to diet. *Hum Nutr Clin Nutr* 1983;37C:237–254.
10. Knuiman JT, West CE, Katan MB, et al. Total cholesterol and high density lipoprotein cholesterol levels in populations differing in fat and carbohydrate intake. *Arteriosclerosis* 1987;7:612–619.
11. Lee J, Lauer RM, Clarke WR. Lipoproteins in the progeny of young men with coronary artery disease: children with increased risk. *Pediatrics* 1986;78:330–337.
12. Schrott HG, Clarke WR, Wiebe DA, et al. Increased coronary mortality in relatives of hypercholesterolemic school children: the Muscatine Study. *Circulation* 1979;59:320–326.
13. Moll PP, Sing CF, Weidman WH, et al. Total cholesterol and lipoproteins in school children: prediction of coronary heart disease in adult relatives. *Circulation* 1983;67:127–134.
14. Freedman DS, Srinivasan SR, Sher CL, et al. The relation of apolipoproteins A-1 and B in children to parental myocardial infarction. *N Engl J Med* 1986;315:721–726.
15. Morrison JA, Namboodiri K, Green P, et al. Familial aggregation of lipids and lipoproteins and early identification of dyslipoproteinemia. The Collaborative Lipid Research Clinics Family Study. *JAMA* 1983;250:1860–1868.
16. Goldstein JL, Brown MS. Familial hypercholesterolemia. In: Scriver CR, Beaudet AL, Sly WS, et al, eds. *The Metabolic Basis of Inherited Disease.* 6th ed. New York, NY: McGraw-Hill; 1989:1215–1250.
17. Kostner GM, Czinner A, Pfeiffer KH, et al. Lipoprotein (a) concentrations as risk indicators for atherosclerosis. *Arch Dis Child* 1991;66:1054–1056.
18. Srinivasan SR, Berenson GS. Serum apolipoproteins A-I and B as markers of coronary artery disease risk in early life: the Bogalusa Heart Study. *Clin Chem* 1995;41:159–164.
19. Burns TL, Moll PP, Lauer RM. Increased familial cardiovascular mortality in obese school children: the Muscatine Ponderosity Family Study. *Pediatrics* 1992;89:262–268.
20. Srinivasan SR, Bao W, Wattigney WA, et al. Adolescent overweight is associated with adult overweight and related multiple cardiovascular risk factors: the Bogalusa Heart Study. *Metabolism* 1996;45:235–240.
21. Williams DP, Going SB, Lohman TG, et al. Body fatness and risk for elevated blood pressure, total cholesterol, and serum lipoprotein ratios in children and adolescents. *Am J Public Health* 1992;82:358–363.
22. Folsom AR, Burke GL, Byers CL, et al. Implications of obesity for cardiovascular disease in blacks: the CARDIA and ARIC Studies. *Am J Clin Nutr* 1991;53(suppl):1604–1611.
23. Strong WB. Physical activity and children. *Circulation* 1990;81:1697–1701.
24. Second Task Force on Blood Pressure Control in Children. *Pediatrics* 1987; 79:1–25.
25. Bao W, Threefoot SA, Srinivasan SR, et al. Essential hypertension predicted by tracking of elevated blood pressure from childhood to adulthood: the Bogalusa Heart Study. *Am J Hypertens* 1995;8:657–665.
26. Craig WY, Palomaki GE, Johnson AM, et al. Cigarette smoking-associated changes in blood lipid and lipoprotein levels in the 8- to 19-year-old group: a meta-analysis. *Pediatrics* 1990;85:155–158.

27. Muhtaseb N, Yousuf A, Bajaj JS. Apolipoprotein A-I, A-II, B, C-II and C-III in children with insulin-dependent diabetes mellitus. *Pediatrics* 1992;89:936–941.
28. Burke GL, Webber LS, Srinivasan SR, et al. Fasting plasma glucose and insulin levels and their relationship to cardiovascular risk factors in children: Bogalusa Heart Study. *Metabolism* 1986;35:441–446.
29. Jiang X, Srinivasan SR, Webber LS, et al. Association of fasting insulin level with serum lipid and lipoprotein levels in children, adolescents, and young adults: the Bogalusa Heart Study. *Arch Intern Med* 1995;155:190–196.
30. Myers L, Coughlin SS, Webber LS, et al. Prediction of adult cardiovascular multifactorial risk status from childhood risk factor levels. The Bogalusa Heart Study. *Am J Epidemiol* 1995;142:918–924.
31. Reaven GM. Banting lecture 1988. Role of insulin resistance in human disease. *Diabetes* 1988;37:1595–1607.
32. Bao W, Srinivasan SR, Wattigney WA, et al. Persistence of multiple cardiovascular risk clustering related to syndrome X from childhood to young adulthood. The Bogalusa Heart Study. *Arch Intern Med* 1994;154:1842–1847.
33. Williams RR, Hunt SC, Hopkins PN, et al. Familial dyslipidemic hyper tension: evidence from 58 Utah families for a syndrome present in approximately 15% of patients with essential hypertension. *JAMA* 1988;259:3579–3586.
34. DISC Collaborative Research Group. The efficacy and safety of lowering dietary intake of total fat, saturated-fat, and cholesterol in children with elevated LDL-cholesterol: the Dietary Intervention Study in Children (DISC). *JAMA* 1995;273:1429–1435.
35. Kwiterovich PO Jr. Diagnosis and management of familial dyslipoproteinemia in children and adolescents. *Pediatr Clin North Am* 1990;37:1489–1523.
36. Cortner JA, Coates PM, Gallagher PR. Prevalence and expression of familial combined hyperlipidemia in childhood. *J Pediatr* 1990;116:514–519.
37. Kwiterovich PO Jr. Pediatric implication of heterozygous familial hypercholesterolemia. Screening and dietary treatment. *Arterioscler Thromb Vasc Biol* 1989;9(suppl):1111–1120.
38. Sprecher DL, Schaefer EJ, Kent KM, et al. Cardiovascular features of homozygous familial hypercholesterolemia: analysis of 16 patients. *Am J Cardiol* 1984;54:20–30.
39. Celermajer DS, Sorensen KE, Gooch VM, et al. Non-invasive detection of endothelial dysfunction in children and adults at risk of atherosclerosis. *Lancet* 1992;340:1111–1115.
40. Hobbs HH, Brown MS, Goldstein JL. Molecular genetics of the LDL receptor gene in familial hypercholesterolemia. *Hum Mutat* 1992;1:445–466.
41. Utermann G, Hoppichler F, Dieplinger H, et al. Defects in the low density lipoprotein receptor gene affect lipoprotein (a) levels: multiplicative interaction of two gene loci associated with premature atherosclerosis. *Proc Natl Acad Sci U S A* 1989;86:4171–4174.
42. Wiklund O, Angelin B, Olofsson SO, et al. Apolipoprotein A and ischemic heart disease in familial hypercholesterolemia. *Lancet* 1990;I:1360–1363.
43. Myant NB, Gallagher JJ, Knight BL, et al. Clinical signs of familial hypercholesterolemia in patients with familial defective apolipoprotein B-100 and normal low density lipoprotein receptor function. *Arterioscler Thromb* 1991;11:691–703.
44. Goldstein JL, Schrott HG, Hazzard WR, et al. Hyperlipidemia in coronary heart disease. II. Genetic analysis of lipid levels in 176 families and delineation of a new inherited disorder, combined hyperlipidemia. *J Clin Invest* 1973;52:1544–1568.

45. Kwiterovich PO Jr. *Beyond Cholesterol. The Johns Hopkins Complete Guide for Avoiding Heart Disease.* Baltimore, MD: The Johns Hopkins University Press; 1989:1–395.
46. Kwiterovich PO Jr. Genetics and molecular biology of familial combined hyperlipidemia. *Curr Opin Lipidol* 1993;4:133–143.
47. Glueck CJ, Mellies MJ, Srivastava L, et al. Insulin, obesity and triglyceride interrelationships in sixteen children with familial hypertriglyceridemia. *Pediatr Res* 1977;11:13–19.
48. Third JLHC, Montag J, Flynn M, et al. Primary and familial hypoalphalipoproteinemia. *Metabolism* 1984;33:136–146.
49. Breslow JL. Genetic basis of lipoprotein disorder. *J Clin Invest* 1989;84:373–380.
50. Kwiterovich PO Jr. The role of fiber in the treatment of hypercholesterolemic children and adolescents. *Pediatrics* 1995;96:1005–1010.
51. Becque MD, Katch VL, Rocchini AP, et al. Coronary risk incidence of obese adolescents: reduction by exercise plus diet intervention. *Pediatrics* 1988;81:605–612.
52. Lifshitz F, Mosez N. Growth failure as a complication of dietary treatment of hypercholesterolemia. *Am J Dis Child* 1989;143:537–542.
53. Sabate J, Lindsted KD, Harris RD, et al. Attained height of lacto-ovo vegetarian children and adolescents. *Eur J Clin Nutr* 1991;45:51–58.
54. Hoeg JM. Pharmacologic and surgical treatment of dyslipidemic children and adolescents. *Ann N Y Acad Sci* 1991;623:275–284.
55. Farah R, Kwiterovich PO Jr, Neill CA. A study of the dose-effect of cholestyramine in children and young adult with familial hypercholesterolemia. *Lancet* 1977;I:59–63.
56. Ducobu J, Brasseur D, Chaudron J-M, et al. Simvastatin use in children. *Lancet* 1992;339:1488.
57. Stein EA, Gormley D, Illingworth DR, et al. A one-year placebo-controlled trial of Lovastatin in adolescent males with severe FH: lipid and safety chemistry data. *Circulation* 1995;92:I-126.
58. Lambert M, Jupien P-J, Gagne C, et al. Treatment of familial hypercholesterolemia in children and adolescents: effect of Lovastatin. *Pediatrics* 1996;97:619–628.
59. Kwiterovich PO Jr, Farah JR, Brown WV, et al. The clinical, biochemical, and familial presentation of type V hyperlipoproteinemia in childhood. *Pediatrics* 1977;59:513–525.

Chapter 9

Preventive Cardiology in Women
The Gender-Specific Aspects of Coronary Risk

Fredric J. Pashkow, MD
JoAnne Micale Foody, MD
and Corinne Varin-LeBreton, MD

Introduction

The risks for coronary heart disease (CHD) are similar in men and women, but the impact of gender is quite profound. Risk factors for CHD have unique characteristics in women and as such require unique strategies for their diagnosis and management.

Epidemiological, clinical, and experimental studies demonstrated a profound effect of estrogen on the risk factor profile in women. Yet estrogen plays only a partial role in distinguishing the characteristics of cardiovascular disease (CVD) in women.

Genetics and environmental factors such as obesity, smoking, and lack of physical exercise all have a profound effect on the lipids and the formation of atherosclerotic plaque. The metabolic and pathophysiological mechanisms, vascular response, and clinical gains of lipid-altering interventions clearly differ between the sexes. There are important other considerations besides the direct effect of lipids, however, related to risk

From Robinson K, (ed): *Preventive Cardiology.* Armonk, NY: Futura Publishing Company, Inc. © 1998.

that are profoundly influenced by gender. Some relate to other essential metabolic processes such as insulin resistance and endothelial function, but differences in risk result from gender dissimilarities in psychology and sociology as well.

The development of strategies for the successful diagnosis and treatment of the coronary risks requires an appreciation of these significant gender differences.

Coronary Disease Risk Factors in Women

"Men are from Mars, women are from Venus," one best-selling contemporary American author tells us (John Gray, *Men are from Mars, Women are from Venus*. Harpercollins, New York, 1992). The fact that gender profoundly affects our biology and psychology is well recognized. The extent to which this influences our thinking with respect to the diagnosis and management of coronary disease was an area of intense interest in recent years.[1]

CVD is the leading killer of women in the United States. It claims the lives of over 500 000 women each year. Nonetheless, a myth persists that coronary artery disease (CAD) is a more common affliction of men. Although it is true that men experience an excess of CAD morbidity and mortality through middle age as compared to women, the gender difference decreases with advancing age, and CAD becomes the major cause of morbidity and mortality in women over age 55. Although women are generally viewed as being relatively protected from CAD, they rapidly develop a risk equivalent to their male counterparts after menopause. The prevention of cardiovascular events in women, either primary or secondary, is critical to the development of sound public health strategies.

Case-control and cohort studies examined the effect of various risk factors on CAD in men, but only a few prospective investigations included sufficient female subjects to adequately assess gender-related differences in risk factors. Recent emphasis on women's health in general led to increasing research focused on gender that led to increasing evidence that gender differences do exist in CAD incidence and risk factors. We will examine the gender issues related to the classical risk factors shared by men and women of cholesterol, hypertension, cigarette smoking, diabetes, and lack of physical exercise as well as risks that are uniquely feminine: the use of oral contraceptive agents, menopause, and postmenopausal hormones.

The Role of Estrogen in Cardiovascular Disease

Epidemiological, clinical, and experimental studies suggest that estrogen confers protection against CVD in premenopausal women and that, in the absence of estrogen, women no longer enjoy this advantage. Furthermore, estrogen replacement therapy was shown to slow the progression of atherosclerosis in experimental studies. In large epidemiological studies, postmenopausal women on estrogen replacement therapy experience 50% fewer coronary events with particular benefit to those women diagnosed with CAD. Furthermore, estrogen use appears to be protective in women with and without risk factors for heart disease. For example, among smokers and nonsmokers, women using estrogen have a lower occurrence of CHD compared to nonusers.[2]

The protective effect of estrogen appears to be strongest among women who are currently using this therapy, that is, former users have a higher risk of heart disease than current users, although lower than women who never took estrogen. Estrogen appears to provide protection against many forms of CVD, including heart attack, stroke, and blockage of coronary blood vessels.[3,4]

These observations led researchers to hypothesize that estrogen may directly or indirectly retard the development of arterial plaques, favorably affect the vulnerability of existing plaques, or reduce the risk of coronary occlusion by preventing the formation of an occlusive thrombus, a consequence of plaque rupture. In addition, estrogen may alter endothelial function and attenuate vasomotor dysfunction, possible triggers of plaque rupture.

Estrogen may protect women through modification of the lipid profile. Postmenopausal women have reduced low-density lipoprotein cholesterol (LDL-C) and elevated high-density lipoprotein cholesterol (HDL-C) compared to men. After menopause, women develop a more atherogenic lipid profile as LDL-C rises, HDL-C levels fall, and lipoprotein (a) [Lp(a)] levels increase.[5] Estrogen replacement reverses these adverse changes in lipoprotein profile and diminishes cardiovascular risk.[6,7] However, multiple regression analyses of large-scale clinical trials indicate that the beneficial changes in lipoprotein levels resulting from estrogen replacement therapy account for only 25% to 50% of the observed risk reduction, suggesting that mechanisms unrelated to lipid lowering are involved.[3] Cardioprotective mechanisms unrelated to lipid lowering are evident in women with heterozygous familial hypercholesterolemia. Despite the higher levels of total cholesterol (TC) and LDL-C, these women have a reduced incidence and a markedly delayed onset of the clinical manifestations of CHD compared to their male counterparts.

The epidemiological observation that women are relatively protected from the clinical manifestations of CAD prior to the menopause focused contemporary research on estrogen as a protection against CAD. However, estrogen may explain only a portion of the difference in cardiovascular risk between men and women.[8] As women age and pass through the menopause, they develop a more atherogenic lipid profile typified by a rise in LDL-C and a fall in HDL-C levels.[9,10] Our assumption that the primary protective effect of estrogen from the development of atherosclerosis is through this modification of the lipid profile is most likely an oversimplification.[3] This assumption extends from the observation that estrogen replacement reverses the proatherogenic lipid profile and reduces cardiovascular risk.[7,11]

Estrogens produce their characteristic responses in target tissues by associating with an intracellular protein moiety called the estrogen receptor. This molecular receptor binds female hormones with great specificity and affinity and is a prerequisite to the occurrence of any estrogenically mediated biologic response, whether of developmental or metabolic significance. The activity of the estrogen receptor varies with the specific nature of the tissue, a woman's age, and her endocrine and metabolic status. The linkage of the estrogen to the receptor triggers the formation of a binding complex that results in the formation of mRNA molecules, which in turn direct the synthesis of many proteins. Characteristically, these proteins are associated with female development and reproduction; however, they account as well for the differential effects of estrogen on virtually all cells, particularly relevant to our interest on liver parenchyma and endothelium.

In addition to the effects of estrogen on absolute levels of LDL-C and HDL-C, estrogen probably mediates protection from CVD via other means: lowering of the very-low-density lipoprotein cholesterol (VLDL-C)/triglyceride (TG) ratio, increasing clearance of intermediate-density lipoprotein and LDL-C via an up-regulated LDL-C receptor, diminished infiltration and degradation of LDL-C in the arterial wall, and inhibition of LDL-C oxidation. In the dynamic process of ischemia, estrogen appears to modulate responses of atherosclerotic coronary arteries such as a reversal of inappropriate acetylcholine (EDRF)-mediated vasoconstriction in afflicted vessels and potentially important estrogen-influenced hemostatic effects.[12] Estrogen modifies directly the functions of the endothelium and vascular smooth muscle. In health the vascular endothelium provides a surface that is vasodilatory, anticoagulating, and antiadhesive for leukocytes and that inhibits proliferation of vascular smooth muscle cells.[13]

Since estrogen (estradiol) is only one of several hormonal constituents that change with menopause and the biological activity of estrogen appears much more complex than initially supposed, it is quite likely that we are far from a complete understanding of the gender-specific differences involved in both the development and clinical manifestations of CAD.

Classical Risk Factors

Hyperlipidemia

Lipid subfractions change predictably with aging in both men and women, but not at all in the same way. The effects of endogenous gonadal hormones in life-cycle changes in women is evident. Furthermore, compositional differences in lipid particles between men and women were observed. TC is a risk factor, but for higher absolute levels in women because their levels of HDL-C are higher. HDL-C, which correlates negatively with CHD, appears to be a better predictor of risk in women than in men and the strongest lipid predictor in women.[14] LDL-C seems to be a less important risk factor at least in premenopausal women, most likely because of a higher level of HDL-C and the protecting effect of estrogen against LDL-C deposition in the arterial wall. Because of its level and the presence of small, dense LDL-C particles, LDL-C is a stronger predictor of CHD in postmenopausal women. TG was recently shown to be an independent predictor for CHD risk in women but not in men.[15,16]

Menopause alters the lipid profile and major lipoprotein risk factors in women. There is not only a decrease of the HDL-C level but also a compositional modification, with a lower level of HDL_2-C, the protective fraction of HDL-C, and a greater level of HDL_3-C, the atherogenic fraction of HDL-C.[17,18] LDL-C levels rise sharply after menopause, and, above all, postmenopausal women have a greater percentage of the more-atherogenic, smaller, denser LDL-C.[19] TG levels are higher in older postmenopausal women. They represent a predictive factor probably, again, because of their association with smaller, denser LDL-C.

Total Cholesterol

Plasma TC level is similar up to 20 years of age in both sexes. Then TC level increases progressively but at a slower rate for women until the sixth decade. Thus men's level generally remains slightly higher. After the sixth decade, women's TC levels generally increase faster, exceeding those of men of similar age.[19] This is attributable to the rise in LDL-C in women postmenopause and the persistent discrepancy in HDL-C. Whereas TC, HDL-C, and LDL-C levels were demonstrated to be independent predictors of CAD in men,[20–23] less is known about the effect of lipid concentrations on CAD in women.

When comparing data by gender, serum cholesterol is associated with CAD in women similarly to men. At each level of cholesterol, however, men have higher rates of disease than do women; thus women may be at high risk for CAD at different levels of cholesterol than men.[24] For example, the Framingham investigators found that women with TC levels >295 mg/dL had only 60% the rate of myocardial infarction (MI) compared with men with TC <204 mg/dL.[9]

However, the data convincingly show that women who have a total serum cholesterol >260 mg/dL are two or three times at risk of developing CAD than are women whose TC level is <200 mg/dL. Only the Lipid Research Clinics (LRC) found increased mortality at lower cholesterol levels (>235 mg/dL). Table 1 summarizes some of the major studies that implicate cholesterol as a coronary disease risk for women.

In the Evans County Study, TC is predictive of CVD mortality in white women younger than 65.[29] Among black women, cholesterol was negatively associated with all-cause mortality. In a study published the same year, the Charleston Heart Study, a lack of consistency of results by different statistical analyses in black women make conclusions concerning the nature of the relation between cholesterol and CHD mortality less strong in black women than in white women. White women having a cholesterol value one standard deviation above the mean (s = 52.5 mg/dL) had a 60% higher CHD mortality rate [hazard ratio = 1.6, 95% confidence interval (CI): 1.2–2.1]. In black women, the estimated hazard ratio for a SD (s = 47.8 mg/dL) increase in cholesterol is 1.4 (95% CI: 1.03–1.8). The results suggest that the relation of cholesterol to CHD mortality is different in white and black women.[30]

Some studies demonstrate gender differences in the elderly for TC as a risk factor for death from CAD. Serum TC level predicted fatal CAD outcomes in middle-aged (<65 years) and older (≥65 years) men and women, although the strength and consistency of these relations in older women were diminished.[31] Analysis of the Rancho Bernardo Study[8] data suggests that, in the elderly, TC level predicts fatal coronary events in men but not in women. These results are not unexpected, given that the TC value is calculated from HDL-C, LDL-C, and TG (TC = HDL-C + LDL-C + TG/5) and that LDC level was found to be no better a predictor

---

Table 1

Major Studies that Implicate Cholesterol as a Coronary Disease Risk for Women

Studies	Women (n)	Ages (ys)	Results
Framingham Heart Study[9]	2 873	35–94	TC >265 mg/dL: twofold risk of CHD compared with women with TC <205 mg/dL
Dono-Tel Aviv[25,26]	1 325	25–69	TC >265 mg/dL: threefold increase compared with TC <200 mg/dL
Rancho-Bernardo[27]	2 048	59–79	TC >260 mg/dL: 2.5-fold increase in risk
Nurses' Health Study[28]	120 343	30–55	Self-reported hypercholesterolemia increases risk of nonfatal MI two times and fatal CHD three times
Lipid Research Clinics[3]	2 270	40–69	Women with TC >235 mg/dL had a 70% higher risk of CAD death than women with TC <200 mg/dL

of fatal CHD than TC in either gender and that women had higher levels of HDL than men, explaining the usually higher TC levels.

The Donolo-Tel Aviv study also noted that the adverse effects of a high TC level may be balanced by a high HDL-C level: women with high HDL-C had similar low rates of CHD regardless of their level of TC. No such relation was observed in the male participants. In the same way, the investigators demonstrated a two- to fivefold higher risk of CHD in women whose HDL-C level was <23% of their TC, even in those individuals whose TC was <200 mg/dL.[25]

High-Density Lipoprotein Cholesterol

Levels of HDL-C in male children are slightly higher than those of female children until puberty, but, as girls pass through puberty, HDL-C levels do not fall as they do in boys of the same age. After puberty, HDL-C levels in women increase slowly until before menopause, whereas they remain constant in men. Thus the average HDL-C values in adult women are approximately 20% higher than those of men.[19] Women prospectively followed through menopause demonstrate a decline in the mean HDL-C levels of approximately 3.5 mg/dL. However, HDL-C levels generally remain higher in women than men throughout life.[5]

Compositional differences in HDL-C between men and women also were observed. HDL-C, which seems to exert a protective effect on the development of atherosclerosis, has two subfractions, HDL_2-C and HDL_3-C. Most studies show that high HDL_2-C levels are associated with reduced risk of CHD,[32] whereas high levels of another component, HDL_3-C (HDL_3-C-B), might be associated with increased CAD risk. Women have higher HDL_2-C and lower HDL_3-C than men.[33,34] In 1988, Ohta et al[35] showed that, in women, HDL-C has a higher content of apolipoprotein A-1 (apo A-1), cholesterol, and phospholipid, particularly in the so-called apo A-1-ontaining fraction. This fraction is roughly equivalent to HDL_2-C, which is thought to be the protective fraction of HDL-C.

The effects of endogenous gonadal hormones during normal life-cycle changes for HDL-C was elucidated. In pregnancy, HDL-C rises (as well as LDL-C and TG) until the 24th week, and then it begins to fall. Interestingly, this fall in HDL-C is not accompanied by a fall in apo A-1 levels, implying a change in HDL-C composition during the last period of pregnancy. After menopause, HDL-C declines again, but the decline occurs gradually over the 2 years preceding cessation of menses.[36] This decline is accompanied by a rise in apo A-1 levels, implying again a change in HDL-C composition.[37] Reductions in HDL_2-C subfractions were reported in relation to a reduced estradiol level after menopause.[5,38]

HDL-C is one of the most powerful negative predictors of CAD mortality and morbidity. Stensvold et al,[39] in a screening for CVD performed in three Norwegian counties on a population of 23 680 men and 23 425 women (6.8 years mean follow-up), showed that CVD mortality decreased with increasing HDL-C. The inverse association between mortality and HDL-C was stronger in women than in men. An analysis of data from the LRC follow-up study by Jacobs and colleagues[20] demonstrated a strong inverse relation between HDL-C level and CHD mortality in women, even after adjustment for multiple other risk factors.

Manolio et al[31] analyzed 22 US and international cohort studies and concluded that HDL-C level inversely predicts CHD in middle-aged women and in older women but not in older men. HDL-C appears to have greater relative predictive value as well. Not only are total HDL-C levels higher, but there is a greater difference in CAD risk per milligram difference in HDL-C in women.[40] Data from the Framingham study also demonstrate that HDL-C level is a more powerful predictor in women: for every 10-mg/dL change in HDL-C, a 40% to 50% change in coronary risk was noted, and the Framingham investigators suggest that the protective effect of HDL-C in women is approximately twice the atherogenic effect of LDL-C.[14] In a more recent review of data from the Framingham population, Kannel and Wilson confirmed that, among men and women, the risk of CHD-related events increases steeply with each increment in the

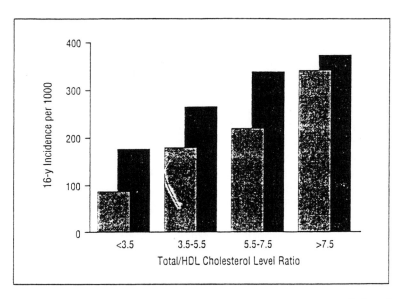

Figure 1. *Risk of CHD by total HDL-C level ratio among women (**lighter bars**) and men (**darker bars**) aged 50–90 years. Reproduced with permission from Reference 41.*

ratio TC/HDL-C, and, in women, a ratio higher than 7.5 appears to attenuate greatly the risk advantage over men, resulting in almost the same incidence rate observed in males (Figure 1).[41]

Bass et al[16] recently reported on a population of 1405 women aged 50 to 69 years selected from the LRC's follow-up data (Figure 2). Higher CVD death was seen at elevated levels of TC in women with low HDL-C levels but not among women with high HDL-C levels. Women with high HDL-C levels had similar CVD mortality rates at all levels of TC. Women with low HDL-C levels had a threefold increased risk of CVD death when compared with women with high HDL-C levels. Hong et al studied the usefulness of the ratio TC/HDL-C in predicting angiographic artery disease in women.[42] TC levels did not correlate with the presence of CAD. However, TC/HDL-C was higher among women with, than without, CAD, and this ratio was the most predictive factor of the presence, extensiveness, and severity of CAD.

It is important to consider the absolute value of the HDL. Most women have mean HDL-C levels of 50 mg/dL or higher.[16,21,23,25] Both the Framingham study and the Donolo-Tel Aviv study documented increased CVD incidence and mortality in women whose HDL-C levels are >35 mg/dL but <50 mg/dL. Considering these data, Bass defined a low HDL-

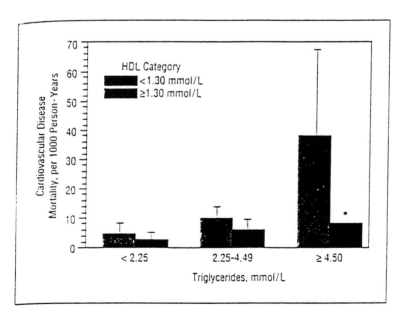

Figure 2. *Age-adjusted CVD mortality rates (per 1000 person-years) with upper 95% CIs (**vertical lines on top of bars**) by TG and HDL levels in women aged 50–69 years. * Upper CI is undefined for TG levels of ≥399 mmol/L and HDL levels of ≥4.5 mmol/L. Reproduced with permission from Reference 16.*

C level for values <50 mg/dL and a high HDL-C level for values ≥50 mg/dL, resulting in an increased mortality relative risk (RR) of 1.7 with an HDL-C level <50 mg/dL in women (compared to an HDL-C >50 mg/dL). Thus the cutoff of 35 mg/dL for HDL-C levels as recommended in the National Cholesterol Education Program Adult Treatment Panel II (NCEP ATP-II) Report[43] to identify individuals at high risk of CVD appears to be appropriate for men but not for women.

Low-Density Lipoprotein Cholesterol

The NCEP ATP-II Report indicates an LDL-C level of 130 mg/dL or higher as a risk factor for CHD in both men and women. In fact, the role of LDL-C as a risk factor in women is somewhat controversial. Few prospective studies examined LDL-C and CHD risk in women.

LDL-C levels are lower in women than in men throughout the first two-thirds of the life span. After the midde of the fifth decade, as a result of evolving menopause, LDL-C levels in women rise abruptly, whereas LDL-C levels in men remain stable. In the last third of life, women generally have higher LDL-C levels.[44] Again, compositional differences in LDL-C exist between pre- and postmenopausal women: postmenopausal women tend to have increasing levels of a smaller, denser type of LDL-C,[45] which is thought to be particularly atherogenic because it may be more susceptible to oxidation.[46] It is interesting to note that high HDL$_3$-C is often associated with higher concentrations of small, dense LDL-C particles and a low LDL-C peak particle diameter.[47] This association characterizes the recently described LDL-C subclass phenotype B, which is a coronary risk factor.[48]

The Framingham Study found LDL-C to be a significant positive predictor of coronary decease in women, although less powerful than HDL-C.[14] In contrast, the LRC study did not find LDL-C to be a significant independent predictor of CVD in women.[3,20]

LDL-C was not evaluated in the Donolo-Tel Aviv study.[25] LDL-C level was a poor predictor of CVD mortality in female participants in the LRC's follow-up study after adjustment for other CVD factors. In fact, after stratification by HDL-C category, the highest CVD deaths rates were noted among women with low HDL-C and normal LDL-C level.[16] This finding is contrary to what is observed in men, where CVD risk increases with levels of either TC or LDL-C.

Very high LDL-C concentrations carry the same poor prognosis in both sexes. Men and women who are homozygous for familial hypercholesterolemia have a similar increased risk for CHD.[49] However, women who are heterozygous have a lower risk attributable to LDL-C compared with heterozygous men.[50] This finding may be merely due to the higher

HDL-C levels found in women. Another possibility is supported by at least one animal study.[51] In this investigation, the arterial wall LDL-C content of estrogen-treated monkeys was considerably lower than that of non-estrogen-treated controls, implying that estrogen may in some way inhibit the arterial wall uptake of LDL-C. This possibility is especially relevant to premenopausal women and could explain why LDL-C level is a less stronger predictor of CHD for them.

Postmenopausal women with high levels of LDL-C are not protected by either estrogen or the generally higher level of HDL-C. The higher levels of LDL-C are most likely associated with a greater percentage of small, dense LDL-C particles. Premenopausal women are relatively protected by estrogen and high level of HDL-C, but, for postmenopausal women, LDL-C level might be a stronger and perhaps more independent risk factor.

Triglycerides and Very-Low-Density Lipoprotein Cholesterol

TG is secreted together with cholesterol and phospholipid in the form of VLDL-C such that 60% to 70% of VLDL-C is TG and 20% cholesterol. Little difference in TG concentrations is noted between genders until puberty. Then, TG increases in both sexes with increasing age, although at a much slower rate in women. TG levels in men actually decrease in middle age, whereas they continue to increase gradually in women. Thus mean levels in women equal those of men by age 70.[19] There are age and gender-related compositional differences in VLDL-C as well. In middle-aged women, the VLDL-C is larger, lighter, and lower in free cholesterol content than the VLDL-C in men of comparable age.[52] The VLDL-C precursors in postmenopausal women are relatively protein and cholesterol poor and richer in TG and thus potentially more atherogenic.

The role of TG in the development of CHD is still the subject of some debate. For the most part, TGs did not show to be a statistically independent predictor of CAD risk when HDL-C and LDL-C are considered in a multivariate analysis.[53] However, studies demonstrated TG as a strong and independent risk factor for women,[15,16] and some experts feel they should be conscientiously addressed.[54]

Previous analysis of data from the LRC follow-up study and the Rancho-Bernardo study demonstrated TG levels to be strong predictors of CVD mortality in women in univariate analysis, but the association is not significant after adjustment for other CVD risk factors.[4,8]

However, Lapidus et al[15] demonstrated the continued importance of TG levels as risk factor for CVD, even after adjustment for multiple risk factors, including TC levels in a longitudinal study involving more than 1400 women. Several other studies support these findings. A large study involving 25 058 middle-aged men and 24 535 middle-aged women over 15 years of follow-up showed that a high level of TG is an independent risk factor for mortality from CHD after adjustment for other risk factors in women but not in men.[55] In the LRC's follow-up study reported by Bass and colleagues,[16] age-adjusted mortality RR in women was 1.6 for TG levels of 200–300 mg/dL and 3.4 for levels >400 mg/dL compared to levels <200 mg/dL. CVD death rates in women with high TG levels were more than 11 times the rates of women with normal TG levels. The risk was stronger if HDL-C level was low (<50 mg/dL).

These findings are consistent with an analysis reported by Castelli[56] from the Framingham study. Castelli points out that patients with high TG and low HDL-C may have TC levels close to normal and may be neglected by most cholesterol screenings. Here again hormonal status may have an important impact. Elevated TG levels are likely to be prevalent in older postmenopausal women where they may be markers for the presence of other atherogenic lipoproteins. We see that, as women age and as they progress through menopause, the percentage of smaller, denser LDL-C rises,[45] and the occurrence of small, dense LDL-C was associated with hypertriglyceridemia.[53] We know that small, dense LDL-C may be more susceptible to oxidation and thus more atherogenic,[46] and its association with TG may explain the predictive power of TG in older postmenopausal women.[57]

Lipoprotein (a)

Lp(a) consists of two components: an LDL-C-like particle with apoprotein B-100 and a hydrophobic protein moiety known as apolipoprotein (a) [apo(a)] linked by a disulfide bond.[58] Apo(a) is synthesized in the liver and is about 80% analogous to plasminogen. Thus Lp(a) is a molecule with both lipoprotein and clotting potential. Lp(a) can be bound by LDL-C receptors and apparently also by plasminogen receptors. Lp(a) is now felt to be an atherogenic lipoprotein.[59,60] A prospective investigation of elevated Lp(a) detected by electrophoresis in the Framingham Heart Study revealed that elevated plasma Lp(a) was a strong, independent predictor of MI in women.[61]

Regarding potential gender-differences in Lp(a) levels and coronary risk, the published studies are inconsistent. Age and sex were not found to influence the plasma levels of Lp(a) according to Maeda et al.[62] No gender differences in Lp(a) levels were observed between men and women, and stepwise discriminant analysis revealed that Lp(a) was a risk factor for the presence of CAD only in men.[60] Another study indicates than Lp(a) levels are higher in women than in men throughout most of the life span, particularly during the postmenopausal period. Steinmetz et al[63] noted that menopause as a factor correlated with increased Lp(a), but this increase was not significant. Solymoss and associates[64] documented that Lp(a) was a significant risk in older women, particularly when it was associated with a high TC to HDL-C-ratio.

All these data suggest women not only manifest age-related alterations in their lipid profile but that menopause additionally contributes to the more atherogenic lipid profile. Jensen et al[36] noted a 6% increase of TC level, an 11% increase of TG level, and a 10% increase of LDL-C within 6 months of menopause and HDL-C levels decreased gradually by 6% within 2 years of menopause. Similarly, Stevenson and colleagues[10] documented that postmenopausal women have significantly higher concentrations of TC, TG, LDL-C, and HDL$_3$-C, whereas those of HDL-C and HDL$_2$-C are significantly lower. These differences were found to be independent of age and body mass index (BMI). Moreover, as noted above, postmenopausal women have higher levels of smaller, denser-type LDL-C, which is particularly atherogenic and higher Lp(a) levels.

Diabetes Mellitus and Hyperinsulinemia

Diabetes mellitus (DM) is the single, most powerful risk factor for CAD in women. Women with diabetes were found to have twice the risk of MI as nondiabetic women of the same age; the risk of MI in diabetic women was found to be equal to that of nondiabetic men of the same age.[65,66] In diabetic women, the incidence of CAD is almost three times that of nondiabetic women as compared with a twofold increase in incidence in men. The relative impact of diabetes on CAD is greater in women. The impact is greater in women than in men, such that a diabetic woman had the same risk of CAD as a nondiabetic man, the diabetes canceling the female hormonal advantage over males. There is also some indication that DM in women predisposes to more lethal coronary events, almost doubling the case fatality rates. In addition to accelerating the pace of CAD, DM may also directly damage the myocardium, predisposing to cardiac failure. Again, this propensity to cardiac failure is more pronounced in diabetic women (Figure 3).

Compared with nondiabetic individuals, diabetics have an adverse lipid profile. TC, LDL-C, and TG levels are higher. HDL-C levels are lower. Interestingly, these differences in lipoprotein levels between diabetics and controls are much more dramatic in women than in men.[67] Numerous other studies confirm Walden's[67] observations.[68–71] Moreover, compared with gender-matched nondiabetics, diabetic women have a greater risk of CAD than do diabetic men.[72] Thus diabetes seems to neutralize much of the protection against CAD conferred in women by their initially favorable lipoprotein profile.

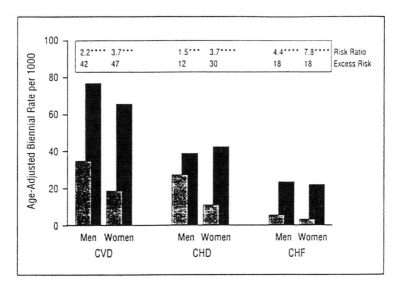

Figure 3. *Risk of cardiovascular events by diabetic status in men and women aged 35–64 years. Data are from the 36-year follow-up of the Framingham Study. Lighter bars, nondiabetic subjects; darker bars, diabetic subjects; CVD, cardiovascular disease; CHD, coronary heart disease; and CHF, congestive heart failure. *** P < 0.001; **** P < 0.0001. Reproduced with permission from Reference 41.*

This is largely explained by insulin activity. In men and women, insulin promotes lipoprotein lipase-mediated TG removal. Thus a deficiency of insulin results in hypertriglyceridemia. Diabetes increases endogenous hepatic VLDL-C secretion. Activity of the LDL-C-receptors is also insulin dependent and is down-regulated in the absence of insulin. Concentrations of HDL-C are increased by insulin administration in men and women with insulin-dependent diabetes.[67,73,74]

Walden and associates[67] concluded that diabetes has a greater adverse effect on TG and lipoprotein cholesterol concentrations in diabetic women than in diabetic men and that this may explain the greater increase in risk of arteriosclerosis for diabetic women. Rates of lipoprotein turnover from the circulation are more rapid in women than in men.[75] These effects are probably sex-hormone mediated. Thus, when lipoprotein processing is impaired by an equivalent loss of insulin efficacy yielding equivalent degrees of hyperglycemia, a greater plasma accumulation of VLDL-C and LDL-C as well as a greater decrease in HDL-C is expected in women than in men.

Hypertension

It was known for decades that hypertension is associated with premature death in both genders. Morbidity due to hypertension occurs either predominantly as a direct consequence of elevated intravascular pressure or via acceleration of atherosclerosis.

The relation between hypertension and atherosclerosis is complex. Hypertension in the presence of other risk factors, in particular hypercholesterolemia, clearly accelerates the progression of atherosclerosis.[76] Among participants of the Second National Health and Nutritional Examination Survey (NHANES II),[77] 40% of persons with hypertension had blood cholesterol levels of >240 mg/dL, and 46% of those with blood cholesterol levels of >240 mg/dL had hypertension. Persons with hypertension and dyslipidemia often have glucose intolerance and upper body obesity. This constellation of risk factors variously referred to as syndrome X, the deadly quartet, familial dyslipidemic hypertension, confers a markedly increased risk of CAD.

In the Walnut Creek Contraceptive Study[78] women between ages 18 and 54 were followed for up to 7 years ($n = 16\ 759$). Hypertension was an independent risk factor for MI, resulting in a threefold increase in risk.

Johnson et al[79] examined 10-year survival rates in 2033 individuals aged 40–69 years in Evans County, Georgia, by sex, race, age, and blood pressure (BP) levels. Survival rates were consistently lower in those who had a systolic BP (SBP) >139 mm Hg or a diastolic BP (DBP) >94 mm Hg. The hypertension-attributable risk for systolic and diastolic hypertension was lower in white women than in black women or in men of both races. For both systolic and diastolic hypertension, the population-attributable fraction in each subgroup was highest for black women. White women had fractions similar to men of both races for systolic hypertension and the lowest fraction for diastolic hypertension among all four gender-race groups.

More recent data are available from NHANES I epidemiological follow-up study. The survival analysis included 2616 white men, 2923 white women, 451 black men, and 509 black women. Twelve year follow-up survival rates for those participants aged 50 years and older were lower in individuals with hypertension than in those with normal BP. This decrease in survival was statistically significant among whites but not among blacks, in part due to the relatively small sample size.

Thus hypertension is a significant risk factor for excess mortality in both sexes. Systolic hypertension is an important predictor of mortality in both black and white women, whereas diastolic hypertension appears to have much greater impact on mortality in black women.

Obesity

Obesity was shown to be an independent risk factor for the development of CAD in women.[80] In a 26-year follow-up of participants in the Framingham Heart Study, relative weight in women was positively and independently associated with coronary disease and coronary and CVD death. For each pound above ideal weight gained over the first 26 years of the Framingham Study, the death rate increased by 2%. Weight gain after the young adult years conveyed an increased risk of CVD in both genders that could not be attributed either to the initial weight or the levels of the risk factors that may have resulted from weight gain.[80] Based upon other epidemiological studies, 30% of the CAD occurring in obese women can be attributed to the excess weight alone, and even mild to moderate overweight increases the risk of coronary disease in middle-aged women.[81]

Obesity was been strongly associated in women with three major risk factors for CAD: non-insulin-dependent DM, hypercholesterolemia, and hypertension.[82] In multiple studies, obesity was found to be associated with significant modifications of the lipid profile, especially higher TG and LDL-C levels.[83–85] These modifications appear relatively more important in women.[84,86] Moreover, HDL-C was also shown to be negatively associated with obesity.[240] Some cross-sectional studies, however, suggest that a higher relative weight[80] or percentage body fat[87] must be present in women, relative to men, to observe these abnormalities in the serum lipids.

In fact, more than generalized obesity, an increase in truncal fat (also called "android" or male pattern obesity) is manifested as a rise in the waist-to-hip ratio and correlates with higher LDL-C and lower HDL-C levels.[87] Central or truncal obesity is associated with both higher BP and hyperinsulinemia, which is thought to result in increases in atherogenic lipoproteins and decreases in HDL-C.[88] The mechanism for this is unclear, although it was hypothesized that it may somehow be related to an increase in peripheral insulin resistance: the portal venous drainage of abdominal fat may induce hepatic insulin resistance, elevated circulating insulin, higher TG levels, and lower HDL-C levels.[89]

Here again, sexual hormones may play an important role. Whereas obese premenopausal women tend to have "gynecoid" or gluteal-femoral fat distribution, menopause was found to promote the development of android or truncal obesity.[90–92] This may be another mechanism by which menopause further influences the atherogenic potential of the lipid profile. In young men, but not in younger women, waist-to-hip ratio correlated with an increase in insulin and was inversely related to HDL-C.[93] This relation appeared to be largely independent of BMI and TGs. The more-efficient, insulin-mediated glucose homeostasis in females imparts a distinct advantage to child-bearing women that is lost in the diabetic state and at least partly explains the gender differential in the atherosclerotic process.[93]

Evidence suggests that the distribution of body fat may be a more determining factor of cardiovascular risk than absolute weight.[92,94] The distribution of adiposity as assessed by waist-to-hip ratio is significantly related to coronary atherosclerosis in both females and males and waist-to-hip ratio was significantly greater in females with CAD.[94] Other investigators similarly observed that individuals with a truncal (android) distribution are at higher risk than those with a gynecoid or peripheral distribution of body fat.[95,96] Lapidus et al[97] showed that an increased waist-to-hip ratio correlates with increased risk of both MI and CVD death in women.

However, the modification of blood lipid levels is not the only factor involved for CAD risk in truncal obesity because the waist-to-hip ratio remains positively correlated with CAD, even after controlling for smoking, hypertension, glucose intolerance, BMI, and especially blood lipids.[95] Perhaps it simply reflects the relative accessibility of omental and peritoneal abdominal fat to the circulation in truncal obesity. For males, the close proximity of the intestinal fat to the circulation can give rapid access to TG-rich lipoproteins such as the chylomicrons, which can be efficiently metabolized for muscle energy, providing an important survival advantage for the otherwise less metabolically efficient male.

Smoking

Whereas diabetes is the most biologically gender-differentiated risk factor for coronary disease in women,[68,98] cigarette smoking may be the most psychologically and sociologically distinguishing risk behavior for men and women. A dose-response relation exists between the number of cigarettes smoked per day and increasing levels of plasma cholesterol for both men and women under age 60.[99] The increase is significantly greater in women; on average, TC increases by 0.33 mg/dL for each cigarette smoked in men and by 0.48 mg/dL in women. Possible mechanisms include enhanced lipolysis, increased levels of plasma free fatty acids, and an antiestrogenic effect of cigarette smoking.[99]

That cigarette smoking increases hepatic reesterification of free fatty acids has been confirmed.[100] This explains the observed smoking-induced increases in serum free fatty concentrations and helps clarify the atherogenic effects of smoking on serum lipids. Insulin-resistance syndrome (IRS) is likely to be an important reason for the increased atherogenicity observed in smokers.[101] Chronic cigarette smokers are insulin resistant, hyperinsulinemic, and dyslipidemic compared with nonsmokers. Furthermore, normotriglyceridemic smokers exhibit an abnormal postprandial lipid metabolism consistent with lipid intolerance. The postprandial hyperlipidemia is characteristic of the IRS, and Axelsen et al[102] suggest that the defect in lipid removal could be related to the low HDL-C in this syndrome.

Finally, it appears that smoking enhances lipid peroxidation. Lipid peroxidation by-products were increased in smokers and fell in those withdrawn from cigarettes.[103] It is quite possible that smoking can cause the oxidative modification of important biological molecules in vivo. Thus, through multiple mechanisms, it appears that smoking impacts the lipid profile and the pathophysiological alteration of lipid. From the gender perspective, smoking neutralizes the advantage of increased HDL-C in both premenopausal and postmenopausal women. Furthermore, the insulin resistance attributable to smoking has profound implications for the woman who has the combination of truncal obesity, glucose intolerance, hypertriglyceridemia, and hypertension.[92]

Sedentary Lifestyle

Increasing evidence shows that inactivity and a sedentary lifestyle may be independent risk factors for the development of CAD in both men and women. Sedentary lifestyle is now recognized as a major risk for CAD.[104] Studies that specifically address the effects of increased physical activity on coronary disease risk factors beyond lipids are uncommon, and up until recently the findings were equivocal.[105] Few studies have addressed the relation of physical fitness or habitual activity level to CVD in women. Powell et al[105] found that only five of 43 studies examining the relation between activity and CAD included and reported data on women. Of these, three reported an increased relative risk of low activity compared with high activity for the end points of angina, MI, and CAD death. However, two large cohort studies, Framingham and Goteburg, failed to find a statistically significant relation between the level of physical activity and subsequent CAD death. Goteburg failed to find a relation between physical activity and either angina or MI.

Even moderately fit women demonstrate significantly better blood sugars, BPs, and anthropometric indices in addition to improvement in the lipid profile when compared to women in the lowest-fitness category.[106]

Women who reported low physical activity at work had a significantly increased age-specific 12-year incidence of overall mortality, as did those who reported low physical activity during leisure hours.[107] The incidence of MI and electrocardiographic changes indicating ischemic heart disease were also increased.

Blair and colleagues[104] studied the effect of physical fitness on all-cause mortality as measured by maximal exercise capacity on treadmill testing in 3120 women. Age-adjusted all-cause mortality rates declined across physical fitness quintiles from 39.5 per 10 000 person-years to 8.5 per 10 000 person-years (slope = −5.5). Whereas the absolute impact on all-cause mortality was greater in men, the negative slope was greater in the females studied (−4.5 vs −5.5, respectively). To influence mortality, the continuance of physical activity may be important. Physical activity was associated with decreased relative risks of MI and sudden coronary death in both women and men but only in those subjects who were exercising for 5 or more years.[108]

Leisure-time physical activity decreases the risk of MI in postmenopausal women.[109] In a population-based, case-control study among women members of an Health Maintenance Organization, after adjusting for confounding factors, the odds ratio for nonfatal MI for women in the fourth (highest) quartile of energy expenditure was 0.40 (95% CI, 0.25–0.63). Interestingly, there was little difference in risk reduction between women in the third and fourth quartiles (1183 vs 3576 kcal per week, respectively), implying that moderate exercise such as 30–45 minutes of walking for exercise is sufficient to impact the risk for acute MI.

Exercise is generally accepted as a mechanism to increase HDL-C and to lower LDL-C levels in men.[40,110] Two large reviews of the literature addressed the impact of exercise on the lipid profile in women.[111,112]

Cross-sectional studies comparing active and sedentary women report a positive association between exercise and HDL-C in both pre- and postmenopausal women. Significant differences between groups remained for HDL-C values when results were adapted for differences in percent body fat. Two studies compared plasma lipids with menopausal status in females runners.[113,114] They showed no differences in HDL-C between pre- and postmenopausal women who exercised, but, when inactive and exercising women were compared, it appeared that younger premenopausal women responded with lipoprotein changes less strongly than older postmenopausal women. Hence, exercise appeared to attenuate the age-related increase in LDL-C and decrease in HDL-C. Otherwise, in these cross-sectional studies, women on hormonal replacement therapy (HRT) who reported exercising had higher HDL-C than sedentary women not on HRT (Table 2).

Results from longitudinal training studies are more difficult to interpret because of experimental design, inadequate type, duration, and intensity of the exercise interventions, or lipid measurements made without regard to the phase of the menstrual cycle or when studies were carried out in women with high baseline HDL-C. Since lipids vary approximately 10% to 25% through the course of the menstrual cycle, menstrual phase should be controlled in premenopausal women when determining lipid changes after an exercise intervention.

Generally, intervention studies suggest that exercise training programs in the absence of other interventions attenuate the age-related increase in TC level but do not cause HDL-C levels to rise appreciably in older women. In younger women, high volumes of exercise (accompanied by decreased body fat) may increase HDL-C. Given the results in the

Table 2

Propsective Studies of the Effect of Exercise Training on HDL-C in Women

Studies	Women (n)	Ages (ys)	Mode	Time	Results
Blumenthal et al[157]	25	45–55	Walk/jog 70% max, 3 times/wk	10 wk	No change, decrease in TC, decrease in body weight
Brownell et al[158]	37	20–57	Aerobic 70% max, 3 times/wk	12 wk	No change, decrease in TC, decrease in body weight
Cauley et al[115]	110	Mean 58, no ERT	Walking 11 km/wk	24 mo	No change
Duncan, et al[159]	59	20–40	Walk/jog 5 km, 5 times/wk	24 wk	Increase in high and low exercise intensity groups, no change in moderate intensity group
Hardman et al[160]	28	Mean 45	Walking 60% max, 55 min/wk	12 mo	Increase, small decrease in TC
Rotkis, 1984	19	24–37	Running 5–6 d/wk	8–15 mo	Increase, no decrease in TC or body weight
Shephard, 1980	65	Mean 34 years	Aerobic 70% max, 3 times/wk	6 mo	No change, decrease in TC, decrease in percent body fat

cross-sectional studies, we note that two of the longitudinal investigations do not compare pre- and postmenopausal women but focus on post-menopausal women. In one study the exercise intensity was low.[115] The other study included few early postmenopausal women.[116]

All of the above mentioned studies concentrated on women. Studies including both men and women could provide some insight about the contribution that sex hormones provide for the regulation of the lipopro-tein-regulating response to exercise. One review of several cross-sectional and longitudinal studies indicated a consistently weaker lipoprotein re-sponse to exercise in premenopausal women compared to men of the same age.[117] Similar results were reported by Donahue et al.[93] In this study, self-reported exercise levels correlated less well with both HDL-C and TG levels in women than in men. Recent data published by Lavie and Milani[118] support a similar conclusion. They studied the effects of cardiac rehabilitation and exercise training on exercise capacity, coronary risk fac-tors, behavioral characteristics, and quality-of-life measures in women. A subgroup of 83 women was compared with 375 men. All patients were referred after a major ischemic CHD event (patients taking lipid-lowering medications were excluded). Female patients had statistically significant improvements in percent body fat ($P < 0.001$) and exercise capacity ($P < 0.0001$), although improvement in BMI and lipids were not significant. For men, improvements were statistically significant for all parameters, (TG, $P < 0.01$; HDL-C, $P < 0.0001$; LDL-C/HDL-C, $P < 0.001$). Within the framework of cardiac rehabilitation, similar results regarding exercise response were reported by Cannistra et al,[119] who found that women have similar rates of exercise compliance and achieve similar improvement in functional capacity with training as men. Neither study addressed the specific issue of hormonal status in the female subjects.

Nonclassical Risk Factors

Psychosocial Issues Related to Gender

Socioeconomic factors, including educational attainment, are an im-portant contributing factor to coronary disease risk. Lapidus and Bengts-son[107] reported a significant age-specific correlation between low socio-economic status according to the husband's occupation, but not between the socioeconomic status of the women themselves, and MI. Women with a low educational level had a significantly increased age-specific incidence of angina pectoris. There was no significant correlation between marital status or number of children and incidence of ischemic heart disease or overall mortality. Multivariate analyses showed that the association be-tween low educational level and incidence of angina pectoris was independent of socioeconomic group itself, cigarette smoking, SBP, indices of obesity, serum TGs, and serum cholesterol.[107]

Matthews et al[120] investigated the association between educational attainment and biological and behavioral risk factors for CHD in a community sample of 2138 middle-aged, perimenopausal women. Among 541 eligible participants, the lower the education level the women reported, the more atherogenic was their risk factor profile, including higher SBP, LDL-C, apo B, TGs, fasting and 2-hour postprandial glucose values, body mass indices, and lower HDL-C and HDL-C/LDL-C ratio. The attainment of lower educational level also correlated with being a cigarette smoker, participating in little physical exercise, and consuming alcohol less than 1 day per week. They more often reported on standardized psychological tests being type B, angry, pessimistic, depressed, and dissatisfied with their jobs and having little social support and self-esteem. Similar associations were obtained between educational attainment and risk factors reported by the 1588 nonparticipants during the telephone screening interview. These results suggest many biological and behavioral factors by which women with little education are at elevated risk for CHD; thus education may be a potentially important public health intervention for women.[120]

These findings were corroborated by Tenconi et al,[121] who studied 2871 women, aged 20–59 years, from nine different Italian communities. The relation between educational level and several lifestyle factors at risk for CHD, including smoking, alcohol consumption, dietary fat intake, sedentary behavior at work and leisure, and the association between education and certain CHD risk factors (ie, TC, HDL-C, TGs, SBP and DBP, and BMI) were compared. The data were analyzed separately according to location in northern, central, and southern Italy. The results show that educational level is often associated with the lifestyle factors considered. The association was positive for both men and women for leisure-exercise activity but only for women with respect to smoking. The age-adjusted mean levels of the CHD risk factors did show some significant differences among subjects with different educational levels, although geographical location influenced this, except for BMI in women, which appears negatively associated to education in all areas. These differences weakened after adjustments were made for cigarette smoking, wine consumption, and dietary fat intake. Education seems to play a determining role in lifestyle; however, its direct and indirect effects on some major CHD risk factors are somewhat different according to geographic locale and different socioeconomic conditions.[121]

Menopause as a Risk Factor

No risk factor is as specific for women as hormonal status. Multiple studies show that a direct relation does exist between menopause and risk of CAD in women.[5,28,122–126] In the Framingham study, the incidence of CHD was twice as high in postmenopausal women compared with pre-menopausal women of the same age.[122] In a number of other studies, the hormonal change that occurs as a result of menopause increases signifi-cantly the risk of CAD, and above all the relation exists even after con-trolling for age. Rosenberg et al,[28] in a study of 121 964 nurses who com-pleted a mailed questionnaire, found 2.8 times the risk of MI in women who had natural menopause before age 35 compared with age-matched controls. The impact of menopause was greater if women were younger when experiencing the change; the risk decreased to 1.1 for natural menopause between age 35 and 39 and was 0.9 for those going through menopause at age 45 or over (Figure 4).

As well as the overall risk for CAD, the severity of CAD is increased in postmenopausal women. Data from the Framingham study showed a rise in CAD incidence and a dramatic increase in severity.[123] In a cohort of 2873 women who were followed up for 24 years, no premenopausal women developed an MI or died of CAD, but such events were common in postmenopausal women even under 55 years of age. Forty percent of the patients presented with these serious manifestations of CAD, whether menopause was either natural or surgically induced. Some authorities feel

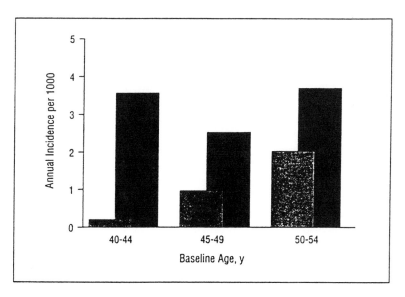

Figure 4. *The annual incidence of CHD according to menopausal status at the bi-ennial examination in women aged 40–54 years at study entry. Data from the 18-year follow-up of the Framingham Study. **Lighter bars,** premenopausal women; **darker bars,** menopausal women. The overall RR is 4.17; P < 0.001. Reproduced with permission from Reference 41.*

it is difficult to establish a cause and effect relation because the incidence of ischemic heart disease does not peak in women until they reach their 70s or 80s, ie, approximately 15–25 years after menopause.[127] Gorodeski[126] noted that, although the menopause denotes the cessation of menses, it can be ascertained only in retrospect by the termination of menstrual periods for at least a year. However, the hormonal processes associated with spontaneous menopause precede the event itself by several years. Thus defining the time course of menopause is difficult due to lack of a specific biological marker. Although some of the attributable risk correlates to the age of menopause, it does not necessarily follow that the risk correlates with the hormonal changes themselves.

Modification of Risk Factors in Women

Primary Prevention or Prevention Before a Coronary Event

The NCEP provided guidelines for identification of persons at high risk of CHD because of lipid abnormalities.[128] Primary prevention focuses on reducing risk factors in large populations of women who have no evidence of disease but who have dyslipidemia. Primary prevention of CVD in women is problematic and faces obstacles to its implementation for several reasons. Women themselves have difficulty recognizing the benefits of the recommendations. The issue is often raised that there is insufficient clinical trials data to justify cholesterol-lowering interventions in women, since most studies were performed in male subjects. The NCEP recommendations may be less appropriate for women in that some who are screened may have TC levels in the desirable range but LDL-C or HDL-C levels that put them at risk.[129]

The guidelines provide for the detection, evaluation, and treatment of hypercholesterolemia and related disorders. In these recommendations, TC and HDL-C are the primary screening parameters. Patients are categorized by age, gender, hormonal status, number of risk factors, and fasting LDL-C level.[43] Patients with two or more risk factors are considered to be at "high risk." Evaluation beyond TC and HDL-C measurement is recommended for those with screening TC levels >240 mg/dL or TC levels of 200–239 mg/dL associated with other risk factors or established CAD. An HDL-C level >60 mg/dL allows "credit" of one risk factor; on the other hand, individuals with low levels of HDL-C (<35 mg/dL) are considered to have an additional risk factor, and lipoprotein analysis is recommended. Neither TC nor HDL-C are parameters actually targeted for intervention; only LDL-C is specifically targeted. Little consideration for gender is present in the guideline as originally published, and the normal values for lipoproteins are considered to be the same for men and women.

Dietary modification is recommended for low-risk patients (one risk factor) with LDL-C levels >160 mg/dL and high-risk patients (two or more risk factors) with LDL-C levels <160 mg/dL. Low-risk patients whose LDL-C levels reach 190 mg/dL or high-risk patients whose LDL-C levels reach 160 mg/dL are recommended to start drug therapy. Drug therapy is not recommended in men under age 35 or in premenopausal women unless LDL-C levels are >220 mg/dL. The guidelines set higher LDL-C thresholds for drug intervention in premenopausal women (LDL-C >220 mg/dL) than in postmenopausal women (LDL-C <190 mg/dL). HRT is currently recommended by NCEP as an option for postmenopausal women with hypercholesterolemia.

The NCEP guidelines prove problematic in women for the following reasons. First, treatment is based on LDL-C levels, which are probably less important in women than other lipoproteins.[16] Second, a cutoff of 35 mg/dL is used for HDL-C, instead of the more-relevant level of 45 mg/dL or 50 mg/dL in womenm, considering that 50 mg/dL is in fact an average HDL-C value for women. Third, TG levels (and for that matter, diabetes) are not considered to be independent risk factors, where they were demonstrated to be a risk in certain subsets of women. Nonpharmacologic therapy (weight reduction, alcohol restriction, and increased physical activity) is recommended for all patients with elevated TG. Drugs are started to lower TG only if other lipoprotein abnormalities are present, if TGs are very high (>1000 mg/dL) to prevent acute pancreatitis, or if there is a personal family history of CHD or other manifestations of atherosclerosis.

Secondary Prevention or Prevention After a Coronary Event

Secondary prevention is aimed at individuals who already have CAD and are therefore at highest risk for developing progressive disease. Women in this group generally accept treatment to reduce risk. Lipoprotein analysis is required in all patients, but again classification is based on LDL-C. For these patients, the optimal LDL-C is 100 mg/dL or less. Above this value, a cholesterol-lowering therapy must be initiated: a nonpharmacologic approach between 100 mg/dL and 130 mg/dL, drug therapy when LDL-C is 130 mg/dL despite a trial of dietary therapy, and physical activity.

Lowering LDL-C below 100 mg/dL will result in a 25% reduction in risk of recurrent MI and 9% reduction in CHD mortality.[130] Drugs to lower TG are recommended for all patients with elevated TG (>200 mg/dL) in the context of secondary prevention. Finally, HRT maintains its position between diet and lipid-lowering drugs. However, HRT has an even greater benefit in secondary prevention than in primary prevention of CHD. There is a 73% reduction in CHD mortality in users of postmenopausal estrogen who have CAD at baseline, compared to the 55% reduction seen in all women regardless of baseline CAD status.[4]

The NCEP recommendations abound with gender discrepancies, but so do virtually all of the standard therapies prescribed to improve the lipid profile in women.

Diet

The NCEP dietary intervention should occur in two steps. Step I involves an intake of saturated fat of 8% to 10% of total calories, 30% or less of the total calories should be derived from fat, and <300 mg of cholesterol per day. If this diet proves inadequate to achieve the goals, the patient should proceed to the step-II diet. Step II calls for further reductions in saturated fat intake to <7% of calories and in cholesterol to <200 mg/day. The polyunsaturated/saturated fat ratio should thus be increased.

All reduced fat diets have a beneficial effect on LDL-C but consistently also reduce HDL-C, which is disadvantageous for women.[131–133] Furthermore, the literature observes specific gender differences for diet responsiveness.[134,135]

TC and LDL-C response to diet appear relatively similar for both sexes in multiple studies.[135–138] Two studies in women who switched from a "typical American diet" to the NCEP step-I diet showed that LDL-C levels fell by 32% and 29%, respectively, and HDL-C levels decreased by 16% and 20%.[134,139] Two similar studies in men showed decreases in LDL-C of 24% and 26% and either no change or a nonsignificant 12% fall in HDL-C, respectively.[140,141] These results suggest that LDL-C falls comparably in men and women with dietary modification, but that the decrease of HDL-C is more drastic in women. However, for HDL-C, a more significant decrease was demonstrated in women.[136,137] Prospective studies that compare men and women following a comparable dietary protocol are necessary for a real gender analysis.

Furthermore, menopausal status may affect dietary responsiveness. In one small study, a similar response to diet was observed in both pre- and postmenopausal women.[142] A large study of 2222 postmenopausal women compared men of corresponding ages and found a greater decline in LDL-C and TG levels in men than in women and a greater decline in HDL-C levels in women than in men when all subjects followed a very low-fat diet.[136] Jenkins et al[143] made a similar observation in men and postmenopausal women who followed a low-fat diet high in soluble fiber.

From the woman's perspective, the most important problem with diet therapy appears to be the accompanying decrease of HDL-C. The decrease is more severe in women and even more extreme in postmenopausal women. Given that the inverse relation of HDL-C to cardiac events may be more emphatic in women than the adverse risk imparted by LDL-C, the conclusion is that diet may have opposite the desired effect. As suggested by Crouse,[144] for women with a very high LDL-C and who are at risk for CHD, all available techniques must be used to lower LDL-C. For low-risk women, unless they have a weight problem, the benefits of a low-fat diet are far from clear.

A monounsaturated-fat diet may avoid the decrease in HDL-C caused by a diet high in polyunsatured fat or restriction of total fat calories.[141,145] Furthermore, the addition of exercise to the dietary regimen may resist the inevitable fall in HDL-C.[146]

Two primary prevention studies conducted more than two decades ago assessed the efficacy of diet on CHD morbidity and mortality in women. In the study by Miettinen et al,[147] institutionalized men and women were fed a low-cholesterol diet for 6 years. In the men, TC decreased 12% to 18% and resulted in a significant reduction in CHD mortality. In the women, TC decreased similarly and CHD mortality tended to be lower in comparison to the control group. In a similar study conducted by Frantz et al,[148] TC levels decreased significantly in response to a 2-year dietary intervention, although coronary mortality was unchanged, perhaps because of the relatively short duration of the study. Thus the data for women are limited concerning the impact of diet on CHD morbidity and mortality.

Weight Loss

As with those involving dietary compositional changes, studies of weight loss suggest that the desirable intervention may not necessarily be associated with favorable changes in lipoproteins.

Dattilo and Kris-Etherton[149] analyzed 70 studies of the effects of weight reduction on blood lipids. They noted that 30% of studies included only women, 27% included only men, and 44% did not specify the gender. Overall, HDL-C increased twofold in both males and females, but TG showed a greater decrease in males. Other studies also indicate that serum lipid responses to weight loss differ for women compared to men. Brownell and Stunkard[150] showed that approximately a 10% reduction in body weight caused HDL-C to rise in men, but to fall slightly in women, and LDL-C levels declined in both men and women but to a greater extent in men. Wood et al[146] reported a decrease in HDL-C in overweight women but not in overweight men. HDL-C levels remained about the same in women who exercised and dieted and were higher than in the women who only dieted but not higher than in the controls. Why this difference? LaRosa[152] suggests that the presence of excess truncal fat in both men and women correlates with increases in LDL-C and decreases in HDL-C, accounting for the increase risk of CHD observed in central obesity.[90,97] We saw that postmenopausal women have a tendency for truncal fat disposition. Adipose tissue in postmenopausal women can serve as a source of estrogen synthesis.[151] Thus the benefits of weight reduction in older women may be offset by the loss of estrogen-producing adipose tissue. As an additional consequence, the expected increases in HDL-C and decline in LDL-C with weight loss may be less evident than in men.

Exercise

Exercise is generally accepted as a mechanism to increase HDL-C and to lower LDL-C levels in men.[110,153] Although a number of studies were carried out in women, they unfortunately failed to consider potential confounders such as hormonal status and body composition. Two large reviews of the literature addressed the impact of exercise on the lipid profile in women.[111,112]

Exercise improves the lipid profile but probably less strongly for women than for men. Again, hormonal status may influence the response. Postmenopausal women seem to exhibit a greater response to exercise, even if some training studies are controversial. Exercise at least seems to attenuate the age-related modifications in the lipid profile. Another interesting finding is that exercise programs of moderate intensity appear to modify the HDL-C lowering effect of a hypocaloric fat-restricted diet.[146] These two nonpharmacologic therapies should be strongly encouraged for women needing primary or secondary prevention measures.

The physiological reasons for differences between men and women and their lipoprotein response to diet, weight loss, and exercise are not well defined. The role of circulating estrogen could be involved. LaRosa[152] proposes that further investigations should include studies of different responses to these therapeutic modalities in postmenopausal women with and without exogenous hormone replacement.

In reviews on the effects of cardiac rehabilitation on morbidity and mortality, reductions in all-cause mortality of 20% to 24% and in CHD mortality by 23% to 25% among rehabilitation-program participants were demonstrated.[154,155] Only three of the 22 studies that were reviewed included women, however, and, in these three studies, women made up only 3% (143 of 4554 patients) of the entire sample. No separate analyses were performed related to the effect of participation in cardiac rehabilitation programs on clinical outcomes in women. Thus inadequate data exist for determining whether women experience reductions in CVD similar to those in men who participate in formal cardiac rehabilitation.

Generally, intervention studies suggest that exercise training programs in the absence of other interventions attenuate the age-related increase in TC level but do not cause HDL-C levels to rise appreciably in older women. In younger women, high volumes of exercise (accompanied by decreased body fat) may increase HDL-C. Given the results in the cross-sectional studies, we note that two of the longitudinal investigations do not compare pre- and postmenopausal women but focus on post-menopausal women. In one study the exercise intensity was low.[115] The other study included few early-postmenopausal women.[116]

All of the above mentioned studies concentrated on women. Studies including both men and women could provide some insight about the contribution that sex hormones provide for the regulation of the lipoprotein-regulating response to exercise. One review of several cross-sectional and longitudinal studies indicated a consistently weaker lipoprotein response to exercise in premenopausal women compared to men of the same age.[117] Similar results were reported by Donahue et al.[156] In this study, self-reported exercise levels correlated less well with both HDL-C and TG levels in women than in men. Recent data published by Lavie and Milani[118] support a similar conclusion. They studied the effects of cardiac rehabilitation and exercise training on exercise capacity, coronary risk factors, behavioral characteristics, and quality-of-life measures in women. A subgroup of 83 women was compared with 375 men. All patients were referred after a major ischemic CHD event (patients taking lipid-lowering medications were excluded). Female patients had statistically significant improvements in percent body fat ($P < 0.001$) and exercise capacity ($P < 0.0001$), although improvement in BMI and lipids were not significant. For men, improvements were statistically significant for all parameters, (TG, $P < 0.01$; HDL-C, $P < 0.0001$; LDL-C/HDL-C, $P < 0.001$). Within the framework of cardiac rehabilitation, similar results regarding exercise response were reported by Cannistra et al,[119] who found that women have similar rates of exercise compliance and achieve similar improvement in functional capacity with training as men. Neither study addressed the specific issue of hormonal status in the female subjects.

Cholesterol-Altering Drugs

Few of the interventional studies include women, and very few analyze women in a separate group. Recent data suggest a significant decrease in coronary morbidity and mortality with the aggressive lowering of cholesterol levels in women.

Primary Prevention

Howes and Simons[161] recently reviewed the benefit of drug intervention for hypercholesterolemia. They retained as pivotal only those of sufficient size and duration and those achieving sufficient cholesterol reduction to likely have a statistically significant outcome. In four such primary prevention studies,[162–165] CHD morbidity was reduced in the range 19% to 45%, but women were included in only one.[162] It is of interest that the latter study evaluated the effects of Colestipol in similar doses on both males and females with similar initial cholesterol levels and achieved a like reduction in cholesterol levels over a similar period of time. A significant reduction in both CHD morbidity and mortality was demonstrated in men, but in women no significant change in either morbidity or mortality was observed. The women in this study were older than the male subjects (57 vs 50). The women who received the placebo had a CAD mortality rate of 5.1/1000 per year, compared to 14.6/1000 per year for the men; furthermore, nearly 20% of the women in this study had CAD at entry, and analysis of morbidity and mortality were not done separately for this subgroup.[162]

Two other studies included women and involved a substantial number of patients, but CHD morbidity and mortality were not analyzed.[166] In a randomized study on 431 elderly patients (mean age was 71) with hypercholesterolemia, 71% of whom were women, two doses of lovastatin were compared to placebo. TC fell 17% to 20%, LDL 24% to 28%, and TG 4.4% to 9.9%. HDL-C levels rose 7.0% to 9.0%. No changes were observed in the placebo group. Gender, race, and age did not significantly affect responses. However, in another study of 1815 patients, 43.1% of whom were women, a more-favorable impact on lipid profile was observed in women taking fluvastatin compared to placebo than in men.[167] Although a similar impact of therapy was observed for TG, there was stronger effect on LDL-C and HDL-C in women than in the men; in women, the change from baseline was −26.7% for LDL-C and +5.3% for HDL-C.

Thus, whereas the impact of drug therapy appears comparable or even more effective in altering lipid levels in women compared with men, the evidence is not completely certain, and further investigation will be required before it can be concluded that primary treatment reduces CAD morbidity or mortality similarly in men and women.

Secondary Prevention

Howes also identified four pivotal studies that addressed secondary prevention. These studies are of smaller size than those performed before the event, but they suggest that drug therapy produces a beneficial reduction in CHD morbidity and mortality in patients with established CAD.[168–171] In two of these studies, women were analyzed separately, and clofibrate therapy appeared to lead to a reduction, although it did not achieve statistical significance.[170,171] A study of serial coronary angiograms in patients with familial hypercholesterolemia who were treated aggressively with drugs showed that, for a similar degree of reduction of LDL-

C and rise of HDL-C, the women appeared to have more regression of coronary atherosclerosis than the male subjects.[172]

The Scandinavian Simvastatin Survival Study of 4444 patients, 18% of whom were women, was designed to evaluate the effect of cholesterol lowering with simvastatin on mortality and morbidity in patients with CHD.[173] Over the 5.4-year median follow-up period, simvastatin produced mean changes in TC, LDL-C, and HDL-C of −25%, −35%, and +8%, respectively. The probability that a woman avoided a major coronary event was 77.5% in the placebo group and 85.1% in the treatment group. Total mortality and risk for a major coronary event were similar for both genders. Other benefits of treatment included a 37% reduction ($P < 0.00001$) in the risk of undergoing myocardial revascularization procedures.

Of particular importance is the Cholesterol and Recurrent Events (CARE) Study. CARE was specifically designed to address the question of whether LDL-C lowering in patients with CHD and normal or only mildly elevated LDL-C concentrations provided clinical benefit. Mean baseline LDL-C in the CARE study was 139 mg/dL. A 24% reduction in the study's primary end point of CHD death or nonfatal MI was observed ($P < 0.002$). Because a large portion of the population with CAD does not have severely elevated cholesterol, risk reduction in this group could have major public health implications. Significantly, a greater reduction in CHD death and nonfatal MI was observed in the subset of women in this study compared to men. Formal subset analysis on women is pending. These data corroborate the findings from other trials that the benefits of lipid-lowering therapy start to appear relatively soon after the initiation of therapy. Of particular significance is the applicability of these results to patients with lipid levels representative of the general population and the implication that women may in fact have a greater benefit from cholesterol-reduction interventions.

All in all, there is relatively little information about the effects of cholesterol-lowering drug therapy in women with known CAD when compared to data in men. Large-scale studies with sufficient numbers of female subjects are warranted. Furthermore, it would be interesting to see greater focus on HDL-C and TG modification, which may be relatively more important parameters in women, and to study more precisely the impact of drugs on lipoprotein composition.

Two small studies looked at LDL-C, LDL-C/HDL-C ratios, and HDL-subtypes. In a study by Clifton and associates,[135] 12 men and 13 women with hypercholesterolemia participated in a 20-week controlled crossover trial to assess the interaction among dietary fat intake, gender, and a 3-hydroxy-3-methylglutaryl coenzyme A-reductase inhibitor, simvastatin. Gender differences were noted with men demonstrating only a 27% fall in LDL-C with simvastatin while consuming a high-fat (40% of caloric intake as fat) diet compared to women with a 35% reduction. In men, the lowest LDL-C/HDL-C ratio was achieved with simvastatin on a low-fat diet (22% of caloric intake as fat).

Gender differences in the effect of simvastatin on HDL-C were confined to HDL_3-C, although the drug raised HDL_2-C in both men and women on the low-fat diet. Simvastatin was responsible for an 11% increase in HDL_3-C in men, particularly when on a low-fat diet, but did not affect HDL_3-C in women. An important diet-drug interaction was seen in TG response, with a 17% to 20% lowering when the subjects were on a low-fat diet. There was also a gender-specific difference in response to dietary fat change, with men demonstrating a 19% decrease in TGs with dietary fat reduction while on simvastatin, whereas women showed a 9% increase (not statistically significant). Men also responded more favorably to a reduction in dietary fat intake with at least twofold greater fall in plasma cholesterol than was seen in women.

Gemfibrozil could be particularly advantageous in postmenopausal women according to a study by Yuan et al[174] that demonstrates a significant alteration in the composition and distribution of LDL subspecies including a shift from small, dense LDL-C particles to large, less-dense particles in hypertriglyceridemic patients. The study was performed as a randomized, double-blind, crossover design with 12-week periods of placebo and gemfibrozil with an intervening washout period. The study unfortunately only involved a small number of patients, and the men and women were not analyzed separately.

Antioxidant Therapy

Antioxidants may suppress the formation of oxidized LDL and thereby influence the formation of atherosclerotic plaque. Both epidemiological and laboratory studies suggest that antioxidants can provide a protective effect on coronary arteries.

The Nurses' Health Study assessed the relative risk of a major CAD event in 87 245 female nurses followed for up to 8 years.[175] Relative risk of major coronary disease of those in the lowest quintile of vitamin E intake was compared with risk in the highest quintile (RR = 0.66 after adjustment for age and smoking). Adjustment for a variety of other coronary risk factors and nutrients, including other antioxidants, had little effect on the results. As the authors point out, "Although these prospective data do not prove a cause-and-effect relation, they suggest that among middle-aged women the use of vitamin E supplements is associated with a reduced risk of coronary heart disease."

No large randomized clinical trials of antioxidants were yet reported, albeit two such trials, the Women's Health Initiative (WHI) and an ancillary Trial of Antioxidant Therapy, are in progress.

Hormonal Replacement Therapy

Of much greater potential significance is the use of exogenous gonadal hormones, an intervention that should be unique to women that affects both lipoproteins as well as CHD risk.[176,177] These drugs are among the most commonly prescribed in women today. Ironically, the first clinical trial that addressed the issue was performed in men and demonstrated an adverse effect of HRT in males with prior MI. Postmenopausal women may be prescribed HRT, either as unopposed estrogen or, increasingly, as combinations of estrogen and progestin.

Impact on the Lipid Profile

Several cross-sectional and longitudinal studies assessed the influence of HRT on plasma lipoprotein concentrations. These were recently reviewed.[178] Estrogens and progestins appear to affect circulating lipoproteins differently.

Estrogens generally have favorable effects on lipoprotein levels: LDL-C generally decreases anywhere from 6% to 20%; thus the magnitude of the LDL-C response appears to be variable. Estrogen was not reported to effect any significant change in LDL-C particle size, however.[179] HDL-C levels (principally HDL_2-C), increases from 10% to 18% with or without an apparent dose effect.[7]

Oral administration of estrogen replacement may be more effective than cutaneous absorption or gel administration. In fact, the estrogen-associated increase in HDL-C may require a nonphysiological first pass through the liver to induce lipid-related enzymes. When estrogen is administered transcutaneously, the LDL-C levels are lowered, but the HDL-C levels are not changed significantly.[180–182] Unfortunately, TG and VLDL-C levels increase in a dose-dependent manner (mean value 24%). Thus women with primary hypertriglyceridemia may develop severe hyperlipemia on estrogen replacement therapy.[183] In such patients, estrogens should be used with caution after therapeutic reduction of TG levels to <500 mg/dL.

Progestins have opposite effects from estrogens and thus may limit the desirable effects of estrogens. The addition of a progestin to estrogen replacement regimens to prevent uterine hyperplasia is now widely accepted as necessary in women with an intact uterus.[184] Furthermore, the effects of added progestins is a function of the dose and androgenicity of the particular preparation. The C-21 progestins, including medroxyprogesterone, which is the most commonly used noncontraceptive progestin in the United States, are less androgenic than the 19-NOR agents. The stronger the progestin, the less the LDL-C decrease and HDL-C increase induced by the estrogen.[185] Nabulsi et al[186] showed that a progestin combined with estrogen may have minimal pernicious effect on LDL-C and HDL-C concentrations compared to estrogens used alone (Table 3).

Haarbo et al[188] note that "while the addition of a progestin agent may partially influence the beneficial effects of estrogens on lipid levels, it was proved that most progesterone containing hormonal replacement regimens were shown to produce favorable change in the lipid profile." Progestin has its own desirable effect: it opposes the increase of TG up to 30% that is induced by estrogen when used alone.[189,190]

One year of therapy with an estrogen-progestin combination (conjugated equine estrogen and medroxy progesterone acetate) substantially reduced plasma levels of Lp(a) according to a preliminary report from Soma and colleagues.[191] If this result is confirmed, HRT may prove to be one of the more-effective methods available for reducing Lp(a) concentrations in women.

With regard to mechanisms of action, estrogen positively influences the rate of removal of chylomicron remnants from the liver and

Table 3

Adjusted Physiological CVD Risk Factors in Women Using Different Postmenopausal Replacement Hormones

	Nonusers		Current		P
	Past	Never	Estrogen	E_2 + Pg	Users vs. Nonusers
TG	123	120	141	131	<0.001
LDL-C:	141	141	125	127	<0.001
HDL-C	58	58	67	66	<0.001
HDL_2-C	17	16	21	21	<0.001
Apo A-I	141	140	159	156	<0.001
Apo B	95	95	91	92	<0.015
Lp(a)	114	116	101	101	<0.006
Fibrinogen	3.1	3.2	3.0	3.0	<0.001
Factor VII	126	125	136	127*	<0.001
Factor VIII	133	136	134	132	NS
von Willebrand factor	119	121	119	118	NS
Antithrombin III	114	115	110	113	<0.001
Protein C	3.3	3.3	3.5	3.3	NS
Glucose	99	99	97	95	<0.001
Insulin	11.7	11.3	10.0	10.5	<0.001
BP					
Systolic	121	122	121	120	NS
Diastolic	72	72	72	72	NS

* $P < 0.001$ estrogen versus estrogen + progestin.

NS, not significant.

Reproduced with permission from Reference 187.

increases the rate of hepatic uptake of VLDL-C remnants and LDL-C uptake by the estrogen up-regulated LDL-C receptors.[192] The susceptibility of LDL-C to oxidation was recently demonstrated to be reduced in postmenopausal women taking estrogen.[193] There is little information about the estrogen-mediated metabolic effects on HDL-C. However, two mechanisms seem to be involved: an increased apo A-1 production and reduced hepatic lipase activity. These two mechanisms induce a preferential increase of HDL_2-C.[194,195] Gerhard and Ganz[196] propose that the decrease in cardiovascular events seen in men who experience lipid-profile modifications in several large-scale studies indicate that the beneficial changes in lipoprotein levels resulting from estrogen replacement therapy should account for a 25% to 50% risk reduction, suggesting that additional factors are involved. The effect of estrogen as a secondary prevention of CHD is rapid, on the order of weeks to months rather than years. Since a benefit is seen before the lipid levels have an opportunity to cause specific regression of coronary artery lesions, it is likely that the improvement are in part due to faster-acting nonatherogenic effects.

Gerhard and Ganz reviewed several of the potential mechanisms in their recent editorial.[196] Estrogen appears to influence endothelially mediated vasoregulatory activity. Long-term estrogen replacement therapy was shown to improve endothelium-dependent vasodilatation in hypercholesterolemic postmenopausal women.[197] Administration of estrogen to postmenopausal women attenuates abnormal coronary endothelium-dependent relaxation.[198] Serum nitrate and nitrite levels are higher in postmenopausal women receiving long-term estrogen therapy, suggesting enhanced production of nitric oxide, which is an endothelium-derived vasodilator.[199] In addition, estrogen appears to modulate the reactivity of vascular smooth muscle by increasing potassium conductance.[200] Recently, Gilligan and associates[201] demonstrated that estrogen acutely and selectively potentiates coronary endothelium-dependent vasodilatation in postmenopausal women.

Collins et al[202] report that coronary vasodilatation in response to acetylcholine administration is restored 20 minutes after administration of estradiol-17β in postmenopausal women with coronary disease but not in men. They conclude that an enhancement of endothelium-dependent relaxation by natural estrogen may be important in postmenopausal women with established CHD.

Extracellular matrix composition may be modified by estrogen therapy, affecting its contribution to vessel wall stability.[203] Under in vitro conditions, estrogen treatment enhances migration and proliferation of endothelial cells and facilitates their organization into tubular networks, steps that are critical for angiogenesis.[204] This in vitro model suggests that estrogen potentiates the angiogenic effect of fibroblast growth factor. The applicability of these findings in patients with clinical coronary disease must be further investigated.

The beneficial effects of HRT on CHD morbidity and mortality are starting to be appreciated.[205] A number of prospective, mostly observational studies were published. Several, encompassing many thousands of women, were reviewed by Kuhn and Rackley.[206] The studies suggest that the risk of CHD is reduced by about 35% to 50% among healthy postmenopausal women who take estrogen. Among women who already have CHD, the degree of protection appears to be even more substantial— several studies reported up to an 80% reduction in the risk for subsequent CAD events. Although one of the earliest reports from the Framingham study noted that the relative risk of cardiovascular events was increased in estrogen users,[207] a reanalysis of these data that corrected for errors in reporting of estrogen use, a nonsignificant protective effect of estrogen (RR = 0.40) was noted in younger women, whereas there was a nonsignificant adverse effect (RR = 1.8) in women aged 50–59 years.[127]

In the Nurses' Health Study, the largest prospective study published to date involving more than 48 000 postmenopausal women, a highly significant reduction in MI or death was noted (RR = 0.56) among postmenopausal estrogen users.[205] Significant reductions were noted even after adjustment for other risk factors and regardless of cause of menopause (natural or surgical), duration of estrogen use, or age. Indeed, several studies suggest that postmenopausal estrogen use may be associated with lower risk of CHD in women well into the eighth decade of life. In both the LRC[3] and in the Leisure World Study,[208] the relative risk of CHD was lower in hormone-using women in each age group compared with nonusers.

Most recently, Ettinger and associates[209] produced evidence that long-term estrogen replacement therapy reduces the rate of death from all causes and provides even greater benefit with respect to reducing cardiovascular events. They studied the health outcomes of 454 women, one-half of whom started HRT, and an age-matched control group, one-half of whom did not. Among those women in the control group, there were 87 deaths from all causes and, in the half using HRT, there were 53 deaths.

A beneficial effect of HRT was observed in angiographic studies as well. Sullivan,[210] in a study of more than 2000 women, showed that postmenopausal estrogen use significantly reduced the risk of angiographically significant CAD. Similar results were noted by McFarland et al[211] in 345 postmenopausal women who underwent coronary angiography for suspected CAD. Gruchow et al[212] observed that estrogen nonusers were twice as likely as users to have moderate or severe occlusion. Furthermore, in nonusers, the likelihood of occlusion increased with age, whereas in users no age trend was evident. Kuhn and Rackley[206] reported significant CAD in only 22% of women taking estrogens compared with 68% of those who were not. HRT was associated with a significantly higher mean HDL-C level and lower mean TC/HDL-C ratio and an 87% reduction in the prevalence of CHD.

Critics of these studies point out that they are not randomized and that some of the benefits are likely related to selection bias.[2] However, these trials, conducted at various centers in different countries using various designs, involving thousands of women, yielded remarkably consistent results. One randomized, placebo-controlled, long-term, clinical trial that examines HRT and CHD is the study performed by Nachtigall and colleagues.[213,214] The relative risk of heart attack in the group treated with estrogen and progestin in combination was one-third that in the placebo group. This difference, although not statistically significant given the numbers studied (84 subject pairs), is consistent with the results of most of the prospective but less stringently designed trials.

It is true that the vast majority of reports on HRT were based on observational and not randomized clinical trial data; that is, women in most of the studies reported to date were using or not using estrogen for a variety of clinical and socioeconomic reasons. Women who took estrogen in such studies likely differ from those who did not in important risk characteristics that associated with CHD, including social class, education, access to basic health care, smoking, etc. Hopefully, important ongoing trials such as the WHI, which will follow 1400 women prospectively for approximately 9 years, or the Heart and Estrogen/Progestin Replacement Study, which will follow 350 women about 5 years, will clarify the impact of HRT on both mortality and events related to CHD in women as well as possible negative outcomes associated with HRT.

An unequivocal association between unopposed estrogen use and endometrial cancer was established.[215] The increased risk is about three- to fivefold,[216] but uterine cancer that occurs in the setting of postmenopausal estrogen use is usually well-differentiated adenocarcinoma associated with a more-favorable prognosis than spontaneously occurring tumors.[217] Evidence suggests that the risk of estrogen-induced endometrial cancer can be substantially reduced by periodic cycling with a progestational agent and periodic uterine sampling.[218] Although the addition of a progestational agent may partially affect the beneficial effects of estrogen on lipid levels, it was shown that most progesterone-containing hormone replacement combinations can produce favorable change in the lipid profile.[188]

Several studies suggest that postmenopausal estrogen use may increase the risk of breast cancer.[219,220] However, four recent meta-analyses failed to demonstrate an overall increased risk of breast cancer among estrogen users,[221–224] while a fifth meta-analysis showed a small but statistically significant association in "ever users" (RR = 1.63) in current hormone users.[225] Thus routine breast cancer screening is advisable for women receiving postmenopausal HRT because of the physiological plausibility of a link between estrogen therapy and breast cancer and the lack of adequate data on the effects of long-term estrogen use.

As Grady et al[226] note in their meta-analytic review of the English language literature since 1970 on the effects of estrogen therapy and estrogen and progestin therapy on endometrial cancer and CHD, "There is evidence that estrogen therapy decreases risk for CHD, but long term HRT increases risk for endometrial cancer and may be associated with a small risk for breast cancer. The increase in uterine cancer can probably be avoided by adding a progestin to the estrogen regimen for women who have a uterus, but the effects of combination hormones in risk for CHD have still to be adequately studied."

The final decision about HRT to reduce risk of CHD should be based on a careful analysis of all potential risks and benefits for an individual patient. HRT should be recommended for women who had a hysterectomy, particularly for those with CHD or at high risk for CHD. For women with cardiovascular risk factors and with a uterus, the decision is more difficult since it requires the addition of progesterone and an annual endometrial biopsy. Women with a personal or family history of breast cancer should probably refrain from estrogen use for primary prevention, but, depending on the circumstances of their disease and the presence of other compelling risk factors, it should be considered carefully in those with already established CHD.

Smoking Cessation

Cigarette smoking in women is an especially serious risk.[227,228] There are both important biological and social implications. In the Cleveland Clinic's series of young women with infarction ≤30 years of age, 71.8% smoked.[229] This serious possible association was reported even earlier by others.[230,231] Cigarette smoking carries an especially increased hazard for young women because it is often accompanied by oral contraceptive use, a combination that promotes thrombogenesis.[232,233] The specific issue of smoking and smoking cessation in women who are pregnant was recently reviewed comprehensively by Ockene.[234]

Young women constitute the major increasing smoking group. The reasons for this are complex. First, more than one-third of women perceive that they must smoke to maintain their weight,[227] and more than two-thirds believe they will gain weight if they quit.[235–237] Hellerstein et al[100] recently offered a metabolic explanation for this.

Almost any magazine marketed toward women, except the very few that restrict advertising for cigarettes, contains large numbers of advertisements that seek to equate smoking with physical attractiveness, social desirability, and even feminine self-assertion and independence.[238–240]

Cigarette advertising in magazines downplays the hazards of smoking, and this is particularly true for women's-interest publications.[241] "Low-yield" cigarettes are specifically targeted at women, with the implication that the lower levels of tar and nicotine are safer, but they were shown not to lower the risk of a first, nonfatal MI than were higher-yield brands.[242]

Cigarette smoking is a good example of a modifiable risk, where there is strong interplay between the biology of gender and social/psychological behavior and where the risk of CAD associated with an apparently inherited predisposition may be substantially modifiable.[243] This interplay may be relevant to other risks, including socioeconomic factors, educational attainment, social roles, physical activity, and stress. Although much appears in the popular literature, and stress appears a major health concern of women,[244] very little prospective research was published that characterizes the nature of stress as a CAD risk for women, but several authorities characterize women as "negative-effect" smokers, meaning they smoke in response to emotional discomfort and for reducing tension.[245]

However, the perceived benefits of smoking (such as appetite suppression) seem to be of greater concern to women than the health hazards, despite the fact that women appear as knowledgeable as men about the risks.[246] Intensive smoking-intervention programs have a limited effect on the general population, since the programs reach relatively few smokers, and women are reported to have a more-difficult time than men in stopping smoking.[234] The vast majority of smokers who stop prefer to do so on their own.[247] Moreover, researchers suggest that women are more resistant than men to formal programs for smoking cessation.[248]

In general, women are less likely to contemplate smoking cessation than men and are likely to smoke to reduce tension and control weight. Although women quit smoking at the same rate as men, they are less able to maintain cessation over the long term. The clinical implications of the past research findings are that smoking-cessation programs for women may have to emphasize strategies to help them develop confidence to stop smoking, to make a commitment to quitting, and to develop strategies for maintaining cessation for extended periods of time. Smoking-cessation programs for women should emphasize techniques for reducing tension and for weight control.

Conclusion

CVD is the leading cause of morbidity and mortality in women, with the vast majority of cardiovascular events occurring in the postmenopausal years. Most of our knowledge of CVD comes from studies in middle-aged men. Recent emphasis on women's health in general and in cardiovascular health in particular led to increasing evidence that significant gender differences do exist in CAD incidence, in risk factors, and in the modification of cardiovascular risk in women.

Health care providers must coordinate their efforts to effectively treat and prevent CVD in women in such a way as to take into account the unique biology, physiology, and epidemiology of CVD in women. There is increasing evidence supporting the unique characteristics of cardiovascular risk factors in women. These distinct characteristics, modified by genetics, feminine physiology, and the environment, lead to the unique clinical characteristics of CVD in women. The challenge to health care providers is to develop new strategies that address these subtle and not-so-subtle differences and to incorporate new evidence of gender difference into the practice of cardiovascular prevention.

References

1. Wenger NK, Speroff L, Packard B. Cardiovascular health and disease in women [see Comments]. *N Engl J Med* 1993;329:247–256.
2. Barrett-Connor E, Bush TL. Estrogen and coronary heart disease in women [see Comments]. *JAMA* 1991;265:1861–1867.
3. Bush TL, Barrett CE, Cowan LD, et al. Cardiovascular mortality and non-contraceptive use of estrogen in women: results from the Lipid Research Clinics Program Follow-up Study. *Circulation* 1987;75:1102–1109.
4. Bush TL, Criqui MH, Cowan LD, et al. Cardiovascular disease mortality in women: results from the Lipid Research Clinics Follow-up Study. In: Eaker E, Packard B, Wenger N, et al, eds. *Coronary Heart Disease in Women*. New York, NY: Haymarket-Doyma; 1987:106–111.
5. Matthews KA, Meilahn E, Kuller LH, et al. Menopause and risk factors for coronary heart disease [see Comments]. *N Engl J Med* 1989;321:641–646.
6. Walsh BW. Estrogen replacement and heart disease. *Clin Obstet Gynecol* 1992;35:894–900.
7. Walsh BW, Schiff I, Rosner B, et al. Effects of postmenopausal estrogen replacement on the concentrations and metabolism of plasma lipoproteins [see Comments]. *N Engl J Med* 1991;325:1196–1204.
8. Barrett-Connor E. Hypercholesterolemia predicts early death from coronary heart disease in elderly men but not women. The Rancho Bernardo Study. *Ann Epidemiol* 1992;2:77–83.
9. Kannel WB. Metabolic risk factors for coronary heart disease in women: perspective from the Framingham Study. *Am Heart J* 1987;114:413–419.
10. Stevenson JC, Crook D, Godsland IF. Influence of age and menopause on serum lipids and lipoproteins in healthy women. *Atherosclerosis* 1993;98:83–90.
11. Hong MK, Romm PA, Reagan K, et al. Effects of estrogen replacement therapy on serum lipid values and angiographically defined coronary artery disease in postmenopausal women [see Comments]. *Am J Cardiol* 1992;69:176–178.
12. Meilahn EN. Hemostatic factors and risk of cardiovascular disease in women. An overview. *Arch Pathol Lab Med* 1992;116:1313–1317.

13. Anderson TJ, Meredith IT, Uehata A, et al. Functional significance of intimal thickening as detected by intravascular ultrasound early and late after cardiac transplantation. *Circulation* 1993;88:1093–1100.

14. Kannel WB. New perspectives on cardiovascular risk factors. *Am Heart J* 1987;114:213–219.

15. Lapidus L, Bengtsson C, Lindquist O, et al. Triglycerides—main lipid risk factor for cardiovascular disease in women? *Acta Med Scand* 1985;217:481–489.

16. Bass KM, Newschaffer CJ, Klag MJ, et al. Plasma lipoprotein levels as predictors of cardiovascular death in women. *Arch Intern Med* 1993;153:2209–2216.

17. Khoo JC, Miller E, McLoughlin P, et al. Prevention of low density lipoprotein aggregation by high density lipoprotein or apolipoprotein A-I. *J Lipid Res* 1990;31:645–652.

18. Van Tol A. Reverse cholesterol transport. In: Steinmetz A, Kaffarnik H, Schneider J, eds. *Cholesterol Transport Systems and their Relation to Atherosclerosis.* New York, NY: Springer-Verlag; 1989:85–91.

19. Rifkind BM, Tamir I, Heiss G, et al. Distribution of high density and other lipoproteins in selected LRC prevalence study populations: a brief survey. *Lipids* 1979;14:105–112.

20. Jacobs D Jr, Mebane IL, Bangdiwala SI, et al. High density lipoprotein cholesterol as a predictor of cardiovascular disease mortality in men and women: the follow-up study of the Lipid Research Clinics Prevalence Study. *Am J Epidemiol* 1990;131:32–47.

21. Gordon T, Castelli WP, Hjortland MC, et al. High density lipoprotein as a protective factor against coronary heart disease. The Framingham Study. *Am J Med* 1977;62:707–714.

22. Kannel WB, Castelli WP, Gordon T. Cholesterol in the prediction of atherosclerotic disease. New perspectives based on the Framingham study. Review. *Ann Intern Med* 1979;90:85–91.

23. Castelli WP, Doyle JT, Gordon T. HDL cholesterol and other lipids in coronary heart disease. The cooperative lipoprotein phenotyping study. *Circulation* 1977;55:767–772.

24. Bush TL, Fried LP, Barrett-Connor E. Cholesterol, lipoproteins, and coronary heart disease in women. *Clin Chem* 1988:34.

25. Brunner D, Weisbort J, Meshulam N, et al. Relation of serum total cholesterol and high-density lipoprotein cholesterol percentage to the incidence of definite coronary events: twenty-year follow-up of the Donolo-Tel Aviv Prospective Coronary Artery Disease Study. *Am J Cardiol* 1987;59:1271–1276.

26. Livshits G, Weisbort J, Meshulam N, et al. Multivariate analysis of the twenty-year follow-up of the Donolo-Tel Aviv Prospective Coronary Artery Disease Study and the usefulness of high density lipoprotein cholesterol percentage. *Am J Cardiol* 1989;63:676–681.

27. Barrett-Connor E, Khaw KT, Wingard D. A ten-year prospective study of coronary artery disease mortality in Rancho Bernardo women. In: Eaker E, Packard B, Wenger N, et al, eds. *Coronary Heart Disease in Women.* New York, NY: Haymarket-Doyma; 1987:117–121.

28. Rosenberg L, Hennekens CH, Rosner B, et al. Early menopause and the risk of myocardial infarction. *Am J Obstet Gynecol* 1981;139:47–51.

29. White AD, Hames CG, Tyroler HA. Serum cholesterol and 20-year mortality in black and white men and women aged 65 and older in the Evans County Heart Study. *Ann Epidemiol* 1992;2:85–91.

30. Knapp RG, Sutherland SE, Keil JE, et al. A comparison of the effects of cholesterol on CHD mortality in black and white women: twenty-eight years of follow-up in the Charleston Heart Study. *J Clin Epidemiol* 1992;45:1119–1129.
31. Manolio TA, Pearson TA, Wenger NK, et al. Cholesterol and heart disease in older persons and women. Review of an NHLBI workshop. *Ann Epidemiol* 1992;2:161–176.
32. Ballantyne FC, Clark RS, Simpson HS, et al. High density and low density lipoprotein subfractions in survivors of myocardial infarction and in control subjects. *Metabolism* 1982;31:433–437.
33. Williams PT, Vranizan KM, Austin MA, et al. Familial correlations of HDL subclasses based on gradient gel electrophoresis. *Arterioscler Thromb* 1992;12:1467–1474.
34. Miller NE, Hammett F, Saltissi S, et al. Relation of angiographically defined coronary artery disease to plasma lipoprotein subfractions and apolipoproteins. *Br Med J Clin Res Ed* 1981;282:1741–1744.
35. Ohta T, Hattori S, Nishiyama S, et al. Studies on the lipid and apolipoprotein compositions of two species of apoA-I-containing lipoproteins in normolipidemic males and females. *J Lipid Res* 1988;29:721–728.
36. Jensen J, Nilas L, Christiansen C. Influence of menopause on serum lipids and lipoproteins. *Maturitas* 1990;12:321–331.
37. Desoye G, Schweditsch MO, Pfeiffer KP, et al. Correlation of hormones with lipid and lipoprotein levels during normal pregnancy and postpartum. *J Clin Endocrinol Metab* 1987;64:704–712.
38. Kuller LH, Gutai JP, Meilahn E, et al. Relationship of endogenous sex steroid hormones to lipids and apoproteins in postmenopausal women. *Arteriosclerosis* 1990;10:1058–1066.
39. Stensvold I, Urdal P, Thurmer H, et al. High-density lipoprotein cholesterol and coronary, cardiovascular and all cause mortality among middle-aged Norwegian men and women. *Eur Heart J* 1992;13:1155–1163.
40. Gordon DJ, Probstfield JL, Garrison RJ, et al. High-density lipoprotein cholesterol and cardiovascular disease. Four prospective American studies. *Circulation* 1989;79:8–15.
41. Kannel WB, Wilson PW. Risk factors that attenuate the female coronary disease advantage. *Arch Intern Med* 1995;155:57–61.
42. Hong MK, Romm PA, Reagan K, et al. Usefulness of the total cholesterol to high-density lipoprotein cholesterol ratio in predicting angiographic coronary artery disease in women. *Am J Cardiol* 1991;68:1646–1650.
43. Summary of the second report of the National Cholesterol Education Program (NCEP) Expert Panel on Detection, Evaluation, and Treatment of High Blood Cholesterol in Adults (Adult Treatment Panel II). *JAMA* 1993;269:3015–3023.
44. Kannel WB. Nutrition and the occurrence and prevention of cardiovascular disease in the elderly. *Nutr Rev* 1988;46:68–78.
45. Campos H, McNamara JR, Wilson PW, et al. Differences in low density lipoprotein subfractions and apolipoproteins in premenopausal and postmenopausal women. *J Clin Endocrinol Metab* 1988;67:30–35.
46. DeGraaf J, Hak LH, Hectors MP, et al. Enhanced susceptibility to in vitro oxidation of the dense low density lipoprotein subfraction in healthy subjects. *Arterioscler Thromb* 1991;11:298–306.
47. Williams PT, Krauss RM, Vranizan KM, et al. Associations of lipoproteins and apolipoproteins with gradient gel electrophoresis estimates of high den-

sity lipoprotein subfractions in men and women. *Chem Thromb* 1992;12: 332–340.

48. Austin MA, Breslow JL, Hennekens CH, et al. Low-density lipoprotein subclass patterns and risk of myocardial infarction. *JAMA* 1988;260:1917–1921.

49. Starzl TE, Bilheimer DW, Bahnson HT, et al. Heart-liver transplantation in a patient with familial hypercholesterolaemia. *Lancet* 1984;1:1382–1383.

50. Slack J. Genetic influences on coronary heart disease in young women. In: Oliver M, ed. *Coronary Heart Disease in Young Women.* Edinburgh, Scotland: Churchill-Livingstone; 1978:24–25.

51. Wagner JD, Clarkson TB, St CR, et al. Estrogen and progesterone replacement therapy reduces low density lipoprotein accumulation in the coronary arteries of surgically postmenopausal cynomolgus monkeys. *J Clin Invest* 1991;88:1995–2002.

52. Kuchinskiene Z, Carlson LA. Composition, concentration, and size of low density lipoproteins and of subfractions of very low density lipoproteins from serum of normal men and women. *J Lipid Res* 1982;23:762–769.

53. Austin MA. Epidemiologic associations between hypertriglyceridemia and coronary heart disease. Review. *Semin Thromb Hemost* 1988;14:137–142.

54. La Rosa JC. Dyslipoproteinemia in women and the elderly. *Med Clin North Am* 1994;78:163–180.

55. Stensvold I, Tverdal A, Urdal P, et al. Non-fasting serum triglyceride concentration and mortality from coronary heart disease and any cause in middle aged Norwegian women. *BMJ* 1993;307:1318–1322.

56. Castelli WP. Epidemiology of triglycerides: a view from Framingham. *Am J Cardiol* 1992;70:3H–9H.

57. Castelli WP. The triglyceride issue: a view from Framingham. *Am Heart J* 1986;112:432–437.

58. Utermann G. The mysteries of lipoprotein (a). *Science* 1989;246:904–910.

59. Scanu AM. Lipoprotein (a). A potential bridge between the fields of atherosclerosis and thrombosis. Review. *Arch Pathol Lab Med* 1988;112:1045–1047.

60. Genest JJ, Jenner JL, McNamara JR, et al. Prevalence of lipoprotein (a) [Lp(a)] excess in coronary artery disease. *Am J Cardiol* 1991;67:1039–1145.

61. Bostom AG, Gagnon DR, Cupples LA, et al. A prospective investigation of elevated lipoprotein (a) detected by electrophoresis and cardiovascular disease in women. The Framingham Heart Study. *Circulation* 1994;90:1688–1695.

62. Maeda S, Abe A, Seishima M, et al. Transient changes of serum lipoprotein (a) as an acute phase protein. *Atherosclerosis* 1989;78:145–150.

63. Steinmetz J, Tarallo P, Fournier B, et al. Reference values of lipoprotein (a) in a French population. *Presse Med* 1994;23:1695–1698.

64. Solymoss BC, Marcil M, Wesolowska E, et al. Relation of coronary artery disease in women 60 years of age to the combined elevation of serum lipoprotein (a) and total cholesterol to high-density cholesterol ratio. *Am J Cardiol* 1993;72:1215–1219.

65. Kannel WB. Lipids, diabetes, and coronary heart disease: insights from the Framingham Study. *Am Heart J* 1985;110:1100–1107.

66. Garcia M, McNamara P, Gordon T, et al. Morbidity and mortality in diabetics in the Framingham population: sixteen year follow-up study. *Diabetes* 1974;23:105–111.

67. Walden CE, Knopp RH, Wahl PW, et al. Sex differences in the effect of diabetes mellitus on lipoprotein triglyceride and cholesterol concentrations. *N Engl J Med* 1984;311:953–959.

68. Barrett-Connor E, Wingard DL. Sex differential in ischemic heart disease mortality in diabetics: a prospective population-based study. *Am J Epidemiol* 1983;118:489–496.
69. Cruickshanks KJ, Orchard TJ, Becker DJ. The cardiovascular risk profile of adolescents with insulin-dependent diabetes mellitus. *Diabetes Care* 1985;8:118–124.
70. Laakso M, Barrett CE. Asymptomatic hyperglycemia is associated with lipid and lipoprotein changes favoring atherosclerosis. *Arteriosclerosis* 1989; 9:665–672.
71. Schernthaner G, Kostner GM, Dieplinger H, et al. Apolipoproteins (A-I, A-II, B), Lp(a) lipoprotein and lecithin: cholesterol acyltransferase activity in diabetes mellitus. *Atherosclerosis* 1983;49:277–293.
72. Kannel WB, McGee DL. Diabetes and cardiovascular disease. The Framingham study. *JAMA* 1979;241:2035–2038.
73. Knopp RH, Van AM, McNeely M, et al. Effect of insulin-dependent diabetes on plasma lipoproteins in diabetic pregnancy. *J Reprod Med* 1993;38: 703–710.
74. Ginsberg HN. Lipoprotein physiology in nondiabetic and diabetic states. Relationship to atherogenesis. Review. *Diabetes Care* 1991;14:839–855.
75. Orchard TJ, Cruickshanks KJ, Becker DJ. Correspondence. Sex differences in diabetes. *N Engl J Med* 1985;312:185.
76. O'Kelly BF, Massie BM, Tubau JF, et al. Coronary morbidity and mortality, pre-existing silent coronary artery disease, and mild hypertension. *Ann Intern Med* 1989;110:1017–1026.
77. National Education Programs Working Group report on the management of patients with hypertension and high blood cholesterol. *Ann Intern Med* 1991;114:224–237.
78. Petetti D, Winegard J, Pelligrin F, et al. Risk of vascular disease in women. Smoking, oral contraceptives, noncontraceptive estrogen and other factors. *JAMA* 1979;242:1150–1154.
79. Johnson JL, Heineman EF, Heiss G, et al. Cardiovascular disease risk factors and mortality among black women and white women aged 40–64 years in Evans County, Georgia. *Am J Epidemiol* 1986;123:209–220.
80. Hubert HB, Feinleib M, McNamara PM, et al. Obesity as an independent risk factor for cardiovascular disease: a 26-year follow-up of participants in the Framingham Heart Study. *Circulation* 1983;67:968–977.
81. Manson JE, Colditz GA, Stampfer MJ, et al. A prospective study of obesity and risk of coronary heart disease in women [see Comments]. *N Engl J Med* 1990;322:882–889.
82. Anonymous. *Plan and Operation of the Second National Health and Nurtition Examination Survey, 1976–1980*. Washington, DC: US Government Printing Office; 1981. National Center for Health Statistics
83. Patterson CC, McCrum E, McMaster D. Factors influencing total cholesterol and high-density lipoprotein cholesterol concentrations in a population at high coronary risk. *Acta Medica Scand* 1988;728(suppl):150–158.
84. Wing RR, Bunker CH, Kuller LH, et al. Insulin, body mass index, and cardiovascular risk factors in premenopausal women. *Arteriosclerosis* 1989;9:479–484.
85. Van Horn LV, Ballew C, Liu K, et al. Diet, body size, and plasma lipids-lipoproteins in young adults: differences by race and sex. The Coronary Artery Risk Development in Young Adults (CARDIA) study. *Am J Epidemiol* 1991;133:9–23.

86. Glueck CJ, Taylor HL, Jacobs D, et al. Plasma high-density lipoprotein cholesterol: association with measurements of body mass. The Lipid Research Clinics Program Prevalence Study. *Circulation* 1980.
87. Despres JP, Allard C, Tremblay A, et al. Evidence for a regional component of body fatness in the association with serum lipids in men and women. *Metabolism* 1985;34:967–973.
88. Dustan HP. Coronary artery disease in women. *Can J Cardiol* 1990;6: 19B–21B.
89. Krauss RM. The tangled web of coronary risk factors. *Am J Med* 1991;90(suppl):36–41.
90. Soler JT, Folsom AR, Kushi LH, et al. Association of body fat distribution with plasma lipids, lipoproteins, apolipoproteins AI and B in postmenopausal women. *J Clin Epidemiol* 1988;41:1075–1081.
91. Razay G, Heaton KW, Bolton CH. Coronary heart disease risk factors in relation to the menopause. *Q J Med* 1992;85:889–896.
92. Kaplan NM. The deadly quartet. Upper-body obesity, glucose intolerance, hypertriglyceridemia, and hypertension. Review. *Arch Intern Med* 1989;149:1514–1520.
93. Donahue RP, Orchard TJ, Becker DJ, et al. Physical activity, insulin sensitivity, and the lipoprotein profile in young adults: the Beaver County Study. Review. *Am J Epidemiol* 1988;127:95–103.
94. Thompson CJ, Ryu JE, Craven TE, et al. Central adipose distribution is related to coronary atherosclerosis. *Arterioscler Thromb* 1991;11:327–333.
95. Larsson B, Bengtsson C, Bjorntorp P, et al. Is abdominal body fat distribution a major explanation for the sex difference in the incidence of myocardial infarction? The study of men born in 1913 and the study of women, Goteborg, Sweden. *Am J Epidemiol* 1992;135:266–273.
96. Martin ML, Jensen MD. Effects of body fat distribution on regional lipolysis in obesity. *J Clin Invest* 1991;88:609–613.
97. Lapidus L, Bengtsson C, Larsson B, et al. Distribution of adipose tissue and risk of cardiovascular disease and death: a 12 year follow up of participants in the population study of women in Gothenburg, Sweden. *BMJ* 1984;289:1257–1261.
98. Barrett-Connor EL, Cohn BA, Wingard DL, et al. Why is diabetes mellitus a stronger risk factor for fatal ischemic heart disease in women than in men? The Rancho Bernardo Study (see Erratum 1991;265:3249). *JAMA* 1991;265:627–631.
99. Muscat JE, Harris RE, Haley NJ, et al. Cigarette smoking and plasma cholesterol. *Am Heart J* 1991;121:141–147.
100. Hellerstein MK, Benowitz NL, Neese RA, et al. Effects of cigarette smoking and its cessation on lipid metabolism and energy expenditure in heavy smokers. *J Clin Invest* 1994;93:265–272.
101. Facchini FS, Hollenbeck CB, Jeppesen J, et al. Insulin resistance and cigarette smoking (published erratum appears in *Lancet* 1992;339(8807):1492) [see Comments]. *Lancet* 1992;339:1128–1130.
102. Axelsen M, Eliasson B, Joheim E, et al. Lipid intolerance in smokers [see Comments]. *J Intern Med* 1995;237:449–455.
103. Morrow JD, Frei B, Longmire AW, et al. Increase in circulating products of lipid peroxidation (F2-isoprostanes) in smokers. Smoking as a cause of oxidative damage. *N Engl J Med* 1995;332:1198–1203.
104. Blair SN, Kohl HD, Paffenbarger R Jr, et al. Physical fitness and all-cause mortality. A prospective study of healthy men and women [see Comments]. *JAMA* 1989;262:2395–2401.

105. Powell KE, Thompson PD, Caspersen CJ, et al. Physical activity and the incidence of coronary heart disease. *Annu Rev Public Health* 1987;8:253–287.
106. Kokkinos PF, Holland JC, Pittaras AE, et al. Cardiorespiratory fitness and coronary heart disease risk factor association in women. *J Am Coll Cardiol* 1995;26:358–364.
107. Lapidus L, Bengtsson C. Socioeconomic factors and physical activity in relation to cardiovascular disease and death. A 12 year follow up of participants in a population study of women in Gothenburg, Sweden. *Br Heart J* 1986;55:295–301.
108. Scragg R, Stewart A, Jackson R, et al. Alcohol and exercise in myocardial infarction and sudden coronary death in men and women. *Am J Epidemiol* 1987;126:77–85.
109. Lemaitre RN, Heckbert SR, Psaty BM, et al. Leisure-time physical activity and the risk of nonfatal myocardial infarction in postmenopausal women. *Arch Intern Med* 1995;155:2302–2308.
110. Fletcher GF, Froelicher VF, Hartley LH, et al. Exercise standards. A statement for health professionals from the American Heart Association. Review. *Circulation* 1990;82:2286–2322.
111. Krummel D, Etherton TD, Peterson S, et al. Effects of exercise on plasma lipids and lipoproteins of women. *Proc Soc Exp Biol Med* 1993;204:123–137.
112. Taylor PA, Ward A. Women, high-density lipoprotein cholesterol, and exercise. *Arch Intern Med* 1993;153:1178–1184.
113. Harting GH, Moore CE, Mitchell R, et al. Relationship of menopausal status and exercise level to HDL-cholesterol in women. *Exp Aging Res* 1984;10:13–18.
114. Rainville S, Vaccaro P. The effects of menopause and training on serum lipids. *Int J Sports Med* 1984;5:137–141.
115. Cauley JA, Kriska AM, LaPorte RE, et al. A two year randomized exercise trial in older women: effects on HDL-cholesterol. *Atherosclerosis* 1987;66:247–258.
116. Boyden T, Parmenter R, Rotkis T. Effect of exercise training on plasma cholesterol, HDL-C, ApoA1, sex steroids levels of early post-menopausal women. In: Eaker E, Packard B, Wenger N, et al, eds. *Coronary Heart Disease in Women.* New York, NY: Haymarket-Doyma; 1987:160–163.
117. Fritz K. Review of several cross-sectional and longitudinal studies. *Perspect Lipid Disorders* 1987.
118. Lavie CJ, Milani RV. Effects of cardiac rehabilitation and exercise training on exercise capacity, coronary risk factors, behavioral characteristics, and quality of life in women. *Am J Cardiol* 1995;75:340–343.
119. Cannistra LB, Balady GJ, O'Malley CJ, et al. Comparison of the clinical profile and outcome of women and men in cardiac rehabilitation. *Am J Cardiol* 1992;69:1274–1279.
120. Matthews KA, Kelsey SF, Meilahn EN, et al. Educational attainment and behavioral and biologic risk factors for coronary heart disease in middle-aged women. *Am J Epidemiol* 1989;129:1132–1144.
121. Tenconi MT, Romanelli C, Gigli F, et al. The relationship between education and risk factors for coronary heart disease. Epidemiological analysis from the nine communities study. The Research Group ATS-OB43 of CNR. *Eur J Epidemiol* 1992;8:763–769.
122. Kannel WB, Hjortland MC, McNamara PM, et al. Menopause and risk of cardiovascular disease: the Framingham study. *Ann Intern Med* 1976;85:447–452.
123. Gordon T, Kannel WB, Hjortland MC, et al. Menopause and coronary heart disease. The Framingham Study. *Ann Intern Med* 1978;89:157–161.

124. Colditz GA, Willett WC, Stampfer MJ, et al. Menopause and the risk of coronary heart disease in women. *N Engl J Med* 1987;316:1105–1110.

125. Bush TL. The epidemiology of cardiovascular disease in postmenopausal women. *Ann N Y Acad Sci* 1990;592:263–271.

126. Gorodeski GI. Impact of the menopause on the epidemiology and risk factors of coronary artery heart disease in women. Review. *Exp Gerontol* 1994;29:357–375.

127. Eaker E, Packard B, Wenger N, et al. *Coronary Heart Disease in Women.* New York, NY: Haymarket-Doyma; 1987.

128. *Report of the Expert Panel on Detection, Evaluation, and Treatment of High Blood Cholesterol in Adults.* Bethesda, Md: National Cholesterol Education Program; 1989. US Department of Health and Human Services publication NIH 87.

129. Bush TL, Riedel D. Screening for total cholesterol. Do the National Cholesterol Education Program's recommendations detect individuals at high risk of coronary heart disease? [see Comments]. *Circulation* 1991;83:1287–1293.

130. Rossouw JE, Lewis B, Rifkind BM. The value of lowering cholesterol after myocardial infarction. *N Engl J Med* 1991;324:922–923.

131. Katan MB. Diet and high density lipoproteins. In: Miller N, Miller G, eds. *Clinical and Metabolic Aspects of High Density Lipoproteins.* Amsterdam, The Netherlands: Elsevier; 1984:103–131.

132. Grundy SM. Cholesterol and coronary heart disease. A new era. Review. *JAMA* 1986;256:2849–2858.

133. Jones DY, Judd JT, Taylor PR, et al. Influence of caloric contribution and saturation of dietary fat on plasma lipids in premenopausal women. *Am J Clin Nutr* 1987;45:1451–1456.

134. Zanni EE, Zannis VI, Blum CB, et al. Effect of egg cholesterol and dietary fats on plasma lipids, lipoproteins, and apoproteins of normal women consuming natural diets. *J Lipid Res* 1987;28:518–527.

135. Clifton PM, Noakes M, Nestel PJ. Gender and diet interactions with simvastatin treatment. *Atherosclerosis* 1994;110:25–33.

136. Barnard RJ. Effects of life-style modification on serum lipids [see Comments]. *Arch Intern Med* 1991;151:1389–1394.

137. Cobb MM, Teitlebaum H, Risch N, et al. Influence of dietary fat, apolipoprotein E phenotype, and sex on plasma lipoprotein levels. *Circulation* 1992;86:849–857.

138. Anderson JW. Diet, lipids and cardiovascular disease in women. *J Am Coll Nutr* 1993;12:433–437.

139. Kohlmeier M, Stricker G, Schlierf G. Influences of "normal" and "prudent" diets on biliary and serum lipids in healthy women. *Am J Clin Nutr* 1985;42:1201–1205.

140. Grundy SM, Nix D, Whelan MF, et al. Comparison of three cholesterol-lowering diets in normolipidemic men. *JAMA* 1986;256:2351–2355.

141. Lewis B, Hammett F, Katan M, et al. Towards an improved lipid-lowering diet: additive effects of changes in nutrient intake. *Lancet* 1981;2:1310–1313.

142. Mata P, Alvarez SL, Rubio MJ, et al. Effects of long-term monounsaturated-vs polyunsaturated-enriched diets on lipoproteins in healthy men and women [see Comments]. *Am J Clin Nutr* 1992;55:846–850.

143. Jenkins DJ, Wolever TM, Rao AV, et al. Effect on blood lipids of very high intakes of fiber in diets low in saturated fat and cholesterol. *N Engl J Med* 1993;329:21–26.

144. Crouse JD. Gender, lipoproteins, diet, and cardiovascular risk. Sauce for the goose may not be sauce for the gander. Review. *Lancet* 1989;1:318–320.
145. Grundy SM. HMG-CoA reductase inhibitors for treatment of hypercholesterolemia. Review. *N Engl J Med* 1988;319:24–33.
146. Wood PD, Stefanick ML, Williams PT, et al. The effects on plasma lipoproteins of a prudent weight-reducing diet, with or without exercise, in overweight men and women. *N Engl J Med* 1991;325:461–466.
147. Miettinen M, Turpeinen O, Karvonen MJ, et al. Cholesterol-lowering diet and mortality from coronary heart-disease. *Lancet* 1972;2:1418–1419.
148. Frantz IJ, Dawson EA, Ashman PL, et al. Test of effect of lipid lowering by diet on cardiovascular risk. The Minnesota Coronary Survey. *Arteriosclerosis* 1989;9:129–135.
149. Dattilo AM, Kris-Etherton P. Effects of weight reduction on blood lipids and lipoproteins: a meta-analysis. *Am J Clin Nutr* 1992;56:320–328.
150. Brownell KD, Stunkard AJ. Differential changes in plasma high-density lipoprotein-cholesterol levels in obese men and women during weight reduction. *Arch Intern Med* 1981;141:1142–1146.
151. Grodin JM, Siiteri PK, MacDonald PC. Source of estrogen production in postmenopausal women. *J Clin Endocrinol Metab* 1973;36:207–214.
152. La Rosa JC. Management of postmenopausal women who have hyperlipidemia. *Am J Med* 1994;96:19S–24S.
153. Gordon DJ, Rifkind BM. High-density lipoprotein—the clinical implications of recent studies. Review. *N Engl J Med* 1989;321:1311–1316.
154. Oldridge NB, Guyatt GH, Fischer ME, et al. Cardiac rehabilitation after myocardial infarction. Combined experience of randomized clinical trials. *JAMA* 1988;260:945–950.
155. O'Connor GT, Buring JE, Yusuf S, et al. An overview of randomized trials of rehabilitation with exercise after myocardial infarction. *Circulation* 1989;80:234–244.
156. Donahue RP, Orchard TJ, Becker DJ, et al. Sex differences in the coronary heart disease risk profile: a possible role for insulin. The Beaver County Study. *Am J Epidemiol* 1987;125:650–657.
157. Blumenthal JA, Matthews K, Fredrikson M, et al. Effects of exercise training on cardiovascular function and plasma lipid, lipoprotein, and apolipoprotein concentrations in premenopausal and postmenopausal women. *Arterioscler Thromb* 1991;11:912–917.
158. Brownell KD, Bachorik PS, Ayerle RS. Changes in plasma lipid and lipoprotein levels in men and women after a program of moderate exercise. *Circulation* 1982;65:477–484.
159. Duncan JJ, Gordon NF, Scott CB. Women walking for health and fitness. How much is enough? *JAMA* 1991;266:3295–3299.
160. Hardman AE, Hudson A, Jones PR, et al. Brisk walking and plasma high density lipoprotein cholesterol concentration in previously sedentary women. *BMJ* 1989;299:1204–1205.
161. Howes LG, Simons LA. Efficacy of drug intervention for lipids in the prevention of coronary artery disease. Review. *Aust N Z J Med* 1994;24:107–112.
162. Dorr AE, Gundersen K, Schneider JJ, et al. Colestipol hydrochloride in hypercholesterolemic patients—effect on serum cholesterol and mortality. *J Chron Dis* 1978;31:5–14.
163. Oliver M, Heady J, Morris J, et al. A cooperative trial in the primary prevention of ischemic heart disease using clofibrate. Report from the Committee of Principal Investigators. *Br Heart J* 1978;40:1069–1118.

164. Anonymous. Lipid Research Clinics Program. Letter. *JAMA* 1984;252:2545–2548.

165. Frick MH, Elo O, Haapa K, et al. Helsinki Heart Study: primary-prevention trial with gemfibrozil in middle-aged men with dyslipidemia. Safety of treatment, changes in risk factors, and incidence of coronary heart disease. *N Engl J Med* 1987;317:1237–1245.

166. La Rosa JC. Cholesterol lowering, low cholesterol, and mortality. *Am J Cardiol* 1993;72:776–786.

167. Peters TK, Muratti EN, Mehra M. Efficacy and safety of fluvastatin in women with primary hypercholesterolaemia. *Drugs* 1994;2:64–72.

168. Carlson LA, Rosenhamer G. Reduction of mortality in the Stockholm Ischaemic Heart Disease Secondary Prevention Study by combined treatment with clofibrate and nicotinic acid. *Acta Med Scand* 1988;223:405–418.

169. Group TCDPR. Clofibrate and niacin in coronary heart disease. *JAMA* 1975;231:360–381.

170. Region GoPftNu-T. Trial of clofibrate in the treatment of ischaemic heart disease. *BMJ* 1971;4:767–775.

171. Physicians RCotSSo. Ischaemic heart disease: a secondary prevention trial using clofibrate. *BMJ* 1971;4:775–784.

172. Kane JP, Malloy MJ, Ports TA, et al. Regression of coronary atherosclerosis during treatment of familial hypercholesterolemia with combined drug regimens [see Comments]. *JAMA* 1990;264:3007–3012.

173. Anonymous. Randomised trial of cholesterol lowering in 4444 patients with coronary heart disease: the Scandinavian Simvastatin Survival Study (4S) [see Comments]. *Lancet* 1994;344:1383–1389.

174. Yuan J, Tsai MY, Hunninghake DB. Changes in composition and distribution of LDL subspecies in hypertriglyceridemic and hypercholesterolemic patients during gemfibrozil therapy. *Atherosclerosis* 1994;110:1–11.

175. Stampfer MJ, Willett WC, Colditz GA, et al. A prospective study of postmenopausal estrogen therapy and coronary heart disease. *N Engl J Med* 1985;313:1044–1049.

176. van der Rijpkema AH, et al. Effects of post-menopausal oestrogen-progestogen replacement therapy on serum lipids and lipoproteins: a review. *Maturitas* 1990;12:259–285.

177. Sacks FM, Walsh BW. The effects of reproductive hormones on serum lipoproteins: unresolved issues in biology and clinical practice. *Ann N Y Acad Sci* 1990;592:272–285.

178. Belchetz PE. Hormonal treatment of postmenopausal women. Review [see Comments]. *N Engl J Med* 1994;330:1062–1071.

179. Campos H, Sacks FM, Walsh BW, et al. Differential effects of estrogen on low-density lipoprotein subclasses in healthy postmenopausal women. *Metabolism* 1993;42:1153–1158.

180. Chetkowski RJ, Meldrum DR, Steingold KA, et al. Biologic effects of transdermal estradiol. *N Engl J Med* 1986;314:1615–1620.

181. Barrett-Connor E. Estrogen and estrogen-progestogen replacement: therapy and cardiovascular diseases. *Am J Med* 1993;95:40S–43S.

182. Lufkin EG, Wahner HW, O'Fallon WM, et al. Treatment of postmenopausal osteoporosis with transdermal estrogen [see Comments]. *Ann Intern Med* 1992;117:1–9.

183. Glueck CJ, Tsang R, Balistreri W, et al. Plasma and dietary cholesterol in infancy: effects of early low or moderate dietary cholesterol intake on subsequent response to increased dietary cholesterol. *Metabolism* 1972;21:1181–1192.

184. The Writing Group for the PEPI. Effects of estrogen or estrogen/progestin regimens on heart disease risk factors in postmenopausal women. The Postmenopausal Estrogen/Progestin Interventions (PEPI) Trial. Trial [see Comments]. *JAMA* 1995;273:199–208.

185. Miller VT, Muesing RA, LaRosa JC, et al. Effects of conjugated equine estrogen with and without three different progestogens on lipoproteins, high-density lipoprotein subfractions, and apolipoprotein A-I. *Obstet Gynecol* 1991;77:235–240.

186. Nabulsi AA, Folsom AR, White A, et al. Association of hormone-replacement therapy with various cardiovascular risk factors in postmenopausal women. The Atherosclerosis Risk in Communities Study Investigators [see Comments]. *N Engl J Med* 1993;328:1069–1075.

187. Knopp RH, Zhu X, Bonet B. Effects of estrogens on lipoprotein metabolism and cardiovascular disease in women. *Atherosclerosis* 1994;110(suppl):83–91.

188. Haarbo J, Hassager C, Jensen SB, et al. Serum lipids, lipoproteins, and apolipoproteins during postmenopausal estrogen replacement therapy combined with either 19-nortestosterone derivatives or 17-hydroxyprogesterone derivatives. *Am J Med* 1991;90:584–589.

189. Granfone A, Campos H, McNamara JR, et al. Effects of estrogen replacement on plasma lipoproteins and apolipoproteins in postmenopausal, dyslipidemic women. *Metabolism* 1992;41:1193–1198.

190. La Rosa JC. Hyperlipidemia: treatment with lipid-lowering agents. *Maryland Med J* 1988;37:401–406.

191. Soma M, Fumagalli R, Paoletti R, et al. Plasma Lp(a) concentration after oestrogen and progestagen in postmenopausal women. Letter. *Lancet* 1991:337.

192. Knopp RH, Walden CE, Wahl PW, et al. Effect of postpartum lactation on lipoprotein lipids and apoproteins. *J Clin Endocrinol Metab* 1985;60:542–547.

193. Sacks FM, Pasternak RC, Gibson CM, et al. Effect on coronary atherosclerosis of decrease in plasma cholesterol concentrations in normocholesterolaemic patients. Harvard Atherosclerosis Reversibility Project (HARP) Group [see Comments]. *Lancet* 1994;344:1182–1186.

194. Schaefer EJ, Foster DM, Zech LA, et al. The effects of estrogen administration on plasma lipoprotein metabolism in premenopausal females. *J Clin Endocrinol Metab* 1983;57:262–267.

195. Tikkanen MJ, Nikkila EA, Kuusi T, et al. High density lipoprotein-2 and hepatic lipase: reciprocal changes produced by estrogen and norgestrel. *J Clin Endocrinol Metab* 1982;54:1113–1117.

196. Gerhard M, Ganz P. How do we explain the clinical benefits of estrogen? From bedside to bench. Editorial [see Comments]. *Circulation* 1995;92:5–8.

197. Lieberman EH, Gerhard MD, Uehata A, et al. Estrogen improves endothelium-dependent, flow-mediated vasodilation in postmenopausal women. *Ann Intern Med* 1994;121:936–941.

198. Reis SE. Oestrogens attenuate abnormal coronary vasoreactivity in postmenopausal women. Editorial. *Ann Med* 1994;26:387–388.

199. Rosselli M, Imthurn B, Keller PJ, et al. Circulating nitric oxide (nitrite/nitrate) levels in postmenopausal women substituted with 17 β-estradiol and norethisterone acetate. A two-year follow-up study. *Hypertension* 1995;21:482–489.

200. Harder DR, Coulson PB. Estrogen receptors and effects of estrogen on membrane electrical properties of coronary vascular smooth muscle. *J Cell Physiol* 1979;100:375–382.

201. Gilligan DM, Badar DM, Panza JA, et al. Acute vascular effects of estrogen in postmenopausal women. *Circulation* 1994;90:786–791.
202. Collins P, Rosano GM, Sarrel PM, et al. 17 beta-Estradiol attenuates acetylcholine-induced coronary arterial constriction in women but not men with coronary heart disease [see Comments]. *Circulation* 1995;92:24–30.
203. Fischer GM, Swain ML. Effects of estradiol and progesterone on the increased synthesis of collagen in atherosclerotic rabbit aortas. *Atherosclerosis* 1985;54:177–185.
204. Morales DE, McGowan KA, Grant DS, et al. Estrogen promotes angiogenic activity in human umbilical vein endothelial cells in vitro and in a murine model. *Circulation* 1995;91:755–763.
205. Stampfer MJ, Colditz GA, Willett WC, et al. Postmenopausal estrogen therapy and cardiovascular disease. Ten-year follow-up from the Nurses' Health Study [see Comments]. *N Engl J Med* 1991;325:756–762.
206. Kuhn FE, Rackley CE. Coronary artery disease in women. Risk factors, evaluation, treatment, and prevention. *Arch Intern Med* 1993;153:2626–2636.
207. Wilson PW, Garrison RJ, Castelli WP. Postmenopausal estrogen use, cigarette smoking, and cardiovascular morbidity in women over 50. The Framingham Study. *N Engl J Med* 1985;313:1038–1043.
208. Henderson BE, Ross RK, Paganini-Hill A, et al. Estrogen use and cardiovascular disease. *Am J Obstet Gynecol* 1986;154:1181–1186.
209. Ettinger WH, Wahl PW, Kuller LH, et al. Lipoprotein lipids in older people. Results from the Cardiovascular Health Study. The CHS Collaborative Research Group (see comments) *Circulation* 1992;86:858–869.
210. Sullivan JM. Coronary arteriography in estrogen-treated postmenopausal women. *Prog Cardiovasc Dis* 1995;38:211–222.
211. McFarland KF, Boniface ME, Hornung CA, et al. Risk factors and noncontraceptive estrogen use in women with and without coronary disease. *Am Heart J* 1989;117:1209–1214.
212. Gruchow HW, Anderson AJ, Barboriak JJ, et al. Postmenopausal use of estrogen and occlusion of coronary arteries. *Am Heart J* 1988;115:954–963.
213. Nachtigall LE, Nachtigall RH, Nachtigall RD, et al. Estrogen replacement therapy I: a 10-year prospective study in the relationship to osteoporosis. *Obstet Gynecol* 1979;53:277–281.
214. Nachtigall LE, Nachtigall RH, Nachtigall RD, et al. Estrogen replacement therapy II: a prospective study in the relationship to carcinoma and cardiovascular and metabolic problems. *Obstet Gynecol* 1979;54:74–79.
215. Bush TL. The adverse effects of hormonal therapy. *Cardiol Clin* 1986;4:145–152.
216. Astedt B. Cancer and other risk factors with estrogen replacement. *Acta Obstet Gynecol Scand Suppl* 1987;140:46–51.
217. Hulka BS. Links between hormone replacement therapy and neoplasia. Review. *Fertil Steril* 1994:48–61.
218. Persson I, Adami HO, Bergkvist L, et al. Risk of endometrial cancer after treatment with oestrogens alone or in conjunction with progestogens: results of a prospective study. *BMJ* 1989;298:147–151.
219. Jick H, Walker AM, Watkins RN, et al. Replacement estrogens and breast cancer. *Am J Epidemiol* 1980;112:586–594.
220. Thomas DB, Persing JP, Hutchinson WB. Exogenous estrogens and other risk factors for breast cancer in women with benign breast diseases. *J Natl Cancer Inst* 1982;69:1017–1025.
221. Dupont WD, Page DL. Menopausal estrogen replacement therapy and breast cancer [see Comments]. *Arch Intern Med* 1991;151:67–72.

222. Steinberg KK, Thacker SB, Smith SJ, et al. A meta-analysis of the effect of estrogen replacement therapy on the risk of breast cancer [see Erratum 1991;266:1362; see Comments]. *JAMA* 1991;265:1985–1990.
223. Henrich JB. The postmenopausal estrogen/breast cancer controversy. Review [see Comments]. *JAMA* 1992;268:1900–1902.
224. Armstrong BK. Oestrogen therapy after the menopause—boon or bane? *Med J Aust* 1988;148:213–214.
225. Sillero AM, Delgado RM, Rodigues CR, et al. Menopausal hormone replacement therapy and breast cancer: a meta-analysis. *Obstet Gynecol* 1992;79:286–294.
226. Grady D, Rubin SM, Petitti DB, et al. Hormone therapy to prevent disease and prolong life in postmenopausal women [see Comments]. *Ann Intern Med* 1992;117:1016–1037.
227. Willett W, Stampfer MJ, Bain C, et al. Cigarette smoking, relative weight, and menopause. *Am J Epidemiol* 1983;117:651–658.
228. Pierce JP, Fiore MC, Novotny TE, et al. Trends in cigarette smoking in the United States. Projections to the year 2000. *JAMA* 1989;261:61–65.
229. Arnold AZ, Moodie DS. Coronary artery disease in young women: risk factor analysis and long-term follow-up [see Comments]. *Cleve Clin J Med* 1993;60:393–398.
230. La Vecchia C, Franceschi S, Decarli A, et al. Risk factors for myocardial infarction in young women. *Am J Epidemiol* 1987;125:832–843.
231. Rosenberg L, Kaufman DW, Helmrich SP, et al. Myocardial infarction and cigarette smoking in women younger than 50 years of age. *JAMA* 1985;253:2965–2969.
232. Goldbaum GM, Kendrick JS, Hogelin GC, et al. The relative impact of smoking and oral contraceptive use on women in the United States. *JAMA* 1987;258:1339–1342.
233. Leaf DA. Women and coronary artery disease. Gender confers no immunity. *Postgrad Med* 1990;87:55–60.
234. Ockene JK. Preventing smoking and promoting smoking cessation among women across the life span. In: Wenger NK, Speroff L, Packard B, eds. *Cardiovascular Health and Disease in Women.* Greenwich, Conn: LeJacq Communications; 1993:247–257.
235. Moffatt RJ, Owens SG. Cessation from cigarette smoking: changes in body weight, body composition, resting metabolism, and energy consumption. *Metabolism* 1991;40:465–470.
236. Williamson DF, Madans J, Anda RF, et al. Smoking cessation and severity of weight gain in a national cohort [see Comments]. *N Engl J Med* 1991;324:739–745.
237. Hall SM, Ginsberg D, Jones RT. Smoking cessation and weight gain. *J Consult Clin Psychol* 1986;54:342–346.
238. Pashkow FJ. The Mona Lisa smiles: impact of risk factors for coronary artery disease in women. Editorial [see Comments]. *Cleve Clin J Med* 1993;60:411–414.
239. Woodbridge M. Why do women smoke? *Nurs Prax N Z* 1992;7:15–20.
240. Amos A, Jacobson B, White P. Cigarette advertising policy and coverage of smoking and health in British women's magazines [see Comments]. *Lancet* 1991;337:93–96.
241. Warner KE, Goldenhar LM, McLaughlin CG. Cigarette advertising and magazine coverage of the hazards of smoking. A statistical analysis. *N Engl J Med* 1992;326:305–309.
242. Palmer JR, Rosenberg L, Shapiro S. "Low yield" cigarettes and the risk of nonfatal myocardial infarction in women. *N Engl J Med* 1989;320:1569–1573.

243. Khaw KT, Barrett-Connor E. Family history of heart attack: a modifiable risk factor? *Circulation* 1986;74:239–244.
244. Walters V. Women's views of their main health problems. *Can J Public Health* 1992;83:371–374.
245. Lazarus RS, Folkman S. *Stress, Appraisal, and Coping.* New York, NY: Springer-Verlag; 1984.
246. Page RM, Gold RS. Assessing gender differences in college cigarette smoking intenders and non-intenders. *J Sch Health* 1983;53:531–535.
247. Fiore MC, Novotny TE, Pierce JP, et al. Trends in cigarette smoking in the United States. The changing influence of gender and race. *JAMA* 1989;261:49–55.
248. Cappotelli HC, Orleans CT. Partner support and other determinants of smoking cessation maintenance among women. *J Consult Clin Psychol* 1985;53:455–460.

Chapter 10

Preventive Cardiology in Minority Groups

Thomas A. Pearson, MD, PhD

Introduction and Overview

Coronary heart disease (CHD) is the leading cause of death among all racial and ethnic subpopulations of the United States, with stroke ranking third or fourth (Figure 1).[1] The heterogeneous racial and ethnic make-up of the United States, however, raises a number of distinct challenges in the prevention of this disease. This chapter will explore these challenges, including an examination of differences in mortality rates among major minority groups, a discussion of possible differences in presentation and natural history among minority groups, and an examination of differences in risk factors for CHD as a possible explanation for some of these differences in mortality and natural history. Also, a review of the scantily available data comparing the benefits of interventions among minority groups and whites will be presented. Finally, differences in access to medical care will also be discussed as a reason for mortality differentials. To a great extent, the discussion will focus on CHD in blacks, though other minority groups will be discussed to illustrate specific points.

A theoretical model illustrates several of the challenges in sorting out the differences in CHD incidence and mortality in minority groups from those of whites (Figure 2). Race and ethnicity are presumed to be related to CHD through at least three possible pathways. First, there may be ge-

Dr. Pearson was supported in part by National Heart, Lung, and Blood Institute Grant HL-49735.

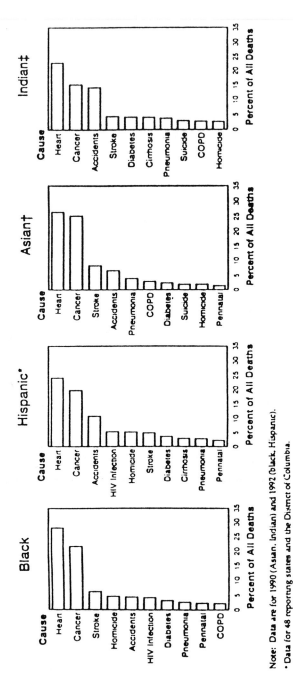

Figure 1. *Ten leading causes of death among minority groups in the United States, 1990–1992. Reproduced with permission from Reference 1.*

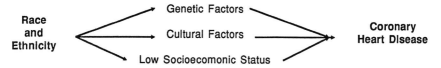

Figure 2. *A theoretical model of mechanisms to explain higher rates of cardiovascular disease in racial and ethnic minorities.*

netic differences that predispose defined subpopulations to disease. For example, French Canadians have a high prevalence of the familial hypercholesterolemia gene (>1%), compared to the rest of Canada or to the United States (0.2%).[2] Persons with such genetic predisposition to CHD may be targets for early identification and preventive intervention. Second, racial and ethnic groups may have distinctive cultural behaviors, such as dietary and eating practices, exercise patterns, use of medical care, etc. These behavioral characteristics may help or hinder efforts to reduce CHD risk and thus must be taken into account in any intervention program.

In the United States, a large number of blacks, Hispanic Americans, and Native Americans are classified as having low socioeconomic status (SES) as defined by income, educational attainment, occupational status, and other related measures.[3] This makes possible the confounding of the

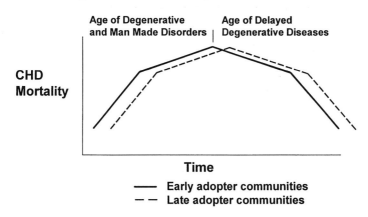

Figure 3. *Theoretical comparison of CHD mortality in early versus late adopter communities.*

relation between race/ethnicity and CHD by low SES. The reason for this is that a steep, inverse gradient exists between SES and CHD, with persons of low income or educational attainment having exceptionally high rates of CHD mortality compared to persons in higher economic or educational strata (Figure 5).[4] This gradient of risk increased over the past 30 years.[5,6] Low SES is strongly related to a poor prognosis after the onset of CHD,[7,8] and was recently associated with the atherosclerotic disease process itself.[9]

The relation between CHD and SES is a paradoxical one, because CHD was a disease of the upper classes in the first half of the 20th century.[10] However, CHD differences between racial and ethnic groups may be explained in the context of the so-called epidemiological transition[11,12] (Figure 3). Early adopter communities with economic resources and high educational attainment become industrialized first and are thus first to be affected by risk factors and rising CHD rates, with late adopter communities of lower economic or educational means lagging behind. At this point, educated, affluent whites would, therefore, have higher rates of CHD. However, as the affluent communities recognize the health problems posed by CHD and adopt hygienic and medical strategies to reduce mortality, their rates begin to fall. CHD rates in less-affluent groups may continue to rise, eventually exceeding those of high-SES white groups and remaining high even after rates among whites actually began to fall. This model may be one explanation for the differences in CHD rates between blacks and whites in the United States in the 1950s to the present, as will be discussed below. The appropriate strategy inferred by this model is to accelerate adoption of hygienic and medical interventions in late adopter communities, namely, racial and ethnic subgroups of low SES.

Coronary Heart Disease and Risk Factors for Coronary Heart Disease in Race/Ethnic Groups in the United States

Coronary Heart Disease Mortality Rates in Selected Racial and Ethnic Groups

The Myth of Invulnerability of African Americans to Coronary Heart Disease

Early reports suggested that blacks, especially men, had much lower rates of CHD incidence and mortality than did whites. The findings were predominantly from studies of whites and blacks in the southern United States in the 1960s, with wide disparities in SES between the racial groups.[13,14] Higher-SES whites in those settings had likely adopted high-risk behaviors, with low-SES blacks lagging behind. However, studies from urban centers, especially in the northeast United States, as well as vital statistics data for the United States as a whole, began to show a different pattern (Figure 4) in the 1970s and 1980s. In general, black males have CHD mortality rates as high as those of white males, with some suggestion that the rates of CHD mortality for white males are decreasing faster than those of black males, again consistent with the theory shown in Figure 3. In addition, recent studies of CHD incidence in the southern United States find similar rates in black and white men.[15] Black women, on the other hand, consistently had higher rates of CHD incidence and death than did white women.

When examining racial differences in CHD mortality rates, it appears important to examine rates by age strata. Often they are presented as single, age-adjusted rates. However, this presentation of a single CHD mortality rate appears to obscure a higher rate of CHD in blacks who are <55 years of age, with similar or higher rates of CHD in whites among those who are >55 years. This predisposition of CHD in younger blacks is especially apparent in men. The finding of similar CHD mortality rates between whites and blacks overall and the fact that there is an actual excess of CHD mortality among black persons in their socially and economically productive years led to a dispelling of the myth of black invulnerability to CHD.[16,17]

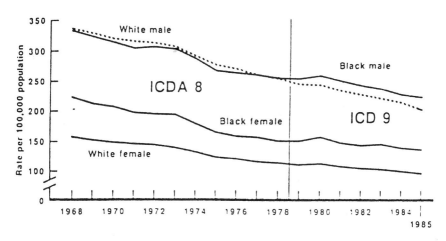

Figure 4. *Death rates for CHD by race and sex in the United States, 1968–1985, from the National Heart, Lung, and Blood Institute. Reproduced with permission from Reference 17.*

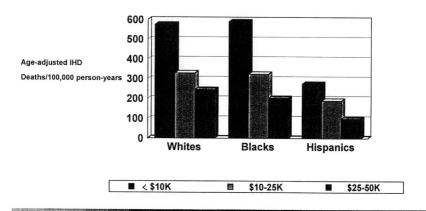

Figure 5. *Coronary heart disease mortality rates (age-adjusted) by income in US men, aged 45–64 years, in the National Longitudinal Mortality Study, 1979–1989. Reproduced with permission from Reference 3.*

Hispanic Americans, Native Americans, and Asian Americans

Hispanic Americans vary in genetic backgrounds and culture, consisting of persons with ancestors from Mexico, Cuba, Puerto Rico, etc. In general, their rates of CHD appear to be lower than those for either whites or blacks, even after adjustment for income (Figure 5).[3,18] Few data are available on groups of Native Americans or Asian Americans other than those of Japanese ancestry. Of those data available, it appears that these groups in general have lower CHD mortality rates.[19]

Asian Indians

One minority group with apparently extraordinary rates of CHD incidence and mortality are persons of Asian-Indian parentage.[20] Migrants from India (and its neighboring countries in southern Asia) have elevated standardized mortality ratios for CHD (1.3- to 4.0-fold increased risk) even when compared to the countries to which they migrate. Interestingly, the three major risk factors of hypertension, smoking, and high blood cholesterol do not explain this predisposition; rather, Asian Indians appear to be predisposed to abdominal obesity, diabetes mellitus (DM), low high-density lipoprotein cholesterol (HDL-C), and high triglycerides (TGs)—the so-called metabolic syndrome.[21] It was hypothesized that Asian Indians may have acquired a predisposition to this syndrome through selection for the "thrifty gene," an inherited trait that imparted a survival advantage during times of famine through efficient use and storage of calories.[22] This trait is deleterious, however, during times of sedentarism and caloric excess. As a variety of disparate groups appear to share this condition, it serves to illustrate the interaction between a genetic predisposition and cultural factors in the determination of CHD risk.

Differences in Coronary Heart Disease Presentation and Natural History In Blacks Versus Whites

An increased CHD mortality rate in young black men could be explained not only by an increased incidence rate but also by a higher case-fatality rate and/or poor prognosis. Again, incidence studies suggest that black men have similar CHD incidence rates as white men.[15] However, a

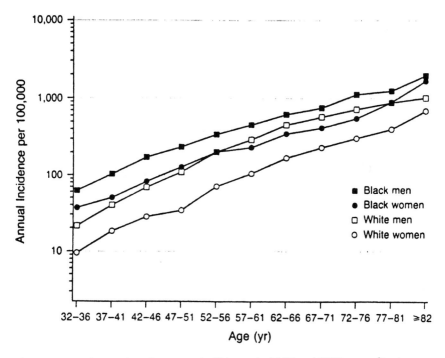

Figure 6. *Incidence of cardiac arrest in Chicago in 1987 and 1988 according to race, sex, and age. Reproduced with permission from Reference 27.*

number of studies suggest that the prognosis after the onset of CHD is much worse in blacks than in whites.[16,23,24] This apparently is especially true in women.[25] At the end of 32 months of follow-up after an acute myocardial infarction in the Multicenter Investigation of the Limitation of Infarct Size (MILIS) Study,[25] 48% of black women died versus only 32% of white women and 21% of white men. Thus black women appear to be at especially high risk for adverse outcomes after the onset of CHD.

One especially important characteristic of CHD presentation in blacks is the high incidence of sudden cardiac death (SCD) and death outside of hospital.[26,27] This is true in both men and women, but especially at ages <55 years (Figure 6).[27] Moreover, blacks are less likely to be successfully resuscitated or, if resuscitated, to survive hospitalization. Thus SCD represents a major public health problem for the black community.

Differences in Risk Factor Prevalence as an Explanation for Differences in Coronary Heart Disease Rates and Natural History

The Relative Importance of Risk Factors Between Racial and/or Ethnic Groups

Even when using the widely accepted paradigm that risk factors cause the development of coronary atherosclerosis and subsequent clinical events, it cannot be assumed that specific risk factors are equally important in all racial and ethnic subgroups. As already mentioned, the US white population risk factor model appears not to fit well in Asian Indians, for example. The relative importance of various risk factors in the causation of CHD in one population subgroup versus another can be described using the population-attributable risk fraction (PARF), which is that proportion of the disease in the population that is attributable to a single risk factor.[28] The PARF is calculated as follows: PARF $(\%) = Pe\,(R - 1) \,/\, [1 + Pe\,(R - 1)] \times 100\%$, where Pe is the proportion of the population with the risk factor and R is the relative risk of developing the disease among those exposed to the risk factor. Therefore, it can be seen that two ways for a single risk factor to account for a larger proportion of disease in one population subgroup is by being more prevalent or by having a stronger association with disease.

A summary of risk-factor differences between whites and blacks illustrates the potential use of the PARF (Table 1).[29] Hypertension might be expected to explain a greater proportion of CHD in blacks than in whites because it is much more prevalent in blacks and also appears to have a

Table 1
Prevalence and Relative Risk of Coronary Risk Factors
in Blacks versus Whites

Risk Factor	Prevalence	Relative Risk
Hypertension	B > W	B > W
Left ventricular hypertrophy	B > W	?
Elevated low-density lipoprotein cholesterol	B = W	B ≤ W
Elevated lipoprotein (a)	B > W	?
Decreased high-density lipoprotein cholesterol	B < W	?
Smoking	B > W	B ≥ W
Diabetes	B > W	B ≥ W
Obesity	B > W	?
Fibrinogen	B > W	?
Sedentary lifestyle	?	?

B > W, blacks' rate greater than whites' rate; B = W, blacks' rate equal to whites' rate; B < W, blacks' rate less than whites' rate; and ?, no definite information.

more deleterious effect when present. This prediction is verified in the Evans County Study, in which hypertension accounted for 10% to 20% of total mortality in whites, but 25% to 45% of total mortality in blacks.[29] Estimates of risk factor prevalences for blacks, Mexican Americans, and whites from the National Health and Nutrition Examination Survey (NHANES) III, 1988–1991, are shown in Tables 2 and 3 for men and women, respectively.

Another observation from Table 1 is that definitive information on the relative risks of a number of risk factors is lacking for blacks as well as for other minority groups. The Charleston Heart Study followed a biracial cohort between 1960 and 1990, measuring relative risks in each race-sex group (Table 4).[15] The relative-risk estimates suggested greater relative risks of CHD for hypertension, smoking, and diabetes in blacks as compared to whites. Similarly, the Meharry-Hopkins study followed two cohorts of medical students, one white and one black, with identical risk-factor assessments in early adulthood (aged 23–27 years) and identical end-point assessments through midlife (28- to 38-year follow-up).[31] That study also showed a significantly elevated relative risk for hypertension in black medical students, with a greater relative risk for serum cholesterol level and smoking in the white medical students. Thus, although available data are still scanty, it appears that the "white" risk-factor model may not be generalizable to other racial and ethnic groups. Such information would be useful in the development of public health programs targeted at minority groups, especially since these programs often need to prioritize their targets and interventions in the utilization of limited resources.

Hypertension and Left Ventricular Hypertrophy: Problems of Special Importance to Blacks

The increased prevalence of hypertension in blacks at all ages above young adulthood is well recognized[32,33] and is not explained by SES (Tables 2 and 3). At least one in three black adults has high blood pressure (BP). Left ventricular hypertrophy (LVH) is associated with hypertension but remains an independent predictor of CHD.[32] LVH is also markedly more prevalent in blacks than in whites, regardless of whether measured on electrocardiogram, echocardiogram, or autopsy.[33]

A variety of theories was presented to explain the predisposition of blacks to hypertension. A full discussion of proposed gene-environment interactions is beyond the scope of this review.[34–36] However, the increased prevalence and severity of hypertension in blacks remains a key variable presumed to explain their predisposition to LVH, excess of SCD, high rates of CHD at young ages, and poor prognosis after the onset of disease.

Table 2

Age-Adjusted Prevalence of Risk Factors by Race and Educational Attainment for U.S. Men from the NHANES III, 1988–1991

	Prevalence (%) by Race/Ethnicity and Education (grade attainment)								
	Blacks			Mexican Americans			Whites		
Risk Factor	<12	12	>12	<12	12	>12	<12	12	>12
Hypertension (>140/90 mm Hg or on medication)	38	36	33	26	27	27	30	27	27
High blood cholesterol (>240 mg/dL)	15	22	22	21	27	15	23	19	22
Current smoking*	56	39	28	35	23	22	43	28	23
Diabetes (self-report)	11	9	6	11	5	9	8	5	5
Overweight**	29	31	36	41	47	42	36	36	31
Sedentary lifestyle*	78	66	66	79	74	42	80	68	52

* Age-specific data for 45- to 64-year-old men. From the National Household Interview Survey, 1993 for smoking and 1990 for sedentarism. Sedentary lifestyle means no self-reported exercise or regular sports.

** Body mass index (kg/m^2) ≥ 27.8.

Reproduced with permission from Reference 3.

Table 3

Age-Adjusted Prevalence of Risk Factors by Race and Educational
Attainment for U.S. Women for the NHANES III, 1988–1991

	Prevalence (%) by Race/Ethnicity and Education (grade attainment)								
	Blacks			Mexican Americans			Whites		
Risk Factor	<12	12	>12	<12	12	>12	<12	12	>12
Hypertension (>140/90 mm Hg or on medication)	38	37	31	25	24	26	27	25	22
High blood cholesterol (>240 mg/dL)	24	22	26	22	26	19	27	25	21
Current smoking*	22	22	21	13	12	8	33	25	20
Diabetes (self-reporting)	14	11	8	15	11	11	8	6	4
Overweight**	54	52	51	53	42	57	38	38	30
Sedentary lifestyle*	81	72	68	80	71	59	77	66	54

* Age-specific data for 45- to 64-year-old women from the National Household Interview Survey, 1990 for smoking and 1990 for sedentarism. Sedentary lifestyle means no self-reported exercise or regular sports.
** Body mass index (kg/m^2) ≥ 27.3.
Reproduced with permission from Reference 3.

Lipids and Lipoproteins

In general, the prevalence of hypercholesterolemia does not differ among whites, Mexican Americans, and blacks (Tables 2 and 3). Likewise, serum low-density lipoprotein cholesterol (LDL-C) levels do not differ considerably between groups. There is no reason to believe that an elevated LDL-C level carries less risk in any single sex-race group.

Other lipoproteins, however, do differ between groups. HDL-C levels are generally higher in blacks than in whites, beginning even in childhood.[37,38] The proportion of HDL-C in subfractions of HDL, namely HDL$_2$ and HDL$_3$, are similar between blacks and whites.[39] Interestingly, black versus white differences in HDL-C seem to disappear with increasing education and/or income,[40] raising doubts about the genetic basis of HDL elevations or suggesting that some other factors, such as obesity or sedentarism, reduce HDL-C levels in both blacks and whites of high SES. HDL-C levels appear to be inversely related to CHD in blacks[41]; differ-

Table 4

Relative Risks for Death from Coronary Heart Disease between 1960 and 1990 for Selected Risk Factors in the Charleston Heart Study, after Adjustment for Age and Other Risk Factors, by Sex-Race Group

Risk Factor in 1960	Relative Risk (±95% CI)			
	White Men	Black Men	White Women	Black Women
Systolic blood pressure (per 28.6 mm Hg)	1.28 (1.02–1.60)	1.71 (1.27–2.29)	1.66 (1.31–2.10)	1.30 (1.02–1.65)
Serum cholesterol (per 48.43 mg/dL)	1.18 (0.98–1.43)	1.15 (0.83–1.58)	1.28 (1.07–1.54)	1.29 (0.99–1.67)
Body mass index* (per 4.88 kg/m²)	0.87 (0.69–1.11)	0.87 (0.62–1.24)	1.09 (0.87–1.36)	0.99 (0.81–1.22)
Years of education (per 0.05 years)	0.79 (0.65–0.96)	1.26 (0.87–1.82)	1.03 (0.79–1.35)	0.79 (0.56–1.13)
Smoking status (yes/no)	1.60 (1.11–2.30)	3.12 (1.66–5.87)	1.94 (1.23–3.06)	0.77 (0.45–1.50)
Diabetes status (yes/no)	1.05 (0.45–2.44)	2.48 (0.33–18.67)	1.25 (0.35–4.47)	2.02 (0.90–4.53)

* Body mass index (kg/m²) ≥ 27.3.
Reproduced with permission from Reference 15.

ences in HDL-C levels do not appear to explain differences in CHD incidence and natural history. This, however, remains to be further defined by longitudinal studies.

Lipoprotein (a) [Lp(a)] remains an enigma as to its role in black-white differences in CHD. Lp(a) appears to be consistently and strongly associated with atherosclerosis and all its clinical sequelae in whites, as documented in both cross-sectional and prospective studies.[42] In terms of biological plausibility, its mechanism of action may be either as an atherogenic particle or as a competitive inhibitor of plasminogen.[43] Of considerable interest is the now well-documented elevation in Lp(a) levels in persons of African descent.[31,42,44-47] The distribution of Lp(a) levels is highly skewed in whites, whereas many more blacks have high levels. In a study comparing black versus white physicians, blacks had median Lp(a) levels three times higher than those of the whites (30 mg/dL vs 10 mg/dL).[45] Lp(a) levels have a strong genetic component related to inherited polymorphisms, which differ between blacks and whites.[46] Black-white differences in serum levels of Lp(a), however, do not appear to be totally explained by these polymorphisms. Finally, since Lp(a) levels are much higher in blacks and are related to CHD in whites, it would seem obvious to infer that Lp(a) may be an important risk factor for CHD in blacks. Evidence to support this, however, has not been forthcoming from one angiography study.[48] Also, elevated Lp(a) levels correlate with a positive family history of CHD in white children but not in black children.[47] Additional prospective studies will be needed to define the role of Lp(a) in racial differences in CHD.

Cigarette Smoking

Strong inverse gradients by education and income characterize smoking rates in all racial and ethnic groups (Tables 2 and 3). In general, the prevalence of cigarette smoking in black men exceeds that of other male groups, whereas white women of low educational attainment have the highest smoking rates of all groups. The figures may be somewhat misleading, however, since there is evidence that white male smokers are more likely to be heavy smokers (25 or more cigarettes per day) than black male smokers. Mexican Americans have the lowest rates of smoking for both men and women.

Diabetes

The prevalence of diabetes in both blacks and Mexican Americans exceeds those of whites in both men and women. The prevalence in women is especially high in these two ethnic groups (Tables 2 and 3). Since diabetes removes the protection from CHD for women, this elevated prevalence of diabetes may explain the higher CHD rates in black women than in white women and may also explain black women's poor prognosis after the onset of CHD.

Obesity and Sedentary Lifestyle

Two related risk factors, obesity and a sedentary lifestyle, show different racial patterns in men and women (Tables 2 and 3). Among men, Mexican Americans have the highest prevalence of overweight, whereas black men have the lowest. Among women, however, both black and Mexican-American women have extremely high rates of overweight. Furthermore, obesity appears to be increasing, especially among women.[49] Because obesity plays a key role in hypertension, diabetes, low HDL-C, etc. in all racial groups, it is an important target for community-based or individual interventions.[50,51] One approach would be to reduce sedentarism, which is highly prevalent among women of low SES (Table 3).

Fibrinogen

Fibrinogen was consistently related to CHD in a number of prospective studies in whites.[52] The Coronary Artery Risk Development in Young Adults Study identified black-white differences even in young men and women, with substantially higher fibrinogen levels found in black women than in white women.[53] Prospective studies of fibrinogen levels in blacks are needed to define whether the relative risks of elevated fibrinogen levels are similar to those of whites.

Preventive Cardiology Interventions

Overview

The selection of interventions for the primary prevention of atherosclerosis[54] and for the management of atherosclerotic disease manifesting as coronary, cerebrovascular, or peripheral vascular disease[55,56] is usually based on the efficacy of the interventions as documented by randomized, clinical trials.[57] Unfortunately, the extent to which minority groups were examined for differences in therapeutic response to these interventions is minimal. Few clinical trials focused solely on a single racial or ethnic group; most of our comparisons of therapeutic response in minorities with those in whites use subgroup analysis within trials in which there was an overall treatment effect.

This section will examine what little we know about specific preventive cardiologic interventions in individuals from minority groups. It should be emphasized, however, that community-wide interventions remain a viable approach to reducing CHD risk in minority populations.[58] Of particular importance here is the recognition of cultural differences in lifestyle behaviors in the way a minority community is organized and in the way health information flows in that community. For example, churches serve as centers for many educational programs for the black community in the United States and were used successfully as a means to implement high BP control[59] and cholesterol screening[60] programs across a wide age spectrum. In the Hispanic community, Spanish-language programs are an obvious requirement if English is not the primary language. Programs that do not recognize, let alone take advantage of, these cultural differences are likely to fall short of their goals.

Antihypertensive Therapies

The importance of the detection and treatment of high BP in the black community cannot be emphasized enough. Moreover, the Hypertension Detection and Follow-up Program suggests that the stepped-care regimen reduced mortality 18.5% and 37.8%, respectively, in hypertensive black men and women, as compared to a reduction of 14.7% in white men and actual increase of 2.1% in mortality in white women.[61] Selection of an antihypertensive agent may also be important since blacks are more likely

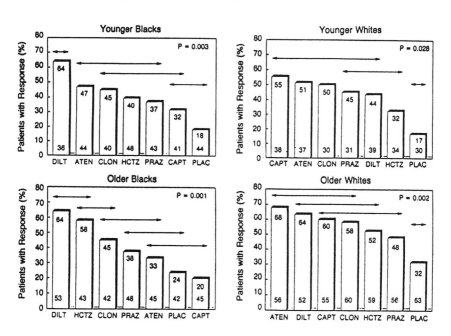

Figure 7. *Percent of male patients responding to various antihypertensive agents by age and race. Reproduced with permission from Reference 63.*

to have low renin hypertension; β-blockers appear to be less effective in general in blacks.[62] Effectiveness of six classes of antihypertensive agents was compared between blacks and whites of younger and older ages (Figure 7).[63] In general, calcium channel blockers and diuretics appear to be more effective in blacks, whereas angiotensin-converting enzyme inhibitor and β-blocker therapies are effective in whites. Finally, there is no evidence that blacks are less aware, compliant, or controllable with regard to high BP. The NHANES II survey actually showed a higher level of awareness of BP status and similar levels of treatment and control among blacks than whites.[64]

Lipid-Lowering Diet and Drug Therapy

The National Cholesterol Education Program's Adult Treatment Panel II recommends that, regardless of race or ethnic group, all Americans aged 18 years and older be screened for lipid disorders with a measurement of serum total and HDL cholesterol level.[65] However, cholesterol awareness in blacks appears to lag behind that of whites. In a study of 15 892 screenees in Hartford, Connecticut, few blacks participated (1.3%), certainly less than their proportion in the population.[66] In the Minnesota Heart Study, blacks were found to be less knowledgeable about CHD in general[67] and significantly less aware of their cholesterol levels—only about 20% of blacks in Minnesota knew their cholesterol levels.[68] It is estimated that approximately 35% of this group would be candidates for diet or drug therapy.[69]

The recommended diet for all Americans should consist of no more than 30% of calories from fat, 10% of calories from saturated fat, and 300 mg of cholesterol per day.[65] Whereas blacks appear to consume similar amounts of fat as whites, blacks' dietary cholesterol intakes appear to be higher.[70] Thus the population-wide dietary recommendations targeted to blacks should emphasize reductions in the consumption of high-cholesterol foods. At the same time, further reductions in fat (20% of calories or less), saturated fat (67% of calories or less), and cholesterol (200 mg per day or less) are recommended for treatment of elevated LDL-C levels. There is no evidence that blacks respond differently to changes in dietary saturated fat. Two clinical trials of cholesterol-lowering diets in which all meals were consumed at the study sites showed similar reductions in serum LDL-C levels in all race-sex groups.[71,72] However, a recent study comparing 32 non-Caucasian men with 52 white men, all aged 25–35 years, suggested that the non-Caucasian men were less sensitive to increases in dietary cholesterol, especially combined with a diet high in saturated fat.[73]

Similarly, there is no evidence that blacks will be less willing to make dietary changes. In the Multiple Risk Factor Intervention Trial (MRFIT) study, there were no differences between races in the changes in nutrient intake or changes in plasma cholesterol among men who received intensive lifestyle counseling.[74] In a study in Chicago, hypercholesterolemic blacks actually had a greater gain in nutrition knowledge and a greater reduction in serum cholesterol level after a 6- to 9-month nutrition education program.[75]

The use of cholesterol-lowering drugs in blacks was not studied to any degree. Little is known about whether cholesterol-lowering drugs of choice may differ in efficacy among racial groups in the way antihypertensive drugs, for example, appear to differ.[63] 3-hydroxy-3-methylglutaryl coenzyme A (HMG-CoA) reductase inhibitors appear to have similar effects in blacks as compared to whites.[76] Niacin is the only drug consistently shown to lower Lp(a) levels; if Lp(a) is an important cause of CHD in blacks, niacin therapy may take on added importance in the treatment of hyperlipidemia in black patients. Bile acid-binding resins appear to be especially effective in prevention of CHD in the presence of a high HDL-C level[77] and may therefore be especially effective in blacks. Unfortunately, many of the large, randomized trials of HMG-CoA reductase inhibitors conducted recently were performed in white populations in Europe. Clearly, clinical trials with sizable numbers of blacks need to be performed to assure that those agents most efficacious in correcting serum lipid abnormalities in whites are also effective in blacks.

Smoking Cessation

Culturally sensitive smoking cessation programs appear effective in reducing the use of tobacco in blacks. There is no reason to believe that the benefits of smoking cessation would be any less spectacular in blacks than in whites. Smoking cessation rates in black men in the MRFIT study were similar to those in whites.[74] A 50% reduction in coronary risk can be expected within 6 months of smoking cessation, both in persons with and without established CHD.

Control of Diabetes with Diet, Drugs, and Insulin

The high prevalence of diabetes, especially among persons with established CHD, makes this an area of potential importance. Unfortunately, little information is available to prove that tight diabetic control yields fewer CHD events. In one study of insulin-dependent diabetics,[78] black women did not improve their lipid profiles with control of blood glucose levels in the same way as white women. Several studies suggested that at least two subpopulations exist within those patients with non-insulin-dependent DM.[79,80] Blacks who are insulin resistant are more obese and have higher LDL-C and TG levels, whereas insulin-sensitive patients have a less atherogenic lipid profile.

Suffice it to say, more research on the extent to which CHD can be prevented with tight diabetic control is needed. Control of other risk factors in diabetes takes on added importance.

Weight Reduction and Physical Activity

Caloric restriction and physical activity will likely remain as the mainstays for maintenance of ideal body weight. Given the central role of obesity in hypertension, diabetes, LVH, etc., every effort to achieve ideal body weight should be used.

Postmenopausal Estrogen Replacement

Little is known about estrogen replacement therapy in black women; moreover, the use of estrogens remains controversial as to its role in the primary or secondary prevention of CHD. Oral estrogen supplements are potent reducers of Lp(a), fibrinogen, and insulin levels in postmenopausal women,[81,82] suggesting a special benefit for postmenopausal black women, especially if these risk factors explain the excess risk of CHD in this race-sex subgroup. Ongoing clinical trials will hopefully clarify the role of estrogen replacement therapy as a preventive cardiologic intervention.

Treatment of Ischemic Heart Disease

A number of therapeutic modalities were compared between racial groups in patients with both acute and chronic CHD. Given the high case-fatality rate for CHD in blacks, it is important to identify interventions that have efficacy in improving these poor outcomes. One established modality in the setting of acute infarction is thrombolysis. The Thrombolysis and Angioplasty in Myocardial Infarction trial examined racial differences in response to thrombolytic therapy.[83] Given the increased levels of fibrinogen, factor VII, and Lp(a) (an inhibitor of plasminogen) in blacks, one might have expected a reduced efficacy of tissue-type plasminogen activation. However, patency rates in the infarct-related artery at 90 minutes were 91% for black patients versus 72% for whites ($P = 0.051$). There was also a greater change in fibrinogen levels and a greater need for transfusions. There was no difference in survival. Thus thrombolysis seems to be at least as effective, if not more so, in blacks as it is in whites.

Other therapies used in patients with established CHD also appear similarly effective. Coronary artery bypass and other revascularization procedures appear to be as effective in blacks as in whites.[84] In the Coronary Artert Surgery Study, black patients treated with bypass surgery had a similar prognosis as whites, whereas black patients treated medically had a significantly worse prognosis.[22] Likewise, in the Beta Blocker Heart Attack Trial (BHAT) trial, reductions in mortality due to the use of β-blockers were similar in both blacks and whites.[85] Given these results, it is likely safe to generalize the joint American Heart Association-American College of Cardiology recommendations for secondary preventive interventions to blacks, at least until data become available to indicate otherwise.[56]

The Problem of Access to Medical Care

When considering differences in case-fatality rates and overall mortality due to CHD, access to medical care must be included in the list of possible explanations. In a study in Alameda County, California, more than one-third of the excess mortality in blacks could be ascribed to potentially preventable causes, suggesting inequalities in health care services as a major part of social inequalities in general.[86] The differential access may be due to several causes—racism on the part of the health care system, patients' SES or educational status, or other geographic or cultural factors. These influences can act on any of several points in the health care-seeking process, including lack of health education messages to reinforce a healthy lifestyle, lack of a primary care provider to assure risk factor detection and management, lack of a primary care provider to detect early signs and symptoms of CHD or to provide advice to the patient soon after the onset of these symptoms, or bias in the use of diagnostic or therapeutic procedures known to reduce cardiac morbidity and mortality.

The lack of health education programs and primary care providers in inner-city and poor rural communities is well known. The lack of health insurance and of a primary care provider are both risk factors for uncontrolled hypertension, leading to severe, symptomatic complications.[87] Poor people tend to have greater severity of illness upon presentation to the hospital for a variety of conditions.[88] Hospital delays after the onset of chest pain are two to three times longer for blacks than whites.[89] Thus the lack of a reliable primary care provider may greatly affect the case fatality rates, both out of hospital as well as among those surviving long enough to be hospitalized.

Moreover, the selection of interventions after the onset of symptomatic CHD appears to be influenced by the race of the patient.[90] The hospitalization and referral rates for further diagnosis and management with such procedures as cardiac catheterization are markedly different between whites and blacks with chest pain.[91] A recent survey by Ford[92] reviewed nine studies, all of which were consistent in the finding that referral rates for cardiac catheterization were 30% to 40% higher in whites than in blacks. Two recent additional studies, including one in Veterans Administration hospitals (which have no financial constraints), found the same differences.[93,94] Furthermore, the same studies showed that subsequent referrals for angioplasty and/or bypass surgery were 1.4 to 4.2 times more likely for whites than blacks.[92]

The cause of these troubling findings is unclear. Blacks may be less trusting of, and satisfied with, the health care system, resulting in fewer visits to physicians and, consequently, fewer referrals to a cardiologist. The mistrust may be reflected in reduced likelihood to agree to bypass surgery, as noted by Maynard et al.[95] Severity of illness and source of care do not appear to explain these results.

Conclusions

The myth that CHD is largely a problem of the white majority was dispelled. In fact, recent trends show that CHD mortality rates continued to fall in white males and, to a lesser extent, white females, whereas CHD mortality in black men and women appears to be leveling off.[96] If these trends continue, CHD will be a relatively more important problem in blacks than in whites.

Excess CHD mortality appears to be due to an equal or modestly increased incidence, a predisposition to presentation as sudden death, and to a poor prognosis after the onset of disease (especially in women). It would appear that established risk factors and differences in SES can explain only part of these differences. One study by Otten et al[97] showed that 31% of the excess mortality of blacks can be explained by the six recognized risk factors (smoking, BP, cholesterol level, body mass index, alcohol intake, and diabetes); 38% can be explained by income; the remaining one-third cannot be accounted for. This leaves open the possibility that newly described risk factors may account for the excess mortality. For example, Lp(a) and the thrombogenic factors (fibrinogen, factor VII, etc.) have higher mean levels in blacks than whites. Other factors, as yet unidentified, may also play a disproportionate role in CHD in minorities. This remains an area for active and fruitful research.

Finally, the benefits of declining CHD mortality rates were enjoyed by all race-sex groups in the United States (Figure 4). The need for further reduction in CHD in blacks leads to questions about public education programs in that community, about access to primary and emergency care, and the use of those secondary prevention interventions shown efficacious against recurrence and death in white CHD patients. Clinical trials should be expanded to include enough patients from minority groups to allow subgroup analyses or should be limited to patients from minority groups. As in the control of hypertension, for example, treatments may be better tailored to specific race-sex-age groups, if clinical trial results support this. Until such data are available, minority groups should receive the appropriately aggressive management of risk factors shown to be efficacious in the prevention of CHD, the leading cause of death in all subsets of the US population.

References

1. American Heart Association. *Heart Facts*. Dallas, Tex: American Heart Association; 1995.
2. Davignon J, Roy M. Familial hypercholesterolemia in French-Canadians: taking advantage of the presence of the "founder effect." *Am J Cardiol* 1993; 72:6–10.
3. *Chart Book of US National Data on Socioeconomic Status and Cardiovascular Health and Disease*. Bethesda, Md: National Heart, Lung and Blood Institute; 1995.
4. Kaplan GA, Keil JE. Socioeconomic factors and cardiovascular disease: a review of the literature. *Circulation* 1993;88:1973–1998.
5. Feldman JJ, Makuc DM, Kleinman JC, et al. National trends in educational differentials in mortality. *Am J Epidemiol* 1989;129:919–933.
6. Preston SH, Elo IT. Are educational differentials in adult mortality increasing in the United States? *J Aging Health* 1995;7:476–496.
7. Weinblatt E, Ruberman W, Goldberg JD, et al. Relation of education to sudden death after myocardial infarction. *N Engl J Med* 1978;299:60–65.
8. Williams RB, Barefoot JC, Califf RM, et al. Prognostic importance of social and economic resources among medically treated patients with angiographically documented coronary artery disease. *JAMA* 1992;267:520–524.
9. Lynch J, Kaplan GA, Salonen R, et al. Socioeconomic status and carotid atherosclerosis. *Circulation* 1995;92:1786–1792.
10. Marmot MG, Shipley MJ, Rose G. Inequalities in death—specific explanations of a general pattern? *Lancet* 1984;1:1003–1006.
11. Omran AR. The epidemiologic transition. A theory of the epidemiology of population change. *Milbank Q* 1971;49:509–538.
12. Olshansky SJ, Ault AB. The fourth stage of the epidemiologic transition: the age of delayed degenerative diseases. *Milbank Q* 1986;64:355–391.
13. McDonough JR, Hanes CG, Stalb SC, et al. Coronary heart disease among negroes and whites in Evans County, Georgia. *J Chron Dis* 1965;18:443–468.
14. Cassel J, Heyden S, Bartel AG, et al. Incidence of coronary heart disease by ethnic group, social class, and sex. *Arch Intern Med* 1971;128:901–906.
15. Keil JE, Sutherland SE, Knapp RG, et al. Mortality rates and risk factors for coronary disease in black as compared with white men and women. *N Engl J Med* 1993;329:73–78.
16. Gillum RF, Grant CT. Coronary heart disease in black populations. II. Risk factors. *Am Heart J* 1982;104:852–864.
17. Watkins LO. Prevention of coronary heart disease in blacks. In: Pearson TA, Criqui M, Luepker R, et al, eds. *Primer in Preventive Cardiology*. Dallas, Tex: American Heart Association; 1994:273–283.

18. Friis R, Nanjundappa G, Prendergast TJ, Jr, et al. Coronary heart disease mortality and risk among Hispanics and non-Hispanics in Orange County, California. *Public Health Rep* 1981;96:418–422.
19. Cooper ES, Kuller LH, Saunders E, et al. Cardiovascular diseases and stroke in African Americans and other racial minorities in the United States. *Circulation* 1991;83:1462–1480.
20. Enas EA, Yusuf S, Mehta JL. Prevalence of coronary artery disease in Asian Indians. Editorial. *Am J Cardiol* 1992;70:945–949.
21. Reaven GM. Banting lecture 1988. Role of insulin resistance in human disease. *Diabetes* 1988;37:1595–1607.
22. Zimmet PZ. Kelly West lecture 1991. Challenges in diabetes epidemiology—from West to the rest. *Diabetes Care* 1992;15:232–252.
23. Maynard C, Fisher LD, Passamani ER. Survival of black persons compared with white persons in the Coronary Artery Surgery Study (CASS). *Am J Cardiol* 1987;60:513–518.
24. Castaner A, Simmons BE, Mar M, et al. Myocardial infarction among black patients: poor prognosis after hospital discharge. *Ann Intern Med* 1988; 109:33–35.
25. Tofler GH, Stone PH, Muller JE, et al. Effects of gender and race on prognosis after myocardial infarction: adverse prognosis for women, particularly black women. *J Am Coll Cardiol* 1987;9:473–482.
26. Gillum RF. Sudden coronary death in the United States: 1980–1985. *Circulation* 1989;79:756–765.
27. Becker LB, Han BH, Meyer PM, et al. Racial differences in the incidence of cardiac arrest and subsequent survival. The CPR Chicago Project. *N Engl J Med* 1993;329:600–606.
28. Cole P, MacMahon B. Attributable risk percent in case-control studies. *Br J Prev Soc Med* 1971;25:242–244.
29. Pearson TA, Jenkins GM, Thomas J. Prevention of coronary heart disease in black adults. In: Saunders E, ed. *Coronary Heart Disease in Blacks.* Philadelphia, PA: FA Davis, 1991:263–276.
30. Deubner DC, Tyroler HA, Cassel JC, et al. Attributable risk, population attributable risk, and population attributable fraction of death associated with hypertension in a biracial population. *Circulation* 1975;52:901–908.
31. Pearson TA, Thomas J. Youthful predictors of midlife coronary artery disease: differences between African Americans and whites in the Meharry-Hopkins Study. Abstract. *Circulation* 1995;92:419.
32. Kannel WB. Prevalence and natural history of electrocardiographic left ventricular hypertrophy. *Am J Med* 1983;75:4–11.
33. Savage DD. Overall risk of left ventricular hypertrophy secondary to systemic hypertension. *Am J Cardiol* 1987;60:8I-12I.
34. Gillum RF. Pathophysiology of hypertension in blacks and whites. A review of the basis of racial blood pressure differences. *Hypertension* 1979;1:468–475.
35. Wilson TW, Grim CE. Biohistory of slavery and blood pressure differences in blacks today. A hypothesis. *Hypertension* 1991;17:122–128.
36. Lang CC. Attenuation of isoproterenol-mediated vasodilatation in blacks. *N Engl J Med* 1995;333:155–160.
37. Glueck CJ, Gartside P, Laskarzewski PM, et al. High-density lipoprotein cholesterol in blacks and whites: potential ramifications for coronary heart disease. *Am Heart J* 1984;108:815–826.
38. Freedman DS, Srinivasan SR, Webber LS, et al. Black-white differences in serum lipoproteins during sexual maturation: the Bogalusa Heart Study. *J Chron Dis* 1987;40:309–318.

39. Brown SA, Hutchinson R, Morrisett J, et al. Plasma lipid, lipoprotein cholesterol, and apoprotein distributions in selected US communities. The Atherosclerosis Risk in Communities (ARIC) Study. *Arterioscler Thromb* 1993; 13:1139–1158.

40. Freedman DS, Strogatz DS, Williamson DF, et al. Education, race, and high-density lipoprotein cholesterol among US adults. *Am J Public Health* 1992; 82:999–1006.

41. Watkins LO, Neaton JD, Kuller LH. Racial differences in high-density lipoprotein cholesterol and coronary heart disease incidence in the usual-care group of the Multiple Risk Factor Intervention Trial. *Am J Cardiol* 1986; 57:538–545.

42. Austin MA, Hokanson JE. Epidemiology of triglycerides, small dense low-density lipoprotein, and lipoprotein (a) as risk factors for coronary heart disease. Review. *Med Clin North Am* 1994;78:99–115.

43. Scanu AM, Lawn RM, Berg K. Lipoprotein (a) and atherosclerosis. *Ann Intern Med* 1991;115:209–218.

44. Guyton JR, Dahlen GH, Patsch W, et al. Relationship of plasma lipoprotein lp(a) levels to race and to apolipoprotein B. *Arteriosclerosis* 1985;5:265–272.

45. Sorrentino MJ, Vielhauer C, Eisenbart JD, et al. Plasma lipoprotein (a) protein concentration and coronary artery disease in black patients compared with white patients. *Am J Med* 1992;93:658–662.

46. Helmhold M, Bigge J, Muche R, et al. Contribution of the apo(a) phenotype to plasma Lp(a) concentrations shows considerable ethnic variation. *J Lipid Res* 1991;32:1919–1928.

47. Srinivasan SR, Dahlen GH, Jarpa RA, et al. Racial (black-white) differences in serum lipoprotein (a) distribution and its relation to parental myocardial infarction in children. Bogalusa Heart Study. *Circulation* 1991;84:160–167.

48. Molitero AJ, Jokinen EV, Miserez AR, et al. No association between plasma lipoprotein (a) concentrations and presence or absence of coronary atherosclerosis in African Americans. *Arterioscler Thromb Vasc Biol* 1995;15:850–855.

49. Kuczmarski RJ, Flegal KM, Campbell SM, et al. Increasing prevalence of overweight among US adults. The National Health and Nutrition Examination Surveys, 1960–1991. *JAMA* 1994;272:205–211.

50. Van Itallie TB. Health implications of overweight and obesity in the United States. *Ann Intern Med* 1985;103:983–988.

51. Folsom AR, Burke GL, Ballew C, et al. Relation of body fatness and its distribution to cardiovascular risk factors in young blacks and whites. The role of insulin. *Am J Epidemiol* 1989;130:911–924.

52. Ernst E, Resch KL. Fibrinogen as a cardiovascular risk factor: a meta-analysis and review of the literature. *Ann Intern Med* 1993;118:956–963.

53. Folsom AR, Qamhieh HT, Flack JM, et al. Plasma fibrinogen: levels and correlates in young adults. The Coronary Artery Risk Development in Young Adults (CARDIA) study. *Am J Epidemiol* 1993;138:1023–1036.

54. Manson JE, Tosteson H, Ridker PM, et al. The primary prevention of myocardial infarction. *N Engl J Med* 1992;326:1406–1416.

55. Pearson T, Rapaport E, Criqui M, et al. Optimal risk factor management in the patient after coronary revascularization: a statement for healthcare professionals from an American Heart Association Writing Group. *Circulation* 1994;90:3125–3133.

56. Smith SC Jr. Preventing heart attack and death in patients with coronary disease: Consensus Panel Statement. *Circulation* 1995;92:2–4.

57. Yusuf S, Lessem J, Jha P, et al. Primary and secondary prevention of myocardial infarction and strokes: an update of randomly allocated, controlled trials. *J Hypertens* 1993;11(suppl):61–73.
58. Mittelmark MB, Hunt MK, Heath GW, et al. Realistic outcomes: lessons from community-based research and demonstration programs for the prevention of cardiovascular diseases. *J Public Health Policy* 1993;14:437–462.
59. Strogatz DS, James SA, Elliott D, et al. Community coverage in a rural, church-based, hypertension screening program in Edgecombe County, North Carolina. *Am J Public Health* 1985;75:401–402.
60. Flack JM, Wiist WH. Cardiovascular risk factor prevalence in African-American adult screenees for a church-based cholesterol education program: the Northeast Oklahoma City Cholesterol Education Program. *Ethn Dis* 1991;1:78–90.
61. Hypertension Detection and Follow-up Program Cooperative Group. Five-year findings of the Hypertension Detection and Follow-up Program. II. Mortality by race-sex and age. *JAMA* 1979;242:2572–2577.
62. Saunders E, Weir MR, Kong BW, et al. A comparison of the efficacy and safety of a beta-blocker, a calcium channel blocker, and a converting enzyme inhibitor in hypertensive blacks. *Arch Intern Med* 1990;150:1707–1713.
63. Materson BJ, Reda DJ, Cushman WC, et al. Single-drug therapy for hypertension in men. A comparison of six antihypertensive agents with placebo. The Department of Veterans Affairs Cooperative Study Group on Antihypertensive Agents. *N Engl J Med* 1993;328:914–921.
64. Subcommittee on Definition and Procedure, 1984. Joint National Commission. Hypertension prevalence and the status of awareness, treatment, and control in the United States. Final report of the subcommittee on definition and prevalence of the 1984 Joint National Committee. *Hypertension* 1985;7:457–468.
65. Summary of the Second Report of the National Cholesterol Education Program (NCEP) Expert Panel on Detection, Evaluation, and Treatment of High Blood Cholesterol in Adults (Adult Treatment Panel II). *JAMA* 1993;269:3015–3023.
66. Wynder EL, Harris RE, Haley NJ. Population screening for plasma cholesterol: community-based results from Connecticut. *Am Heart J* 1989; 117:649–656.
67. Folsom AR, Sprafka JM, Luepker RV, et al. Beliefs among black and white adults about causes and prevention of cardiovascular disease: the Minnesota Heart Survey. *Am J Prev Med* 1988;4:121–127.
68. Sprafka JM, Burke GL, Folsom AR, et al. Hypercholesterolemia prevalence, awareness, and treatment in blacks and whites: the Minnesota Heart Survey. *Prev Med* 1989;18:423–432.
69. Sempos C, Fulwood R, Haines C, et al. The prevalence of high blood cholesterol levels among adults in the United States. *JAMA* 1989;262:45–52.
70. Block G, Rosenberger WF, Patterson BH. Calories, fat and cholesterol: intake patterns in the US population by race, sex and age. *Am J Public Health* 1988;78:1150–1155.
71. Howard BV, Hannah JS, Heiser CC, et al. Effects of sex and ethnicity on responses to a low-fat diet: a study of African Americans and whites. *Am J Clin Nutr* 1995;62:488S–492S.
72. Ginsberg HN, Dennis B, Elmer PJ, et al. Effects of reducing dietary saturated fatty acids on plasma lipids and lipoproteins in healthy subjects: the DELTA study. *J Athero Throm Vasc Dis.* In press.
73. Fielding CJ, Havel RJ, Todd KM, et al. Effects of dietary cholesterol and fat saturation on plasma lipoproteins in an ethnically diverse population of healthy young men. *J Clin Invest* 1995;95:611–618.

74. Connett JE, Stamler J. Responses of black and white males to the special intervention program of the Multiple Risk Factor Intervention Trial. *Am Heart J* 1984;108:839–848.

75. Mojonnier ML, Hall Y, Berkson DM, et al. Experience in changing food habits of hyperlipidemic men and women. *J Am Diet Assoc* 1980;77:140–148.

76. Prisant LM. Extended clinical evaluation of lovastatin (EXCEL) study results: efficacy of lovastatin in blacks. *J Clin Pharmacol* 1991;31:852.

77. Gordon DJ, Knoke J, Probstfield JL. High-density lipoprotein cholesterol and coronary heart disease in hypercholesterolemic men: the Lipid Research Clinics Coronary Primary Prevention Trial. *Circulation* 1986;74:1217–1225.

78. Semenkovich CF, Ostlund RE Jr, Schechtman KB. Plasma lipids in patients with type I diabetes mellitus. Influence of race, gender, and plasma glucose control: lipids do not correlate with glucose control in black women. *Arch Intern Med* 1989;149:51–56.

79. Banerji MA, Lebovitz HE. Coronary heart disease risk factor profiles in black patients with non-insulin-dependent diabetes mellitus: paradoxic patterns. *Am J Med* 1991;91:51–58.

80. Chaiken RL, Banerji MA, Pasmantier R. Patterns of glucose and lipid abnormalities in black NIDDM subjects. *Diabetes Care* 1991;14:1036–1042.

81. Manolio TA, Furberg CD, Shemanski L. Associations of postmenopausal estrogen use with cardiovascular disease and its risk factors in older women. The CHS Collaborative Research Group. *Circulation* 1993;88:2163–2171.

82. Nabulsi AA, Folsom AR, White A. Association of hormone-replacement therapy with various cardiovascular risk factors in postmenopausal women. The Atherosclerosis Risk in Communities Study investigators. *N Engl J Med* 1993;328:1069–1075.

83. Sane DC, Stump DC, Topol EJ, et al. Racial differences in responses to thrombolytic therapy with recombinant tissue-type plasminogen activator. Increased fibrin(ogen)olysis in blacks. The Thrombolysis and Angioplasty in Myocardial Infarction Study Group. *Circulation* 1991;83:170–175.

84. Oberman A, Cutter G. Issues in the natural history and treatment of coronary heart disease in black populations: surgical treatment. *Am Heart J* 1984; 108:688–694.

85. Haywood LJ. Coronary heart disease mortality/morbidity and risk in blacks. I. Clinical manifestations and diagnostic criteria: the experience with the Beta Blocker Heart Attack Trial. *Am Heart J* 1984;108:787–793.

86. Woolhandler S, Himmelstein DU, Silber R, et al. Medical care and mortality: racial differences in preventable deaths. *Int J Health Serv* 1985;15:1–22.

87. Shea S, Misra D, Ehrlich MH, et al. Predisposing factors for severe, uncontrolled hypertension in an inner-city minority population. *N Engl J Med* 1992;327:776–781.

88. Epstein AM, Stern RS, Weissman JS. Do the poor cost more? A multihospital study of patients' socioeconomic status and use of hospital resources. *N Engl J Med* 1990;322:1122–1128.

89. Cooper RS, Simmons B, Castaner A. Survival rates and prehospital delay during myocardial infarction among black persons. *Am J Cardiol* 1986;57: 208–211.

90. Ayanian JZ. Heart disease in black and white. *N Engl J Med* 1993;329: 656–658.

91. Johnson PA, Lee TH, Cook EF. Effect of race on the presentation and management of patients with acute chest pain. *Ann Intern Med* 1993;118:593–601.

92. Ford ES. Implications of race/ethnicity for health and health care use. *Health Serv Res* 1995;30:237–252.

93. Ayanian JZ, Udvarhelyi IS, Gatsonis CA. Racial differences in the use of revascularization procedures after coronary angiography. *JAMA* 1993;269:2642–2646.
94. Whittle J, Conigliaro J, Good CB. Racial differences in the use of invasive cardiovascular procedures in the Department of Veterans Affairs medical system. *N Engl J Med* 1993;329:621–627.
95. Maynard C, Fisher LD, Passamani ER. Blacks in the Coronary Artery Surgery Study (CASS): race and clinical decision making. *Am J Public Health* 1986; 76:1446–1448.
96. Liao Y, Cooper R. Continued adverse trends in coronary heart disease mortality among blacks, 1980–1991. *Public Health Rep* 1995;110:572–579.
97. Otten MW, Jr., Teutsch SM, Williamson DF, et al. The effect of known risk factors on the excess mortality of black adults in the United States. *JAMA* 1990;263:845–850.

Chapter 11

Arterial Gene Transfer as Preventive Therapy

Laurent J. Feldman, MD
and Jeffrey M. Isner, MD

Acute coronary events result from the rupture of an atherosclerotic plaque, leading to formation of an occlusive coronary thrombus. Recent developments in the field of gene transfer provide an opportunity to genetically modify cells involved in plaque rupture as well as thrombus formation and thus prevent acute coronary syndromes. A first approach consists of transferring genes, the product of which may stabilize the vulnerable plaque by reducing the plaque content in lipids and macrophages. Alternatively, the introduction into the atherosclerotic plaque of genes encoding for thrombolytic proteins or growth factors able to restore physiological antithrombotic functions of endothelial cells may inhibit thrombus formation should the plaque rupture. The success of such strategies depends on the efficiency with which the transgene is introduced and expressed into the target cell, the duration of transgene expression, and the ability of the transgene product to ultimately prevent plaque rupture and/or thrombus formation.

Introduction

Rupture of coronary atherosclerotic plaque and subsequent formation of an occlusive intracoronary thrombus are the major events precip-

Dr. Feldman is a recipient of an award from the Fullbright Scholar Program. Dr. Isner is supported by grants HL-40518 and HL-02824 from the National Institutes of Health.

Table 1
Potential Targets for Genetic Interventions to Prevent
Acute Coronary Syndromes

Target Gene	Intervention	Mechanisms
LDL receptor	Augmentation	Plaque stabilizaton
HDL	Augmentation	Plaque stabilization
eNOS	Augmentation	Plaque stabilization
		Inhibition of SMC proliferation
		Inhibition of thrombus formation
sVCAM-1	Augmentation	Plaque stabilization
Metalloproteinases	Inhibition	Plaque stabilization
TPA	Augmentation	Inhibition of thrombus formation
scu-PA	Augmentation	Inhibition of thrombus formation
VEGF	Augmentation	Inhibition of thrombus formation
		Inhibition of SMC proliferation

LDL: low-density lipoprotein; HDL: high-density lipoprotein; eNOS: constitutive endothelial nitric oxide synthase; SMC: smooth muscle cells; sVCAM-1: soluble vascular cell adhesion molecule 1; TPA: tissular plasminogen activator; scu-PA: single-chain urokinase plasminogen activator; VEGF: vascular endothelial growth factor.

itating acute coronary syndromes.[1-6] The vulnerable plaque is smaller in size,[7] richer in lipids,[1,2] and more infiltrated with macrophages[2,3,8-10] than the stable, fibromuscular lesion. Therefore, lowering the lipid and/or macrophage pools stored in the plaque may "stabilize" the plaque and reduce the incidence of plaque rupture.[2,4-6] Indeed, cholesterol-lowering trials yielded a significant reduction in acute cardiac events.[11-18] Antithrombotic therapies may further prevent acute coronary syndromes by altering the consequences of plaque rupture.[4]

Recent advances in the field of molecular biology, combined with the development of efficient vectors to perform in vivo gene transfer, led to the emergence of new therapies to prevent acute coronary syndromes. Because gene therapy, in contrast to drug therapy, implies a variable and currently undetermined time interval for the transgene to be expressed, certain gene therapy approaches ultimately may not prove appropriate for treatment of patients with acute infarction. Genetic interventions that are designed to stabilize the vulnerable plaque and/or inhibit thrombus formation (Table 1), however, hold considerable promise and may ultimately constitute a novel form of preventive therapy.

Gene Therapy for the Vulnerable Plaque

Lowering the level of plasma cholesterol may reduce progression and even induce regression of atherosclerotic lesions.[11-19] This result appears to represent the consequence of reducing plasma low-density lipoprotein (LDL) levels as well as increasing plasma high-density lipoprotein (HDL) levels. Even modest changes in coronary luminal diameter observed in patients, as a result of lipid-lowering interventions, were associated with a significant reduction in the incidence of acute coronary syndromes.[11–18] It is likely that this beneficial effect was due to the regression of plaques rich in cholesterol and macrophages, ie, plaques prone to rupture.[4,19] Therefore, therapeutic strategies aimed at (1) lowering plasma LDL, (2) increasing plasma HDL, and/or (3) mitigating macrophage infiltration hold promise for reducing the mortality and morbidity associated with coronary atherosclerosis.

Familial Hypercholesterolemia: A Model for Low-Density Lipoprotein-Targeted Gene Therapy

Familial hypercholesterolemia (FH) is caused by a genetic deficiency in the hepatic receptors for LDL cholesterol (LDL-C) and is associated with severe hypercholesterolemia and premature coronary artery disease (CAD).[20] The observation that orthotopic liver transplantation from donors who express normal LDL receptor activity may lead to complete correction of the dyslipidemia in homozygotes[21] set the stage for a genetic strategy, first articulated by Goldstein et al,[22] targeted toward introduction into the liver of normal LDL receptor genes.

Two different approaches to gene therapy were developed for FH. In the first approach, referred to as "ex vivo" (or "indirect") gene transfer, cells are removed, transduced ex vivo with the LDL receptor gene, then transplanted back into the liver. In the second approach, referred to as "in vivo" (or "direct") gene transfer, the LDL receptor gene is directly introduced into the liver during a one-step procedure. Although FH accounts for only a small minority of patients, the promise of genetically increasing LDL receptor abundance in the liver may have implications for treating more common forms of hypercholesterolemia and thereby potentially reducing the incidence of acute coronary syndromes in these patients.[23]

Ex Vivo Gene Therapy for Familial Hypercholesterolemia

Wilson et al[24] and Chowdhury et al[25] used an animal model for FH, the Watanabe heritable hyperlipidemic (WHHL) rabbit, to isolate hepatocytes following partial hepatectomy, to transfect these cells ex vivo with replication-defective retroviruses including an LDL receptor cDNA, and to implant the transduced hepatocytes into the liver of recipient WHHL rabbits. Stable expression of the recombinant LDL receptor gene as well as a consistent decrease in serum cholesterol could be detected for several months after autologous transplantation.[25]

On the basis of these encouraging results, the first clinical trial of gene therapy to treat patients with homozygous FH was initiated in 1992.[26] In this protocol, an ex vivo approach similar to the one used in the WHHL rabbit was adopted. After partial hepatectomy, hepatocytes were released and transfected ex vivo with recombinant retroviruses expressing a human LDL receptor cDNA. Transduced hepatocytes were subsequently infused directly into the portal circulation to allow engraftment of LDL receptor-expressing hepatocytes in the liver. Preliminary results on the first patient enrolled in this trial were recently published.[27] The patient tolerated the surgical procedure well, and expression of the transfected LDL receptor gene was documented 4 months after gene transfer in $1:10^3$ to $1:10^4$ liver cells. This was paralleled by a 17% decrease in serum LDL that persisted for at least 18 months.

These results, although remarkable, require further analysis. Brown et al[28] outlined three major concerns that remain to be addressed before the promise of gene therapy for FH can be fulfilled. First, it is unclear whether the observed reduction in serum LDL was due to an actual increase of LDL receptor activity versus a reduction in LDL production in response to liver surgery. Study of LDL clearance, rather than LDL levels, may help to answer this question. Second, it must be established that the reduction in serum LDL resulted from expression of the exogenous LDL receptor gene rather than from up-regulation of the patient's own residual LDL receptor activity induced, in this case, by the surgical procedure itself[29] and/or lovastatin therapy.[28] Third, clinical application of ex vivo gene therapy will be limited by the surgical hazard, the costly and time-consuming procedures required for ex vivo transfection, and by the fact that most hepatocytes lose their capacity for reintroduction following ex vivo transfection.

In Vivo Gene Therapy for Familial Hypercholesterolemia

According to the ideal paradigm for in vivo gene therapy, a vector expressing a normal LDL receptor gene would be directly injected into the liver as an atraumatic, one-step procedure. Efficient gene transfer in vivo, however, was difficult to achieve using retroviral vectors because mitotic activity is required to facilitate retrovirus-mediated transfection,[30] and hepatocytes are typically quiescent under normal physiological conditions. Therefore vectors capable of transducing nondividing cells, namely recombinant adenoviruses and molecular conjugates, were investigated for this purpose.

Several features of recombinant adenoviruses suggest that they might be appropriate vehicles for human gene therapies in general and liver-directed gene therapy in particular.[23] Indeed, recombinant adenoviruses can be rendered defective for replication by deleting early sequences E1A and E1B from their genome; they do not integrate into the genome of transfected cells, thus reducing the risk of insertional mutagenesis; they can be produced at high titers; and they accommodate relatively large cDNA inserts (up to 7.5 kb).

These theoretical considerations were translated into successful experimental studies. Indeed, intravenous or intraportal introduction of adenoviruses expressing a human LDL receptor cDNA—in normal mice,[31] knockout mice lacking functional LDL receptor genes,[32] and WHHL rabbits[33]—results in extremely efficient liver transfection as well as increased LDL clearance and/or decreased LDL levels. This effect, however, was transient, lasting <3 weeks. The relatively rapid diminution in transgene expression may involve a T-lymphocyte-mediated immune response toward certain viral proteins.[34] In the case of hypercholesterolemia, such transient expression of the therapeutic gene is a major drawback of gene transfer strategies based on "first-generation" adenoviruses. Repeated administration of the same vector may not represent a simple solution to more protracted expression, given the additional evidence of antibody-mediated reduction in gene expression upon subsequent exposures to the adenovirus.[33] Recent reports suggest that insertion of a temperature-sensitive mutation within the E2A region of the adenoviral genome results in less immunogenic vectors and prolonged transgene expression at permissive temperatures.[35,36] The effect of further deletions within the E2 and E4 regions on time course of gene expression is currently under investigation.

Molecular conjugates were recently used to perform liver-directed gene transfer in vivo.[37] A DNA-protein complex containing an LDL receptor cDNA complexed to a protein conjugate was injected systemically into WHHL rabbits. The protein conjugate incorporates a ligand (asialoorosomucoid) for the hepatocyte-specific asialoglycoprotein receptor covalently attached to the polycation poly-L-lysine. In this system, referred to as receptor-mediated gene transfer, liver transfection is mediated by the interaction between asialoorosomucoid and its receptor. Total serum cholesterol was decreased significantly after gene transfer but returned to baseline in <6 days. The nonviral nature of the DNA-protein complex, as well as the noninvasive approach for gene delivery, nevertheless, remain attractive features for clinical application. Alternatively, the coupling of molecular conjugates to adenoviral particles were shown to increase the efficiency of in vitro hepatocyte gene transfer as obtained by conjugates alone by promoting DNA escape from lysosomal hydrolysis.[38]

High-Density Lipoprotein Cholesterol: A New Target for Gene Therapy

Previous studies established an inverse correlation between plasma levels of HDL and the incidence of CAD.[39–41] In several lipid-lowering clinical trials, an increase in serum HDL was correlated with a reduction in the incidence of acute coronary syndromes and sometimes with a reduction in progression and/or slight regression of angiographic evidence of coronary atherosclerosis.[12,14,16,42] Taken together, these results suggest that therapies that increase serum HDL may have an antiatherogenic effect. Indeed, Badimon et al[43,44] showed that intravenous administration of HDL not only inhibited the formation but also induced regression of established fatty streaks. More recently, Rubin et al[45,46] developed a transgenic mouse that overexpresses apo A-1, the major protein component of HDL, and is protected from the development of early atherosclerotic lesions. The mechanism of the protective effect of HDL is still unclear. It was postulated that HDL may reduce the amount of cholesterol entering the plaque and promote clearance of cholesterol deposits from the plaque.[47] Alternatively, intravenous injection of apo A-1 in the hypercholesterolemic rabbit reduces intimal thickening induced by arterial injury and is associated with a 50% reduction in neointimal macrophage content.[48,49] Therefore, high serum HDL might be expected to induce regression of lipid- and macrophage-rich plaques and ultimately reduce the risk of plaque rupture. Overexpression of apo A-1 by means of gene therapy was recently reported in mice in which intravenous injection of an apo A-1 expressing adenovirus transiently increased serum HDL to a level comparable to that shown to be protective in humans.[50] Such an approach holds promise for future development of gene therapy strategies targeted toward stabilization of the vulnerable plaque through HDL-mediated lipid and/or macrophage removal.

Future Directions: Targeting the Macrophage

Certain studies suggested that unstable plaque may be comprised of abundant macrophages[10] (Figure 1), especially at the margins of the plaque.[3] Macrophages release lytic enzymes as well as matrix metalloproteinases[51,52] (Figure 2) that may be responsible for fibrous cap weakening and subsequent plaque rupture.[6,10,53] The association between macrophages and plaque rupture was strengthened by the recent observations that activity of a 92-kd metalloproteinase is more frequently found in macrophages from coronary lesions of patients with unstable versus stable angina,[52] and incubation of human atherosclerotic fibrous caps with macrophages in vitro increased collagen breakdown.[54] It is therefore con-

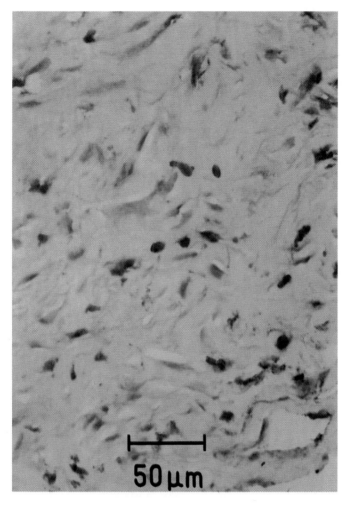

Figure 1. *Immunohistochemical staining with monoclonal antibody to HAM56, a macrophage marker, of an atherectomy specimen from a patient with unstable angina (magnification ×200).*

ceivable that reducing macrophage infiltration may potentially reduce the risk of plaque rupture.

A first approach was developed by Chen et al,[55] in which a recombinant adenovirus expressing a soluble form of the endothelial adhesion molecule VCAM-1 (sVCAM-1) is transferred into porcine vein grafts ex vivo. Vein grafts, interposed as vascular grafts in the carotid arteries, were shown to express high levels of sVCAM-1 3-days postimplantation. These findings suggest the possibility that high-level sVCAM-1 expression may be exploited to competitively inhibit interaction between endothelial

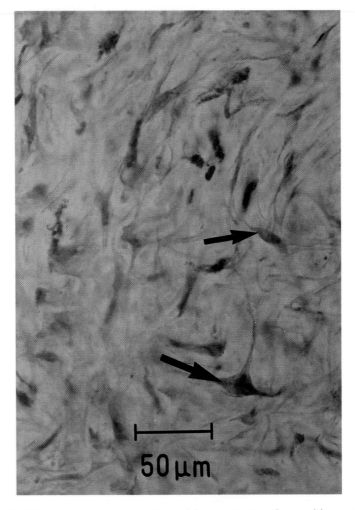

Figure 2. *Atherectomy specimen obtained from patient with unstable angina and immunostained for 92-kd gelatinase. **Arrows**, sites of positive intracellular staining (magnification ×200).*

VCAM-1 and its VLA-4 counterpart at the surface of circulating monocytes and thereby prevent macrophage infiltration of the graft.

Alternatively, preliminary findings indicate that nitric oxide (NO) inhibits monocyte chemotactic activity of the endothelium by down-regulating the cytokine monocyte chemoattractant protein 1 (MCP-1) at the transcriptional level[56]; if these data are confirmed, it is likely that secretion of high levels of NO in the vicinity of an atherosclerotic plaque may reduce macrophage recruitment into the plaque. In this case, the antithrombotic, antiproliferative, and vasorelaxing activities of NO[57] may also facilitate plaque passivation. One way to increase local levels of NO is to transfer into the atherosclerotic lesion the gene encoding constitutive endothelial nitric oxide synthase (eNOS).[58] It was recently reported that the transfer of a eNOS cDNA packaged into a liposome-Sendaï virus carrier inhibits neointima formation after balloon injury of the rat carotid artery.[59] It is still speculative, however, whether such a strategy may limit macrophage recruitment through down-regulation of MCP-1 since many other cytokines as well as oxidized LDLs may act as monocyte chemoattractants and participate in up-regulation of monocyte and/or endothelial cell adhesion molecules.[5] Moreover, the potential toxicity associated with local secretion of high levels of NO in the arterial wall, resulting in further LDL oxidation, remains to be addressed.[5]

Arterial Gene Transfer: Contribution to Antithrombotic Strategies

When plaque ruptures, the development of an occlusive thrombus plays a major part in determining the clinical presentation in acute coronary syndromes.[1,53,60–62] Indeed, antithrombotic agents, such as aspirin, were shown to reduce the risk of myocardial infarction.[63,64] Administration of antithrombotic therapies in the past was conventionally achieved via a systemic route, enhancing the risk of hemorrhagic complications. Because of the focal nature of atherosclerosis, local delivery of antithrombotic agents at the site of the culprit lesion constitutes a logical alternative to systemic antithrombotic therapies. High concentrations of a pharmacologic agent can thus be achieved in the vicinity of the atherosclerotic lesion with a reduced risk of systemic toxicity.[65,66] Pharmacologic agents with antithrombotic activity, however, do not address the biological mechanisms of thrombosis. Certain of these mechanisms involve aberrant endothelial gene expression.[67] Specifically, increased expression of pro-thrombotic molecules, such as plasminogen activator inhibitor type 1 (PAI-1),[68] and/or decreased expression of antithrombotic compound, such as tissue-type plasminogen activator (TPA),[69] by the diseased endothelium may facilitate the development of an occlusive thrombus at the site of plaque rupture. These observations suggest a rationale for the application of gene therapy to restore and/or augment antithrombotic endothelial cell function.[70]

Feasibility of Arterial Gene Transfer Targeted toward the Endothelium

As previously described, in the liver, two different approaches were used to perform arterial gene transfer. Ex vivo gene transfer was used to seed endothelium-denuded arteries, prosthetic vascular grafts, and stents with genetically modified endothelial cells. In vivo gene transfer, in contrast, involves direct introduction of genetic material into the arterial wall.

Ex Vivo Gene Transfer

Ex vivo gene transfer to native arteries

Nabel et al[71] first demonstrated that genetically engineered endothelial cells could be introduced into the arterial wall and express a recombinant gene. In this study, porcine endothelial cells were transfected in vitro with a retroviral vector expressing a recombinant β-galactosidase gene. Successfully transfected cells were then introduced into denuded iliofemoral arteries of syngenic animals using a double-balloon catheter. Following this procedure, 2% to 11% of transduced endothelial cells attached to the arterial wall. Of these cells, 20% to 100% expressed β-galactosidase up to 4 weeks following gene transfer.

Ex vivo gene transfer to vascular prosthetic devices

Conventional use of grafts and stents has been compromised by the risk of acute thrombosis, predominantly during the first weeks following implantation,[72] the time window required for endothelialization of the prosthetic material. Endothelial cells genetically engineered to produce antithrombotic molecules were therefore investigated as a means of favorably influencing the patency of such prosthetic devices.

Wilson et al,[73] for example, employed Dacron grafts coated with genetically modified endothelial cells as carotid interposition grafts in a canine model. In this model, endothelial cells were transfected in vitro using a retroviral vector expressing a β-galactosidase gene prior to graft coating. By 5-weeks postimplantation, the luminal aspect of the graft was covered by a monolayer of endothelial cells, some of which expressed the β-galactosidase gene. On the basis of these results, the authors proposed that endothelial cells may be genetically modified to secrete antithrombotic proteins and thereby improve vascular graft patency. Successful implantation of in vitro endothelialized polytetrafluoroethylene femorotibial grafts in four patients, resulting in 100% patency 3 months following implantation,[74] suggests the feasibility of using this strategy to bypass medium-sized arteries.

The risk of acute or subacute thrombosis after implantation of coronary stents remains a major issue for the interventional cardiologist.[72] Aggressive systemic antithrombotic treatment may not be optimal for prevention of stent occlusion since it is accompanied by increased bleeding complications, extended hospital stay, and increased cost.[75] Seeding of arterial stents with endothelial cells prior to implantation was proposed as an alternative strategy.[76] Because the antithrombotic activity of seeded endothelial cells may be altered, Dichek et al seeded stents with endothelial cells genetically engineered to express a human TPA gene. A significant percentage of transfected endothelial cells remained adherent to the stent after in vitro balloon-mediated stent expansion[77] and subsequent exposure to pulsatile flow.[78] Long-term adherence of the seeded cells under variable in vivo flow conditions, however, remains a concern.

Ex vivo gene transfer to vein grafts

Early vein graft thrombosis as well as accelerated graft atherosclerosis limits the long-term efficacy of aortocoronary bypass surgery.[79] Systemic delivery of antiplatelet agents was shown to reduce by nearly one-half the incidence of graft occlusion.[80] Ex vivo manipulation of vein grafts, however, provides a unique opportunity for local therapy to be applied to the graft prior to implantation. One attractive approach would be to transfect freshly explanted vein grafts with a foreign gene encoding an antithrombotic protein. As indicated previously, ex vivo, adenovirus-mediated vein-graft transfection is feasible and results in relatively high-level recombinant protein secretion.[55] Successful introduction of anti-thrombotic genes in vein grafts, however, was not yet reported.

In Vivo Arterial Gene Transfer

Since the first demonstration by Nabel et al[82] that direct introduction of a foreign gene into a specific arterial segment could be performed in live animals,[81] the field of in vivo arterial gene transfer evolved rapidly. As recently depicted by Leclerc and Isner, strategies aimed at introducing foreign genetic material into the arterial wall in live animals involve a macrodelivery system (the "gun") to transport the foreign gene to the arterial target site, a vector of gene transfer (the "bullet") to facilitate the cellular uptake of the transgene, and a molecular mechanism (the "target") with which the product of the transgene will ultimately interact.

The guns

Earlier techniques designed to perform arterial gene transfer included those that relied on direct introduction of the transgene in a surgically exposed, isolated arterial segment.[83–87] Although this method is likely to optimize the efficiency of gene transfer, the invasive nature of this approach clearly limits its clinical applicability.

An alternative approach involves catheter-based local delivery of the foreign gene to a specific arterial segment. In their seminal work, Nabel and colleagues[81] introduced a double-balloon catheter in porcine iliofemoral arteries via a side branch under direct vision. Sequential inflation of the two balloons isolates an arterial segment in which a solution containing retroviral vectors or liposomes is instilled, allowed to incubate, and then retrieved before restoration of flow. Since these pioneering experiments, other delivery catheters were developed (see Riessen and Isner[66] for review), and different groups reported entirely percutaneous approaches.[88–91]

The bullets

Several vectors were used to facilitate cellular uptake of the transgene into the arterial wall. Cationic liposomes[81,83,92,93] and retroviruses[81,94] were first used to demonstrate that arterial gene transfer was feasible. Transfection efficiencies using these vectors, however, were extremely low (typically, fewer than $1:10^6$ cells expressed the transgene). Similar results were reported when DNA with no vehicle ("naked" DNA) was used (Figure 3).[95]

Replication-defective, recombinant adenoviruses represent an alternative to liposome- or retrovirus-based arterial gene transfer.[23] Several groups recently reported highly efficient adenovirus-mediated arterial transfection, using either an intraoperative route[85,86,96] or a percutaneous

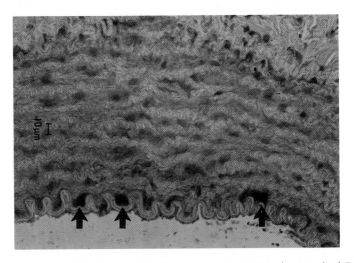

Figure 3. *Gene transfer to the rabbit iliac artery using DNA alone (naked DNA). A plasmid coding for nuclear-specific β-galactosidase was applied onto the surface of a hydrogel-coated balloon and expressed into the arterial wall during balloon inflation. Double labeling for nuclear β-galactosidase (**blue**) and cytoplasmic smooth muscle α-actin (**brown**). Only rare medial smooth muscle cells show evidence of successful transfection (**blue**). Reproduced with permission from Reference 95.*

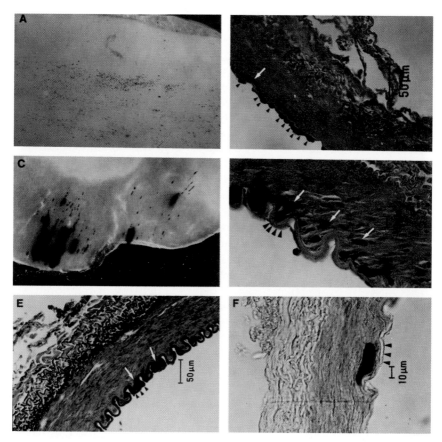

Figure 4. *X-Gal staining of a rabbit iliac artery showing β-galactosidase activity 3 days after adenovirus-mediated transfer of the nlslacZ gene in vivo using the double-balloon technique without (**A** and **B**) or with (**C**, **D**, **E**, and **F**) previous de-endothelialization. (**A**) Normal artery; macroscopic view of the luminal aspect of the artery. Blue staining identifies foci of transfected cells (original magnification ×25). (**B**) Light-microscopic appearance of **A**. X-Gal staining is confined to the nuclei of the endothelial layer (**black arrowheads**). Note the presence of one superficial medial cell expressing β-galactosidase (**white arrow**) just below a site of focal disruption of the endothelium. (**C**) Injured artery. Macroscopic view shows a mottled blue appearance of the luminal aspect of the artery. (**D**) Light-microscopic appearance of **C** after hematoxylin-eosin counterstaining. Sparse medial cells, underlying an apparently intact internal elastic lamina (**black arrowheads**), express β-galactosidase (**white arrows**). (**E**) Photomicrograph of **C** after Richardson's elastic trichrome counterstaining. Note the apparent integrity of the internal elastic lamina (**black arrowheads**). Some superficial medial cells, below the internal elastic lamina, express β-galactosidase (**white arrows**). (**F**) Photomicrograph of **C** after immunohistochemical staining with monoclonal anti-α-actin antibody. **Black arrowheads** indicate internal elastic lamina. Reproduced with permission from Reference 90.*

approach.[88–91,97–99] Transfection efficiencies achieved using adenoviruses are at least three logs higher than those reported using liposomes[93,99] and retroviruses.[81] Important drawbacks of adenoviral vectors, however, include transient transgene expression, typically limited to 2–3 weeks post-gene transfer (see preceding text), and the risk of systemic dissemination facilitated by the amphotropic character of the adenovirus. Reports varied with regard to extraarterial distribution of adenoviral vectors following percutaneous local delivery.[90,91,97–99] These discrepancies may be related to the specific local delivery device used for gene transfer. Indeed extraarterial transfection has been reported with the double-balloon[90,98] and the porous-balloon catheters[97,99] but not with the hydrogel-balloon catheter.[90] Finally, we recently reported that the efficiency of adenovirus-mediated gene transfer is reduced in atherosclerotic versus normal arteries.[91] Transfection efficiency achieved in atherosclerotic arteries with adenoviruses, however, is still several orders of magnitude higher than that achieved using liposomes.[99]

In vivo transfection of the endothelium has been achieved using intraoperative[85,86,88] or catheter-based[81,88–90,100,101] delivery of retroviral[81] or adenoviral[85,86,88–90,101] vectors. Interestingly, exposure of a nondenuded, normal peripheral artery to adenoviral vectors results in gene expression that is limited to the endothelium[85,86,88–90,101] (Figure 4). Conversely, arterial de-endothelialization at the time of adenovirus-mediated gene transfer results in efficient medial smooth muscle cell transfection (Figure 4).[86–88,90,98,102,103] Taken together, these findings suggest that (1) cell-specific gene transfer targeted toward the endothelium is feasible when adenoviruses are used as vectors and (2) an intact endothelium constitutes a potential physical barrier to adenovirus penetration into the media of peripheral arteries. A recent report by Barr and colleagues,[100] suggests, however, that intracoronary infusion of adenoviral vectors results in significant medial as well as myocardial transfection in addition to predominant endothelial transfection. This discrepancy may be due to structural differences between peripheral and coronary arteries. In contrast, very-low-level gene transfer to all the layers of the arterial wall was observed after local delivery of liposomes or retroviral vectors using a double-balloon catheter.[81] Therefore, recombinant adenoviruses appear currently to be the most appropriate vector with which to perform endothelium-specific arterial gene transfer.

Current Approaches for a Genetic Intervention to Prevent Thrombus Formation

The demonstration that site-specific gene transfer to the vascular endothelium is feasible set the stage for the development of genetic strategies aimed at preventing acute coronary syndromes. Dichek et al[104] proposed that arterial thrombosis might be prevented by altering certain endothelial functions at the site of endothelial injury or dysfunction. One approach by which normal antithrombotic activity of the endothelium might be restored involves transfection of the TPA gene.[77,104] In vitro transfection of endothelial cells with a retrovirus expressing a human TPA gene resulted in high-level secretion of TPA.[77,104] One of the main limitations of this strategy, however, is the inactivation of recombinant TPA resulting from binding of TPA molecules to PAI-1. A single-chain urokinase cDNA, which encodes an enzyme that does not bind to PAI-1, was used to circumvent this limitation.[96,105] Taken together, these data suggest that endothelial cells genetically engineered to produce fibrinolytic compounds such as TPA may express high levels of thrombolytic agent in vitro and, presumably, in vivo. Hence, a gene transfer protocol in which endothelial cells would be directly transfected in vivo using catheter-based local delivery of adenoviral vectors expressing fibrinolytic molecules may augment endothelial antithrombotic activity and ultimately prevent thrombus formation at the site of endothelial injury or dysfunction.

Other potential candidates for endothelium-targeted gene therapy await experimental evidence that they may confer protection against arterial thrombosis. For example, secretion of NO contributes to the non-thrombogenic surface of the normal endothelium.[57] Therefore, successful transfection of a vulnerable atherosclerotic plaque with a cDNA encoding the constitutive eNOS (see preceding text and Reference 58) may reduce the likelihood of arterial thrombosis.

Other potential candidates for endothelium-targeted gene therapy await experimental evidence that they may confer protection against arterial thrombosis. For example, local delivery of the endothelium-specific mitogen vascular endothelial growth factor (VEGF) at the site of arterial injury accelerates reendothelialization and attenuates intimal thickening.[106] Therefore it is possible that restoration of a potentially antithrombotic endothelial layer can be facilitated by transferring the VEGF gene to the endoluminal surface of a vulnerable atherosclerotic plaque. Successful transfer to the arterial wall of a VEGF-expressing plasmid from the surface of a hydrogel-coated balloon catheter was recently reported.[107,108] This genetic strategy has several potential advantages over protein therapy. First, the prolonged synthesis and local release of VEGF following gene transfer may constitute a more effective means of stimulating endothelium regrowth than a single bolus of VEGF protein. Second, relatively inexpensive expression plasmids encoding a secreted form of VEGF can be designed that may ultimately reduce the high costs associated with production of recombinant proteins. Direct introduction of DNA with no vehicle (naked DNA) into the arterial wall was shown to be feasible, although with low efficiency.[95] In the case of VEGF, however, even a low efficiency may prove sufficient to induce re-endothelialization, since the VEGF gene product is in this case secreted and therefore capable of modulating neighboring cells via a paracrine effect. Further studies are warranted to investigate whether the favorable effect of VEGF on abluminal endothelial cells is associated with deleterious intraplaque neoangiogenesis that might predispose to plaque hemorrhage.

Conclusions

Prevention of acute coronary syndromes represents a major target for cardiovascular research. Pharmacologic interventions aimed at lowering serum cholesterol or inhibiting thrombus formation proved efficient in reducing mortality related to acute coronary events. Recent progress in the field of gene transfer, as well as a better understanding of the pathophysiology of plaque rupture and thrombus formation, established new avenues for a molecular approach to acute coronary syndromes. Preliminary results of the first ex vivo gene therapy for FH suggest that genetically engineered hepatocytes expressing the human LDL receptor can be introduced into the liver and in some patients induce significant reduction in serum LDL. Development of more practical protocols using direct administration of the LDL receptor gene in vivo are warranted, however, before the promise of this technology can be realized. Genetic modification of endothelial cells to improve endothelial antithrombotic activity is a viable alternative. Ultimately, strategies simultaneously addressing the concepts of atherosclerotic plaque stabilization and restoration of physiological endothelial functions represent an opportune field for future research.

References

1. Richardson PD, Davies MJ, Born GVR. Influence of plaque configuration and stress distribution on fissuring of coronary atherosclerotic plaques. *Lancet* 1989;2:941–944.
2. Falk E. Why do plaques rupture? *Circulation* 1992;86(suppl):30–42.
3. Lendon CL, Davies MJ, Born GVR, et al. Atherosclerotic plaque caps are locally weakened when macrophages density is increased. *Atherosclerosis* 1991;87:87–90.
4. Fuster V, Badimon L, Badimon JJ, et al. The pathogenesis of coronary artery disease and the acute coronary syndromes, II. *N Engl J Med* 1992;326:310–318.
5. Ross R. The pathogenesis of atherosclerosis: a perspective for the 1990s. *Nature* 1993;362:801–809.
6. MacIsaac AI, Thomas JD, Topol EJ. Toward the quiescent coronary plaque. *J Am Coll Cardiol* 1993;22:1228–1241.
7. Nobuyoshi M, Tanaka M, Nosaka H, et al. Progression of coronary atherosclerosis: is coronary spasm related to progression? *J Am Coll Cardiol* 1991;18:904–910.

8. van der Wal AC, Becker AE, van der Loos CM, et al. Site of intimal rupture or erosion of thrombosed coronary atherosclerotic plaques is characterized by an inflammatory process irrespective of the dominant plaque morphology. *Circulation* 1994;89:36–44.

9. Alexander RW. Inflammation and coronary artery disease. *N Engl J Med* 1994;331:468–469.

10. Moreno PR, Falk E, Palacios IF, et al. Macrophage infiltration in acute coronary syndromes. Implications for plaque rupture. *Circulation* 1994;90:775–778.

11. Kane JP, Malloy MJ, Ports TA, et al. Regression of coronary atherosclerosis during treatment of familial hypercholesterolemia with combined drug regimens. *JAMA* 1990;264:3007–3012.

12. Brown G, Albers JJ, Fisher LD, et al. Regression of coronary artery disease as a result of intensive lipid-lowering therapy in men with high levels of apolipoprotein B. *N Engl J Med* 1990;323:1289–1298.

13. Ornish D, Brown SE, Scherwitz LW, et al. Can lifestyle changes reverse coronary heart disease? The Lifestyle Heart Trial. *Lancet* 1990;336:129–133.

14. Blankenhorn DH, Nessim SA, Johnson RL, et al. Beneficial effects of combined colestipol-niacin therapy on coronary atherosclerosis and coronary venous bypass grafts. *JAMA* 1987;257:3233–3240.

15. Brensike JF, Levy RI, Kesley SF, et al. Effects of therapy with cholestyramine on progression of coronary arteriosclerosis: results of the NHLBI Type II Coronary Intervention Study. *Circulation* 1984;69:313–324.

16. Buchwald H, Varco RL, Matts JP, et al. Effect of partial ileal bypass surgery on mortality and morbidity from coronary heart disease in patients with hypercholesterolemia: report of the Program on the Surgical Control of the Hyperlipidemias (POSCH). *N Engl J Med* 1990;323:946–955.

17. Cashin-Hemphill L, Mack WJ, Pagoda JM, et al. Beneficial effects of colestipol-niacin on coronary atherosclerosis. *JAMA* 1990;264:3013–3017.

18. Watts GF, Lewis B, Brunt JN, et al. Effects on coronary artery disease of lipid-lowering diet, or diet plus cholestyramine, in the St. Thomas' Atherosclerosis Regression Study (STARS). *Lancet* 1992;339:563–569.

19. Badimon JJ, Fuster V, Chesebro JH, et al. Coronary atherosclerosis. A multifactorial disease. *Circulation* 1993;87(suppl):3–16.

20. Brown MS, Goldstein JL. A receptor-mediated pathway for cholesterol homeostasis. *Science* 1986;232:34–47.

21. Bilheimer DW, Goldstein JL, Grundy SM, et al. Liver transplantation to provide low-density-lipoprotein receptors and lower plasma cholesterol in a child with homozygous familial hypercholesterolemia. *N Engl J Med* 1984;311:1658–1664.

22. Goldstein JL, Kita T, Brown MS. Defective lipoprotein receptors and atherosclerosis. Lessons from an animal counterpart of familial hypercholesterolemia. *N Engl J Med* 1983;309:288–296.

23. Schneider MD, French BA. The advent of adenovirus. Gene therapy for cardiovascular disease. *Circulation* 1993;88:1937–1942.

24. Wilson JM, Chowdhury NR, Grossman M, et al. Temporary amelioration of hyperlipidemia in low density lipoprotein receptor-deficient rabbits transplanted with genetically modified hepatocytes. *Proc Natl Acad Sci U S A* 1990;87:8437–8441.

25. Chowdhury JR, Grossman M, Gupta S, et al. Long-term improvement of hypercholesterolemia after ex vivo gene therapy in LDLR-deficient rabbits. *Science* 1991;254:1802–1805.

26. Wilson JM. Clinical protocol: ex vivo gene therapy of familial hypercholesterolemia. *Hum Gene Ther* 1992;3:179–222.
27. Grossman M, Raper SE, Kozarsky K, et al. Successful ex vivo gene therapy directed to liver in a patient with familial hypercholesterolaemia. *Nat Genet* 1994;6:335–341.
28. Brown MS, Goldstein JL, Havel RJ, et al. Gene therapy for cholesterol. *Nat Genet* 1994;7:349–350.
29. Dichek DA, Bratthauer GL, Beg ZH, et al. Retroviral vector-mediated in vivo expression of low-density-lipoprotein receptors in the Watanabe heritable hyperlipidemic rabbit. *Somat Cell Mol Genet* 1991;17:287–301.
30. Miller DG, Adam MA, Miller AD. Gene transfer by retrovirus vectors occurs only in cells that are actively replicating at the time of infection. *Mol Cell Biol* 1990;10:4239–4242.
31. Herz J, Gerard RD. Adenovirus-mediated transfer of low density lipoprotein receptor gene acutely accelerates cholesterol clearance in normal mice. *Proc Natl Acad Sci U S A* 1993;90:2812–2816.
32. Ishibashi S, Brown MS, Goldstein JL, et al. Hypercholesterolemia in low density lipoprotein receptor knockout mice and its reversal by adenovirus-mediated gene delivery. *J Clin Invest* 1993;92:883–893.
33. Kozarsky KF, McKinley DR, Austin LL, et al. In vivo correction of low-density lipoprotein receptor deficiency in the Watanabe heritable hyperlipidemic rabbit with recombinant adenoviruses. *J Biol Chem* 1994;269:13695–13702.
34. Yang Y, Nunes FA, Berencsi K, et al. Cellular immunity to viral antigens limits E1-deleted adenoviruses for gene therapy. *Proc Natl Acad Sci U S A* 1994;91:4407–4411.
35. Yang Y, Nunes FA, Berencsi K, et al. Inactivation of E2A in recombinant adenoviruses improves the prospect for gene therapy in cystic fibrosis. *Nat Genet* 1994;7:362–369.
36. Engelhardt JF, Ye X, Doranz B, et al. Ablation of E2A in recombinant adenoviruses improves transgene persistence and decreases inflammatory response in mouse liver. *Proc Natl Acad Sci U S A* 1994;91:6196–6200.
37. Wilson JM, Grossman M, Wu CH, et al. Hepatocyte-directed gene transfer in vivo leads to transient improvement of hypercholesterolemia in low-density lipoprotein receptor-deficient rabbits. *J Biol Chem* 1992;267:963–967.
38. Cristiano R, Smith L, Kay M, et al. Hepatic gene therapy: efficient gene delivery and expression in primary hepatocytes utilizing a conjugated adenovirus-DNA complex. *Proc Natl Acad Sci U S A* 1993;90:11548–11552.
39. Castelli WP, Doyle JT, Gordon T, et al. HDL cholesterol and other lipids in coronary heart disease: the cooperative lipoprotein phenotyping study. *Circulation* 1977;55:767–772.
40. Gordon T, Castelli WP, Hjortland MC, et al. High density lipoprotein as a protective factor against coronary heart disease: the Framingham Study. *Am J Med* 1977;62:707–714.
41. Heiss G, Johnson NJ, Reiland S, et al. The Lipid Research Clinics Program Prevalence Study: summary. *Circulation* 1980;62(suppl):116–136.
42. Frick MH, Elo O, Haapa K, et al. Helsinki heart study primary prevention trial with gemfibrozil in middle-aged men with dyslipidemia: safety of treatment, changes in risk factors, and incidence of coronary heart disease. *N Engl J Med* 1987;317:1237–1245.
43. Badimon JJ, Badimon L, Galvez A, et al. High density lipoprotein plasma fraction inhibit aortic fatty streaks in cholesterol-fed rabbits. *Lab Invest* 1989;60:455–461.

44. Badimon JJ, Badimon L, Fuster V. Regression of atherosclerotic lesions by high density lipoprotein plasma fraction in the cholesterol-fed rabbit. *J Clin Invest* 1990;85:1234–1241.

45. Rubin EM, Krauss RM, Spangler EA, et al. Inhibition of early atherogenesis in transgenic mice by human apolipoprotein A1. *Nature* 1991;353:265–267.

46. Pászty C, Maeda N, Verstuyft J, et al. Apolipoprotein A1 transgene corrects apolipoprotein E deficiency-induced atherosclerosis in mice. *J Clin Invest* 1994;94:899–903.

47. Reichl D, Miller NE. Pathophysiology of reverse cholesterol transport: insights from inherited disorders of lipoprotein metabolism. *Arteriosclerosis* 1989;9:785–797.

48. Ameli S, Hultgardh-Nilsson A, Cercek B, et al. Recombinant apolipoprotein A-1 Milano reduces intimal thickening after balloon injury in hypercholesterolemic rabbits. *Circulation* 1994;90:1935–1941.

49. Soma MR, Donetti E, Parolini C, et al. Recombinant apolipoprotein A-I Milano dimer inhibits carotid intimal thickening induced by perivascular manipulation in rabbits. *Circ Res* 1995;76:405–411.

50. Kopfler WP, Willard M, Betz T, et al. Adenovirus-mediated transfer of a gene encoding human apolipoprotein A-I into normal mice increases circulating high-density lipoprotein cholesterol. *Circulation* 1994;90:1319–1327.

51. Welgus HG, Campbell EJ, Cury JD, et al. Neutral metalloproteinases produced by human mononuclear phagocytes. *J Clin Invest* 1990;86:1496–1502.

52. Brown DI, Hibbs MS, Kearney M, et al. Expresssion and cellular location of 92 kDa gelatinase in coronary lesions of patients with unstable angina. *Circulation* In press.

53. Fuster V, Badimon L, Badimon JJ, et al. The pathogenesis of coronary artery disease and the acute coronary syndromes, I. *N Engl J Med* 1992;326:242–250.

54. Shah PK, Falk E, Badimon JJ, et al. Human monocyte-derived macrophages express collagenase and induce collagen breakdown in atherosclerotic fibrous caps: implications for plaque rupture. Abstract. *Circulation* 1993;88(suppl):I–254.

55. Chen S-J, Wilson JM, Muller DWM. Adenovirus-mediated gene transfer of soluble vascular cell adhesion molecule to porcine interposition vein grafts. *Circulation* 1994;89:1922–1928.

56. Zeiher AM, Schray-Utz B, Busse R. Nitric oxide modulates the expression of monocyte chemoattractant protein 1 in cultured human endothelial cells. *Circ Res* 1995;76:980–986.

57. Moncada S, Higgs A. The L-arginine-nitric oxide pathway. *N Engl J Med* 1993;329:2002–2012.

58. Sessa WC, Harrison JK, Barber CM, et al. Molecular cloning and expression of a cDNA encoding endothelial cell nitric oxide synthase. *J Biol Chem* 1992;267:15274–15276.

59. von der Leyen H, Gibbons GH, Morishita R, et al. Gene therapy inhibiting neointimal vascular lesion: in vivo transfer of endothelial cell nitric oxide synthase gene. *Proc Natl Acad Sci U S A* 1995;92:1137–1141.

60. DeWood MA, Stifter WF, Simpson CS, et al. Coronary arteriographic findings soon after non-Q-wave myocardial infarction. *N Engl J Med* 1986;315:417–423.

61. DeWood MA, Spores J, Notske R, et al. Prevalence of total coronary occlusion during the early hours of transmural myocardial infarction. *N Engl J Med* 1980;303:897–902.

62. Falk E. Unstable angina with fatal outcome: dynamic coronary thrombosis leading to infarction and/or sudden death: autopsy evidence of recurrent mural thrombosis with peripheral embolization culminating in total vascular occlusion. *Circulation* 1985;71:699–708.
63. Steering Committee of the Physicians' Health Study Research Group. Final report on the aspirin component of the ongoing Physicians' Health Study. *N Engl J Med* 1989;321:129–135.
64. Juul-Möller S, Edvardsson N, Jahnmatz B, et al. Double-blind trial of aspirin in primary prevention of myocardial infarction in patients with stable chronic angina pectoris. *Lancet* 1992;340:1421–1425.
65. March KL, Wilensky RL, Hathaway DR. Novel drug and device combinations for targeted prevention of restenosis. *Cardio Intervention* 1992;2:11–26.
66. Riessen R, Isner JM. Prospects for site-specific delivery of pharmacologic and molecular therapies. *J Am Coll Cardiol* 1994;23:1234–1244.
67. Gimbrone MA. Vascular endothelium: nature's blood container. In: Gimbrone MA, ed. *Vascular Endothelium in Hemostasis and Thrombosis*. New York, NY: Churchill Livingstone;1986:1–13.
68. Quax PHA, van den Hoogen CM, Verheijen JH, et al. Endotoxin induction of plasminogen activator and plasminogen activator inhibitor type 1 mRNA in rat tissues in vivo. *J Biol Chem* 1990;265:15560–15563.
69. Loscalzo J, Braunwald E. Tissue plasminogen activator. *N Engl J Med* 1988;319:925–931.
70. Dichek DA. Interventional approaches to the introduction of genetic material into the vasculature. In: Topol EJ, ed. *Textbook of Interventional Cardiology*. Philadelphia, PA: WB Saunders; 1993:989–1005.
71. Nabel EJ, Plautz G, Boyce DM, et al. Recombinant gene expression in vivo within endothelial cells of the arterial wall. *Science* 1989;244:1342–1344.
72. Sutton JM, Ellis SG, Roubin GS, et al. Major clinical events after coronary stenting. The Multicenter Registry of Acute and Elective Gianturco-Roubin Stent Placement. *Circulation* 1994;89:1126–1137.
73. Wilson JM, Birinyi LK, Salomon RN, et al. Implantation of vascular grafts lined with genetically modified endothelial cells. *Science* 1989;244:1344–1346.
74. Kadletz M, Magometschnigg H, Minar E, et al. Implantation of in vitro endothelialized polytetrafluoroethylene grafts in human beings. A preliminary report. *J Thorac Cardiovasc Surg* 1992;104:736–742.
75. Leon MB, Wong SC. Intracoronary stents. A breakthrough technology or just another small step? *Circulation* 1994;89:1323–1327.
76. van der Giessen WJ, Serruys PW, Visser WJ, et al. Endothelialization of intravascular stents. *J Intervent Cardiol* 1988;1:109–120.
77. Dichek DA, Neville RF, Zwiebel JA, et al. Seeding of intravascular stents with genetically engineered endothelial cells. *Circulation* 1989;80:1347–1353.
78. Flugelman MY, Virmani R, Leon MB, et al. Genetically engineered endothelial cells remain adherent and viable after stent deployment and exposure to flow in vitro. *Circ Res* 1992;70:348–354.
79. Fitzgibbon GM, Leach AJ, Kafka HP, et al. Coronary bypass graft fate: long-term angiographic study. *J Am Coll Cardiol* 1991;17:1075–1080.
80. Antiplatelet Trialists' Collaboration. Collaborative overview of randomised trials of antiplatelet therapy—II: maintenance of vascular graft or arterial patency by antiplatelet therapy. *BMJ* 1994;308:159–168.
81. Nabel EG, Plautz G, Nabel GJ. Site-specific gene expression in vivo by direct gene transfer into the arterial wall. *Science* 1990;249:1285–1288.

82. Leclerc G, Isner JM. Percutaneous gene therapy for cardiovascular disease. In: Topol EJ, ed. *Textbook of Interventional Cardiology.* Philadelphia, PA: WB Saunders; 1993:1019–1029.

83. Lim CS, Chapman GD, Gammon JB, et al. Direct in vivo gene transfer into the coronary and peripheral vasculatures of the intact dog. *Circulation* 1991;83:578–583.

84. Barbee RW, Stapleton DD, Perrry BD, et al. Prior arterial injury enhances luciferase expression following in vivo gene transfer. *Biochem Biophys Res Commun* 1993;190:70–78.

85. Lemarchand P, Jones M, Yamada I, et al. In vivo gene transfer and expression in normal uninjured blood vessels using replication-deficient recombinant adenovirus vectors. *Circ Res* 1993;72:1132–1138.

86. Guzman R, Lemarchand P, Crystal RG, et al. Efficient and selective adenovirus-mediated gene transfer into vascular neointima. *Circulation* 1993;88: 2838–2848.

87. Lee SW, Trapnell BC, Rade JJ, et al. In vivo adenoviral vector-mediated gene transfer into balloon-injured rat carotid arteries. *Circ Res* 1993;73:797–807.

88. Willard JE, Landau C, Glamann DB, et al. Genetic modification of the vessel wall. Comparison of surgical and catheter-based techniques for delivery of recombinant adenovirus. *Circulation* 1994;89:2190–2197.

89. Rome JJ, Shayani V, Flugelman MY, et al. Anatomic barriers influence the distribution of in vivo gene transfer into the arterial wall. Modeling with microscopic tracer particles and verification with a recombinant adenoviral vector. *Arterioscler Thromb* 1994;14:148–161.

90. Steg PG, Feldman LJ, Scoazec J-Y, et al. Arterial gene transfer to rabbit endothelial and smooth muscle cells using percutaneous delivery of an adenoviral vector. *Circulation* 1994;90:1648–1656.

91. Feldman LJ, Steg PG, Zheng LP, et al. Low-efficiency of percutaneous adenovirus-mediated arterial gene transfer in the atherosclerotic rabbit. *J Clin Invest* 1995;95:2662–2671.

92. Leclerc G, Gal D, Takeshita S, et al. Percutaneous arterial gene transfer in a rabbit model. Efficiency in normal and balloon-dilated atherosclerotic arteries. *J Clin Invest* 1992;90:936–944.

93. Takeshita S, Gal D, Leclerc G, et al. Increased gene expression after liposome-mediated arterial gene transfer associated with intimal smooth muscle cell proliferation. In vitro and in vivo findings in a rabbit model of vascular injury. *J Clin Invest* 1994;93:652–661.

94. Flugelman MY, Jaklitsch MT, Newman KD, et al. Low level in vivo gene transfer into the arterial wall through a perforated balloon catheter. *Circulation* 1992;85:1110–1117.

95. Riessen R, Rahimizadeh H, Takeshita S, et al. Successful vascular gene transfer using a hydrogel coated balloon angioplasty catheter. *Hum Gene Ther* 1993;4:749–758.

96. Lee SW, Kahn ML, Dichek DA. Control of clot lysis by gene transfer. *Trends Cardiovasc Med* 1993;3:61–66.

97. March KL, Gradus-Pizlo I, Wilensky RL, et al. Cardiovascular gene therapy using adenoviral vectors: distant transduction following local delivery using a porous balloon catheter. Abstract. *J Am Coll Cardiol* 1994;23:177A.

98. Ohno T, Gordon D, San H, et al. Gene therapy for vascular smooth muscle cell proliferation after arterial injury. *Science* 1994;265:781–784.

99. French BA, Mazur W, Ali NM, et al. Percutaneous transluminal in vivo gene transfer by recombinant adenovirus in normal porcine coronary arteries, ath-

erosclerotic arteries, and two models of coronary restenosis. *Circulation* 1994;90:2402–2413.

100. Barr E, Carroll J, Kalynych AM, et al. Efficient catheter-mediated gene transfer into the heart using replication-defective adenovirus. *Gene Ther* 1994;1:51–58.

101. Muller DWM, Gordon D, San H, et al. Catheter-mediated pulmonary vascular gene transfer and expression. *Circ Res* 1994;75:1039–1049.

102. Guzman RJ, Hirschowitz EA, Brody SL, et al. In vivo suppression of injury-induced vascular smooth muscle cell accumulation using adenovirus-mediated transfer of the herpes simplex virus thymidine kinase gene. *Proc Natl Acad Sci U S A* 1994;91:10732–10736.

103. Chang MW, Barr E, Seltzer J, et al. Cytostatic gene therapy for vascular proliferative disorders with a constitutively active form of the retinoblastoma gene product. *Science* 1995;267:518–522.

104. Dichek DA, Nussbaum O, Degen SJF, et al. Enhancement of the fibrinolytic activity of sheep endothelial cells by retroviral vector-mediated gene transfer. *Blood* 1991;77:533–541.

105. Lee SW, Kahn ML, Dichek DA. Expression of an anchored urokinase in the apical endothelial cell membrane. *J Biol Chem* 1992;267:13020–13027.

106. Asahara T, Bauters C, Pastore C, et al. Local delivery of vascular endothelial growth factor accelerates reendothelialization and attenuates intimal hyperplasia in balloon-injured rat carotid artery. *Circulation* 1995;91:2793–2801.

107. Takeshita S, Tsurumi Y, Couffinahe T, et al. Gene transfer of naked DNA encoding for three isoforms of vascular endothelial growth factor stimulates collateral development in vivo. *Lab Invest* 1996;75:487–501.

108. Isner JM, Pieczek A, Schainfeld R, et al. Clinical evidence of angiogenesis after arterial gene transfer of phVEGF$_{165}$ in patient with ischemic limb. *Lancet* 1996;348:370–374.

Chapter 12

Smoking Cessation in Cardiac Preventive Health

Garland Y. DeNelsky, PhD
and Mary E. Bower, PhD

Overview of Smoking Morbidity and Mortality

Smoking is clearly the single, most preventable cause of premature death in our country.[1] An estimated 30% of all cancer deaths, including 87% of lung cancer deaths,[1] and 30% of all cardiovascular deaths[2] are attributable to smoking. Eighty percent of all deaths from chronic obstructive pulmonary disease are due to smoking.[3] In 1990, smoking accounted for 1150 deaths per day—a total 20% of all deaths.[4] An estimated 5 million years of potential life were lost in that year alone due to smoking. In this chapter, we will outline the cardiac effects of smoking and the health benefits of cessation. We will then review the literature on methods of smoking cessation and conclude with an outline of suggested smoking cessation interventions for physicians designed to allow them to maximize their impact within the time constraints of daily practice.

Smokers experience direct reductions in the quality of their lives because of the high morbidity rates associated with smoking. Cigarette smoking is an established cause of lung and laryngeal cancer, chronic bronchitis, oral cancer, esophageal cancer, intrauterine growth retarda-

From Robinson K, (ed): *Preventive Cardiology*. Armonk, NY: Futura Publishing Company, Inc. © 1998.

tion, and low-birth-weight babies.[1] Smoking is considered to be a contributing factor for a variety of other medical conditions, including cancer of the bladder, pancreas, kidney, and stomach.[1] Additionally, the connection between smoking and unsuccessful pregnancy and pediatric morbidity and mortality is becoming increasingly apparent.[4,5]

Although smoking is the chief preventable cause of morbidity and mortality in our society,[3] in 1993 approximately 25% of the US population (46 million Americans) were smokers.[6] The annual cost of smoking-related medical care for this population was $50 billion,[7] amounting to $2.06 for each of the 24 billion packs of cigarettes sold in 1993.[7] Indirect costs of smoking (eg, burn care for cigarette-related fires, care for low-birth-weight babies of mothers who smoke, and medical care for diseases related to passive smoking) that same year totaled approximately $46 billion.[7]

Cardiac Effects of Smoking

In 1983, a report of the Surgeon General concluded that tobacco use constitutes "the strongest preventable cause" of cardiovascular disease (CVD). Smoking is associated with a two- to fourfold increase in coronary heart disease and with increased risk for atherosclerotic peripheral vascular disease and stroke.[1,2,8] Overall, 30% of all cardiovascular deaths are due to smoking.[3] In 1990, more individuals died from cardiovascular consequences of smoking than from smoking-related cancer or smoking-related respiratory disease.[4]

The mechanism by which smoking leads to cardiovascular morbidity and mortality is not fully understood; however, nicotine and carbon monoxide appear to play major roles in the cardiac effects of smoking. When a smoker inhales, nicotine raises systolic blood pressure (BP) and increases heart rate, increasing myocardial oxygen demand. At the same time, the carbon monoxide produced by cigarettes and inhaled by smokers reduces oxygen availability to body tissues, including the myocardium.[9]

Carbon monoxide, nicotine, and smoke potentially cause atherogenic injury by damaging the endothelium in the coronary arteries, carotid arteries, aorta, and peripheral vessels.[9] This endothelial damage increases the likelihood that monocytes and other macrophages will adhere to the vessel wall and that lipoproteins will pass into the subendothelial area. Nicotine increases platelet activation and platelet adhesion to the vessel wall.[10] Following endothelial injury, atherosclerotic plaque develops, with eventual partial occlusion of the vessel. These mechanisms accelerate the development of coronary artery disease (CAD) and precipitate myocardial infarction (MI) in smokers. For those with post-MI, smoking cessation has a more dramatic effect on subsequent outcome than change of diet, weight loss, or exercise.[11]

Health Benefits of Cessation

Smoking cessation has major, immediate health benefits for people of all ages, including those with smoking-related disease.[11] Within 20 minutes after the last cigarette is smoked, BP drops to normal. Within 8 hours, the carbon monoxide level in the bloodstream drops to normal and the oxygen level increases to normal, and within 24 hours the chance of a heart attack decreases significantly.[12] After the first year of cessation, the risks of CVD decrease markedly, and they are nearly normal at 5 years postcessation. Stopping smoking also decreases the risk of lung and other cancers, stroke, and chronic lung disease.[11,13] After 10 to 15 years of abstinence, risk of dying from any smoking-related disease is nearly as low as that of persons who never smoked.[11]

An Overview of Smoking and Quitting

The Behavior of Smoking

People learn to smoke early, or they do not learn at all. Ninety percent of all smokers start by age 19.[14] There is at least a fivefold increase in the likelihood of a teenager smoking if one or both parents smoke and an older sibling smokes.[15]

Smoking is first of all an addiction. This fact is in contrast to earlier views that described tobacco use as "habituating."[16] In 1988, a landmark Report of the Surgeon General provided an exhaustive review of the facts and came up with three major conclusions: (1) cigarettes and other forms of tobacco are addicting, (2) nicotine is the drug in tobacco that causes addiction, and (3) the pharmacologic and behavioral processes that determine tobacco addiction are similar to those that determine addiction to drugs such as heroin and cocaine.[16]

Primary criteria for drug dependence—highly controlled or compulsive use, psychoactive effects, and drug-reinforced behavior—are all present with nicotine.[16] The fact that many smokers continue to smoke despite life threatening, smoking-related illnesses is consistent with assertions that the "core" of addictive behavior is "the inability to regulate behavior, despite contrary desires or significant deleterious consequences."[17] As with other addictive substances, nicotine is a psychoactive drug that has direct effects on the brain. It produces transient alterations in mood, including "dampening" of unpleasant emotional states and, possibly, direct stimulation of "pleasure centers" in the brain.[17] These psychoactive effects are sufficiently rewarding to maintain self-administration.[16] Most regular nicotine users develop some form of withdrawal effects when nicotine use is not sustained.[16,18]

Inhalation of cigarette smoke is an extremely rapid and efficient means of delivering nicotine to the brain. Within 7 seconds of puffing, a quarter of the nicotine in inhaled smoke crosses the blood-brain barrier.[19] Thus nicotine's rapid effects on the brain provide a strong reinforcement of smoking behavior that undoubtedly helps account for nicotine's powerful control over behavior. In fact, 85% of teenagers who smoke two or more cigarettes completely will become regular smokers.[20]

The powerful, addictive properties of nicotine are multiplied by the sheer frequency with which this substance is used. Assuming a smoker takes an average of 10 puffs per cigarette, a pack-per-day smoker will obtain approximately 73 000 nicotine "hits" each year. In less than 15 years—by the time an average smoker who began midway through their teenage years is approximately age 30—a pack-per-day smoker will have experienced over a million such nicotine hits. No other addiction is as frequently practiced.

Associations or linkages play a major role in smoking as well. When a specific behavior (eg, smoking) occurs in a particular situation (eg, while driving an automobile), an association (or "linkage") is formed between the two. Gradually the association is strengthened to the point where the presence of the stimulus (driving) is sufficient to elicit the behavior (smoking). Because of the frequency of smoking, smoking becomes linked in this fashion to many situations: arising in the morning, having a cup of coffee, taking a "break," finishing a task, talking on the telephone, etc. Smoking can also become linked to negative or positive emotional states (eg, boredom, anger, excitement, joy, etc.) and to certain people in a smoker's life with whom smoking occurs (eg, "smoking buddies"). Hence, smoking involves a process in which the use of a powerfully addictive substance (nicotine) is supported by its acute, reinforcing, pharmacologic effects and by the learned association of this behavior with many environmental cues.

Support for smoking behavior may also derive from "psychological meanings" of smoking that smokers derive over their years of tobacco use.[21] Perhaps the most common "meaning" of smoking is an "old friend" or companion that was by the person's side through many rough times. Others consider smoking to be a very special means of handling stress or tolerating and managing emotional upset (probably by dampening their emotions, as noted above). Some people feel that smoking expands their abilities or see it as a means of "buying time," taking a relaxation break, or providing self-reward. These beliefs about smoking may have little validity, but they seem to have a powerful impact on the smoker—especially when the smoker contemplates quitting. In essence, the smoker anticipates a loss of emotional control, coping skills, and pleasures after quitting.

The Process of Quitting Smoking

In theory, quitting smoking is relatively simple. The person quits, goes through withdrawal from nicotine, and gradually weakens and breaks the many associations through the process of extinction (eg, has many cups of coffee without smoking so that eventually drinking coffee is no longer associated with thoughts of, and desires for, smoking). Over time, as the person deals with a variety of life situations and stressors, the realization gradually emerges that the "psychological meanings" of smoking were, in fact, myths. For example, a clearer perspective often develops about smoking as a "friend" when its departure results in the ex-smoker feeling healthier, less stressed, and more vigorous.

In actuality, quitting smoking is considerably more complicated. Although smoking cessation may appear to be a discrete event—one day a person smokes, the next day that person quits—in reality, there is a process involved. Prochaska and DiClemente[22,23] delineate five stages of quitting on the basis of their years of research on addictions. Individuals in the first stage, "precontemplation," do not even consider the possibility of quitting. Those in the next stage, "contemplation," think about quitting but make no active efforts to do so. When people move into the "action" stage, they actually attempt quitting—if only for a few hours or days. Persons move from the action stage to the "maintenance" stage, which is the ultimate goal. However, some persons will go from maintenance to "relapse" by beginning smoking again. Typically, relapsers cycle back to the contemplation stage, then to the action stage, etc.[23]

Data show that 90% of smokers report that they know smoking is hazardous and say that they would quit if they could find a way, indicating that a huge proportion of smokers are in the contemplation stage.[24] Sixty percent of smokers were in the action stage at some point by trying to quit.[24] Notably, by 1993 more than 46 million Americans quit smoking cigarettes and maintained their quitting—one-half of all living adults who ever smoked.[6] In sum, however powerfully addictive and overpracticed smoking is, tens of millions of people already quit, millions more are trying, and most of the rest of those presently smoking are thinking about quitting.

For many, quitting smoking is a "try and try again" matter in which many attempts are made using a variety of methods before complete abstinence is achieved. Persistence, both in terms of the quantity of attempts to quit and the search for an effective method of quitting, seems to be a fundamental characteristic of those who successfully quit.

The only realistic goal for quitting is complete quitting and total abstinence. For some persons, cutting down the amount of smoking may be useful in preparation for quitting. For others, "controlled smoking" — whereby persons decrease the number of cigarettes smoked or switch to a brand with lower tar and nicotine content—may be a useful preparatory step; however, this is not a safe alternative to cessation or a realistic treatment goal.[6,16,25] In our experience with hundreds of smokers in our cessation program at the Cleveland Clinic, individuals who merely decrease their smoking or attempt to be "social smokers" rather than quitting com-

Table 1
Withdrawal Symptoms

Symptom	Cause	Average Duration	Relief
Irritability	Body's craving for nicotine	2–4 weeks	Walks, hot baths, relaxation techniques, nicotine gum
Fatigue	Nicotine is a stimulant	2–4 weeks	Take naps; do not push yourself; nicotine gum
Insomnia	Nicotine affects brain wave function, influences sleep patterns; coughing and dreams about smoking are common	1 week	Avoid caffeine after 6 p.m.; relaxation techniques
Cough, Dry Throat, Nasal Drip	Body getting rid of mucous which has blocked airways and restricted breathing	A few days	Drink plenty of fluids; try cough drops
Dizziness	Body is getting extra oxygen	1 or 2 days	Take extra caution; change positions slowly
Lack of Concentration	Body needs time to adjust to not having constant stimulation from nicotine	A few weeks	Plan workload accordingly; avoid additional stress during first few weeks
Tightness in the Chest	Probably due to tension created by body's need for nicotine; may be caused by sore muscles from coughing	A few days	Relaxation techniques, especially deep breathing. Nicotine gum may help
Constipation, Gas, Stomach Pain	Intestinal movement decreases for a brief period	1 or 2 weeks	Drink plenty of fluids; add fruits, vegetables and whole grain cereals

continues

pletely eventually revert to their previous smoking patterns. In fact, such relapsers often smoke more than before.

When individuals actually quit smoking, most (but not all) experience some type of withdrawal syndrome.[16,17] Table 1, which is adapted from

Table 1 Continued

Symptom	Cause	Average Duration	Relief
Hunger	Craving for a cigarette can be confused with hunger pang; Oral craving, desire for something in the mouth	Up to several weeks	Drink water or low-calorie liquids; be prepared with low calorie snacks
Craving for Cigarette	Withdrawal from nicotine, a strongly addictive drug	Most frequent first 2 or 3 days; can happen occasionally for months or years	Wait out the urge. Urges last only a few minutes. Distract yourself. Exercise; go for a walk around the block

Quitting smoking brings about a variety of symptoms associated with physical and psychological withdrawal. Most symptoms decrease sharply during the first few days of cessation, followed by a continued, but slower rate in decline in the second and third week of abstinence. For some people, coping with withdrawal symptoms is like "riding a roller coaster"—there may be sharp turns, slow climbs, and unexpected plunges. Most symptoms pass within two to four weeks after quitting.

Adapted from materials from the National Cancer Institute.

materials from the National Cancer Institute, describes some common withdrawal symptoms, their suspected causes, their average duration, and suggested ways of obtaining relief from them. Although withdrawal varies from person to person, most withdrawal symptoms appear within the first 24 hours after quitting, "peak" within the first few days of abstinence, and then gradually decline during the next week or two.[16] Patients who have a cigarette or two along the way may report withdrawal symptoms for a considerably extended period of time, perhaps due to the lack of clearance of nicotine from their systems. The use of nicotine replacement therapy also postpones or considerably modifies the course of withdrawal.

As noted previously, the ex-smoker passes through withdrawal and beyond, gradually weakening the many associations (linkages) between situations, emotions, and people in their life and smoking.[16] Somewhat paradoxically, many of the strongest linkages the person has are the more quickly eliminated ones (eg, smoking with a cup of coffee). Because the associated event (drinking coffee) is frequently experienced, the linkage with smoking is quickly broken once an individual becomes a nonsmoker. Other, less frequently experienced linkages (eg, weddings, reunions, and unusual stressors) take much longer to extinguish because they are exposed more slowly to the extinction process. Some particularly strong and/or rarely experienced linkages may continue to elicit brief desires to smoke many months, even years, after quitting.

As individuals progress through the quitting phase, they gradually come to realize that their psychological meanings of smoking were, in fact, myths.[21] These ex-smokers begin to experience increased self-esteem and improved health, and they feel increasingly determined to remain smoke-free.

Methods of Smoking Cessation

With a behavior as ubiquitous and tenacious as smoking, it is hardly surprising that a substantial number of approaches to smoking cessation emerged. This section will briefly review several of the leading methods.

Quitting On One's Own

According to the 1985 Health Interview Survey, approximately 90% of former smokers report that they quit smoking without formal treatment programs or smoking cessation devices.[16] A similar process can and does occur with other addictions; for example, it was estimated that approximately 30% of opioid-dependent persons spontaneously ceased their opioid use.[26] Of course, it is possible that "self-quitters" talked with others, read self-help materials, and listened to media discussions of quitting, which helped their efforts along the way. It is also possible that, for many "self-quitters," urgings to quit from their physicians or other health care professionals played an important role. In terms of sheer success, persons who quit on their own are more likely to be more successful than those who seek help in quitting.[27] The National Cancer Institute[28] provides a summary of self-help materials available to assist individuals who are interested in quitting on their own.

Education

Knowledge acquisition is believed to be the first major step for behavior change in general and smoking cessation in particular.[29] As such, education is postulated to be a necessary, but not sufficient, variable in the smoking cessation process.[30] The strongest motivation for quitting may derive from the specific, tangible benefits to be gained: better health, more attractive appearance, financial savings, better self-image, etc.[31] Fear-arousing education may strengthen intentions to quit and reduce smoking, but it does not by itself lead to quitting.[23] Notably, in a study of ex-smokers, the most common reason listed that precipitated smoking cessation was a general concern about health.[32]

Data suggest that smokers are not necessarily fully aware of the risks that they assume as a result of their tobacco use. According to a study completed in the mid-1980s, one-half of the surveyed smokers did not know that smoking caused most cases of lung cancer, and one-half did not identify smoking as a cause of heart attacks.[33] The 1990 Surgeon General's Report indicated that 30% to 40% of smokers surveyed in 1987 did not believe that smoking increases the risks of developing lung cancer, cancer of the mouth and throat, heart disease, emphysema, and chronic bronchitis or did not believe that smoking cessation decreases the risks from these diseases.[11] Overall, smokers know less about specific health consequences of smoking than nonsmokers.[34] Clearly, continued educational efforts are essential in the ongoing campaign for smoking cessation.

Pharmacologic Approaches

Fifty years of investigation yielded countless attempts to introduce pharmacologic approaches to facilitate smoking cessation. The primary approaches involved use of nicotine antagonists, medications to mimic nicotine effects, and nicotine replacement therapy.

Antagonist therapy was introduced as a means to facilitate cessation via reduction in the pleasurable effects of smoking. Contrary to early expectations, the most commonly used antagonists, mecamylamine and naltrexone, were associated with increased smoking as well as high dropout rates due to side effects.[35-37] In general, the use of antagonists yielded disappointing results.

Medications utilized to mimic nicotine effects include clonidine, anxiolytics, and antidepressants.[36] Clonidine received the strongest research support of the three. It is reported to as much as double quit rates in some meta-analytic reviews, although some users suffer side effects.[38,39] Preliminary research with buspirone and several forms of antidepressants suggest some degree of benefit. However, use of antidepressants was complicated by problems with side effects and long time lags to achieve therapeutic doses.[36,40] The use of medications to mimic nicotine is not typically recommended as a first-line approach to smoking cessation.

During the 1980s, a new and more promising pharmacologic approach emerged: nicotine replacement therapy. Nicotine gum, and later the transdermal patch, comprised the primary alternate delivery systems to enable smokers to minimize or eliminate withdrawal symptoms during smoking cessation. More recently, nicotine replacement via nasal spray or inhalers was considered. Nicotine replacement allows the user to begin to break smoking linkages while remaining addicted to nicotine; the addiction is typically managed through gradual tapering of the replacement nicotine dose. While nicotine is a dangerous toxin, replacement therapy allows the user to avoid many other dangerous carcinogens and other poisons contained in cigarette smoke. The most common forms of nicotine replacement (gum or patch) provide nicotine at a slow rate, eliminating the pleasurable nicotine hit (a few seconds after a smoker inhales) that perpetuates the smoking behavior. Nasal sprays and inhalers have a much faster effect. No form of nicotine replacement therapy is to be used in conjunction with smoking.

Nicotine chewing gum was the first form of nicotine replacement to be introduced. Nicotine is released from the gum (available in 2-mg or 4-mg strength) to be absorbed by the mucous membranes of the mouth.[16] Proper technique involves alternately compressing and parking the gum in the cheek to provide steady nicotine delivery.[41] Used properly, the gum produces nicotine levels sufficient to prevent withdrawal symptoms[24]; however, food and beverage intake (particularly acidic beverages) within the 15 minutes preceding gum use can interfere with nicotine uptake.[42]

Transdermal nicotine systems, introduced in the United States in 1991, use rate-control membrane technology to deliver nicotine for either 16 or 24 hours. Patches provide three doses of transdermal nicotine, estimated to produce high (21–22 mg for 24 hours; 15 mg for 16 hours), medium (14 mg for 24 hours or 10 mg for 16 hours), or low (7 mg for 24 hours or 5 mg for 16 hours) levels of nicotine.[43] Recommended therapeutic programs involve roughly 6–12 weeks of treatment. Nicotine levels provided by the patch are typically about one-half that of smoking,[44] and treatment often includes two taperings to lower-dose patches as treatment progresses.

Use of nicotine replacement proved to be quite safe. Side effects of gum use commonly include hiccoughs, nausea, vomiting, and jaw muscle ache,[31] and tolerance to most side effects usually occurs in the first week.[45] The most common side effects of transdermal replacement were minor skin reactions (35% to 54%) and, less frequently, insomnia or vivid dreams, and nausea.[45,46] Skin reactions can usually be reduced by rotating the patch site.[46] The 14-mg patch was demonstrated to produce no significant medical complications in a population with stable CAD.[47] Nicotine gum and the nicotine patch are currently available without a prescription.

Therapeutic outcomes of nicotine replacement were widely variable, reflecting, in part, inconsistencies in the definition and measurement of smoking cessation, the length of follow-up, and the subject populations. Across studies with varying methodologies, nicotine gum or patch use appears to roughly double successful quit rates at 6–12 months posttreatment, with the patch showing slightly stronger benefit than gum when one compares results across the literature.[48,49] However, outcomes of specific studies vary considerably as a function of the degree of adjunctive treatment (advice, support, or behavior therapy) that is provided.

When minimal adjunctive treatment is provided (eg, no more than brief advice or support, warnings, or booklets) with nicotine replacement, success rates typically range from 10% to 17% at 1 year.[43,49–51] This compares favorably to the 6% or lower cessation rate in control groups receiving no real treatment.[52] Cessation rates using placebo replacement therapy typically fall in the 4% to 15% range for patch[48,50] and 7% to 9% for gum.[49]

The difficulties with maintenance of cessation following replacement therapy are underscored by reports of much higher cessation rates on short-term versus long-term follow-up.[48,50,51] Although patch users experience reductions in withdrawal symptoms and nicotine craving while on the nicotine patch,[53] significant relapse was shown to occur during the periods of down-titration of the nicotine replacement and once the drug is discontinued completely.[50,54] Difficulties with maintenance do not appear to be significantly lessened by tapering of nicotine replacement as opposed to abrupt nicotine withdrawal.[48,55]

Evaluation of treatment outcome for nicotine gum use was complicated by the fact that some individuals continue gum use as long as 2 years postcessation.[56] In one observational study of 538 patients at a smoking cessation clinic, 25% of abstainers at 1 year postcessation were still using the gum.[57] A 1987 review by Schwartz[24] noted that about one-third of patients were using nicotine gum 6 months or longer after cessation, and abstinence dropped by 50% as users ceased gum use from 6 months to 1 year postsmoking cessation. In light of these facts, Schwartz argued that treatment cannot be considered completed until gum use ceases.[24]

Addition of behavioral or multimodal cessation programs to patch or gum use appears to improve treatment effects. In traditional and meta-analytic reviews, when nicotine replacement (gum or patch) was combined with psychosocial treatment (usually behavior therapy), long-term quit rates were increased by an average factor of 1.5–2.0 times compared with nicotine replacement alone.[49,51] Cooper and Clayton[58] and Tonnesen et al[59] combined nicotine replacement with a behavioral group setting and found 1-year quit rates of 33% and 47%, respectively. In one primary care setting in which nicotine gum was combined with 12 weekly sessions of behavioral instruction, 12-month abstinence was as high as 52%![60] These rates clearly exceed cessation rates when either the patch or gum are used alone. Although the effects of both forms of replacement therapy appear to be improved by the addition of a psychosocial component, the data led some to conclude that adjunctive treatment is particularly necessary when nicotine gum is used.[48,61,62]

Attempts continue to identify the populations that may derive most benefit from nicotine replacement therapy and from specific replacement methods. Preliminary research suggests that the patch may be particularly beneficial for patients with pretreatment subclinical dysthymic symptoms,[55] reducing the possibility of depression-related relapses. Although some found the patch to be equally effective with highly dependent or less-dependent smokers,[55] Tang and colleagues[63] found that the patch had little effect with the most highly dependent individuals. They concluded that the patch and gum were roughly comparable in less-dependent smokers and recommended 4-mg nicotine gum as the most effective form of replacement for highly dependent smokers.

Combined use of the transdermal nicotine patch with nicotine gum received increasing attention in recent years. Advocates of combination treatment suggested that smokers may benefit from a constant level of nicotine to alleviate the most prominent withdrawal symptoms (the patch) as well as a self-administered and faster-acting preparation for use with acute withdrawal and craving.[64] The combination approach was demonstrated to reduce quitters' withdrawal and craving to levels experienced by continuing smokers.[65] In one study, the addition of five to seven pieces of 2-mg gum (daily) to the patch in a program with regular medical follow-up contacts increased cessation rates for heavy smokers from 15% to 28% at 24 weeks.[64] More recently, the combination was demonstrated to increase 1-year abstinence from 12% (with patch alone) to 18%.[66] Yet these modest success rates suggest that pharmacologic agents do not provide a complete answer to the challenge of smoking cessation.[18]

Behavioral Methods

Behavioral methods generally include specific techniques designed to engage the patient actively in treatment and facilitate concrete behavior change. In the area of smoking cessation behavioral methods were among the more successful treatment approaches, yielding positive outcomes when used alone and, as noted above, improving outcomes when added as adjuncts to pharmacologic treatments. The most common behavioral methods include aversive procedures, self-monitoring, nicotine fading, stimulus control, and contingency management.

Aversive procedures most commonly attempt to effect cessation by exaggerating some aspect of smoking to the point that it becomes noxious to the smoker. Rapid smoking is the most popular and effective form of aversive treatment. This technique requires the subject to inhale smoke from a cigarette every 6 seconds for the duration of the cigarette or until nauseated.[31] Due to the effects of nicotine on the heart, this method potentially entails medical risk for patients with CAD. However, after careful study, Hall et al[67] concluded that rapid smoking is safe for healthy subjects and for those with mild-to-moderate cardiopulmonary disease and uncomplicated heart attacks. Schwartz[24] found that rapid smoking yielded a median 1-year abstinence rate of 21% alone and 30% when combined with other procedures.

Another behavioral method, self-monitoring, involves recording the frequency of a behavior to establish a "baseline." Not surprisingly, when a behavior is systematically recorded, supposedly to establish a baseline (eg, keeping a record of all foods eaten), the very act of recording can—and often does—alter the behavior in question, even before the change is intended. Recording smoking behavior results in changes in both smoking frequency and duration.[24]

In the Cleveland Clinic's Smoking Cessation Program, patient self-monitoring consists of completing a "smoking diary." The subject records each cigarette smoked, when it was smoked, where it was smoked, what (if any) people were present, and the prevailing emotion or mood the subject felt at the time. Later, the subjects are instructed to review their diaries to determine if their smoking follows any patterns or contains linkages of which they were previously unaware. Self-monitoring is rarely used alone as a cessation technique, but researchers reported quit rates of 26% by the end of treatment and 13% on follow-up when it is combined with other methods.[68] Because self-monitoring can increase dropout rates in smoking programs,[69] encouraging but not requiring monitoring may be most beneficial.

Nicotine fading is another behavioral method, yielding a median rate of 1-year abstinence of 25%.[24] This approach, which typically involves reducing the number of cigarettes smoked each day, may be most useful for getting subjects down to a level at which quitting "cold turkey" is more achievable. Changing to a lower nicotine brand in and of itself yields little health benefit, as smokers tend to modify their smoking behavior to maximize their nicotine intake,[70] thereby exposing themselves to increased levels of carbon monoxide and other toxins.[71]

The stimulus-control method is based on the finding that a wide variety of environmental stimuli (cues) are associated with and tend to trigger smoking (via linkages described previously). A gradual reduction in smoking is achieved by having subjects limit the situations in which they smoke. Most commonly, subjects are instructed to not smoke in certain situations that are strongly associated with smoking (eg, while driving, telephoning, within 20 minutes of ending a meal, etc.). Although evidence does not support stimulus control as an effective means of achieving cessation,[16] it does appear to help smokers reduce their smoking.[24]

Contingency management involves contracting with subjects so that they are rewarded for not smoking, or conversely, punished for returning to smoking. For example, subjects may pledge to donate money to a disliked organization or individual for every cigarette smoked[72] or pay a deposit to be returned at program completion if they do not smoke. One-year abstinence rates in 13 contingency contracting trials ranged from 14% to 38%, with a median of 27%.[24]

Coping Skills Training

When smokers quit smoking, they are in all likelihood bound to have some recurring desires to smoke. As the period of abstinence becomes greater, these desires become less frequent and less intense. Coping skills training is intended to provide the ex-smoker with skills to manage desires to smoke.

As described by Shiffman,[73] who emphasizes the use of coping skills in relapse prevention, coping skills may be behavioral or cognitive. Behavioral coping responses to deal with cravings include behaviors such as eating or drinking, relaxing, exercising, and leaving difficult situations. Cognitive coping responses consist of mental activities that bolster motivation and sustain a focus on abstinence. These include reminding oneself of the health benefits of quitting or the health dangers of smoking, distracting oneself mentally from the desire to smoke, reminding oneself of how others will react to one's resumption of smoking, reminding oneself of one's reasons for quitting, etc. In the Cleveland Clinic's Smoking Cessation Program, participants report that recalling "the basic rule" (repeatedly drummed into the minds of participants) that "smoking is not an option in my life" constituted a useful cognitive coping response. Coping skills training may enhance short-term outcome when combined with other approaches.[24] Coping skills training may be particularly effective for smokers who are less nicotine dependent or who rely more on smoking to cope with emotional stressors.[16]

Hypnosis

Hypnosis showed moderate efficacy in smoking cessation, yielding overall success rates that generally exceed those of medication or education alone.[52] Perhaps the most important consideration is to keep people's expectations realistic. If people are looking for a "magic bullet" that will effortlessly make smoking vanish as though it never existed, hypnosis is not the answer. However, hypnosis may prove to be a useful part of the process of quitting for motivated subjects who do not place all their hopes on this (or any other single) technique.

Multimodal Treatment

Because there is no single, most effective approach to smoking cessation, and because different individuals may benefit from different approaches to treatment, a multimodal approach to smoking cessation appears most advisable. Combinations of nonpharmacologic treatments generally outperform any single constituent of treatment,[74] yielding biochemically validated long-term cessation rates in the range of 30% to 40%.[75] It was speculated that adding pharmacologic adjuncts might make these cessation rates even higher, especially for highly addictive smokers who were unable to achieve even short-term abstinence despite repeated attempts.[16,75] There is little evidence, however, that pharmacologic agents actually increase the efficacy of multimodal cessation programs.

Maintenance

The problem of maintenance is ubiquitous in smoking cessation programs. Although most approaches to smoking cessation produce some initial quitters, there is invariably significant relapse over the first 12 months, and even beyond. If one in three smokers who entered a particular program did not relapse 1 year later, the outcome is considered good.[24] This problem is not limited to formal cessation programs: between 1979 and 1985, 75% to 80% of 1.3 million smokers who quit on their own resumed smoking within 6 months.[70] Those who are highly motivated, in the right frame of mind, less stressed, and more confident in their ability to quit (although most quitters have some doubts) generally are more successful with maintenance.[24] However, by definition, the factor that ultimately distinguishes maintainers from relapsers is the ability to cope with urges, cravings, and linkages without smoking.

Shiffman found that most relapses situations can be classified into one of four categories: (1) social situations marked by alcohol consumption, good feelings, and the presence of smokers; (2) relaxation situations marked by feelings of "unwinding," often after a meal; (3) work pressure marked by tension and frustration; and (4) emotional upset situations marked by negative affect.[76]

Most "relapse crises"—situations where ex-smokers feel a strong desire to return to smoking—occur in the presence of negative emotional states.[73] However, one-third of the relapse crises were linked to positive mood states and were frequently precipitated by other smokers, eating, and alcohol. Ex-smokers who had some type of coping response, either something appropriate to do (behavioral) or something relevant to think (cognitive), were much more likely to survive their relapse crises.[73] Persons who were drinking alcohol were less likely to utilize behavioral coping responses, and depression diminished the effectiveness of coping responses.[77] The situations that precipitated relapse crises could not be reliably predicted from one crisis to another.[78] Similarly, the coping skills that people find effective vary from one situation to another, with behavioral coping skills being more consistently helpful than cognitive coping skills.[78] Support from family, friends, coworkers, and nonsmoking buddies can be very useful.[24] Follow-up treatment contacts and verbal rewards for smoking cessation by physicians can also be extremely helpful.

The Role of the Physician in Smoking Cessation

The physician's advice to quit smoking was described as the most effective means of motivating smokers to make an attempt at quitting.[3] The fact that 70% of smokers see a physician at least once a year suggests that physicians are in a powerful position to influence their patients.[3] Furthermore, physicians are likely to encounter smokers at times when health concerns are already on their mind and they may be most motivated to quit.[8] The enormity of cigarette-related morbidity and mortality and the clear potential for recovery from (or improvement of) many smoking-related problems provides ample reason for physicians to take an active role in altering their patients smoking behavior.[8] Notably, most smokers[79] and 80% to 90% of physicians[24] believe that it is the physician's job to help smokers stop smoking.

At the Cleveland Clinic Foundation patients are frequently reminded that persistence is a pivotal ingredient in successfully quitting and that failure does not occur until one stops trying. In fact, the successful quitter generally "failed" on one or more previous quit attempts.[80] Similarly, the physician's advice to quit is not considered to have failed when it does not convince a smoker to quit; physician "failure" only occurs when the physician stops trying to get patients to quit.

To be of any impact, the physician must, of course, communicate with the patient about smoking. In patient surveys, 40% to 50% of smokers indicate that they were advised to quit by their doctors.[81,82] This advice was given more recently (1989–1990) than earlier (1979–1980)[81] and is given more frequently by nonsmoking than by smoking physicians.[81]

Advising patients to quit smoking takes only a few minutes of physician time. Although this advice alone cannot be expected to produce large cessation rates, it does have an impact. In fact, simple but firm advice to quit smoking by the physician could double the rates reported for spontaneous cessation in this country.[83] In a comprehensive survey of 12 studies of physician advice or counseling over a 16-year period, the quit rate ranged from 3% to 13% with a median of 3.[24] If this success ratio were extended to all 50 million current smokers, 70% of whom see a physician at least once a year, over 2 million smokers would quit each year. That constitutes an effect 17 times greater than saying nothing![84]

When a patient's smoking is addressed, physicians may lack awareness of time-effective means of facilitating quitting. In one study where 85% of physicians addressed the issue of smoking, 34% never gave their patients self-help materials, and 83% never used a quit date contract. Seventy-three percent never made appointments primarily for the purpose of discussing smoking[85]—even though physician counseling about smoking during office visits is reported to be at least as cost-effective as other routinely accepted medical practices such as the treatment of mild hypertension or hypercholesterolemia.[86]

Fiore and Baker[87] suggested that smoking might be viewed as an ongoing disease that, as with other such diseases, is chronic and characterized by periods of remission and relapse. Within this model, smoking requires ongoing attention from the physician and sensitivity to the patient's individual condition. Physician interventions that do not lead directly to cessation attempts may still have the important effect of moving the patient closer to quitting.[88]

It should be noted that a variety of resources are available to assist physicians in dealing with patient tobacco use. For example, the Cancer Information Service (1-800-4-CANCER) provides a wealth of informational booklets and brochures designed for patients and physicians free of charge upon request. Another resource is Richards,[89] which provides a more detailed summary of specific questions that physicians may wish to ask smokers and suggested verbal strategies to deal effectively with patient blockers to discussion of their tobacco use. The DeNelsky-Plesec Smoking Cessation Checklist[90] (Table 2) may be given to patients to assist them in their quitting efforts. It is a simple checklist that provides information on preparing to quit, actual quitting, and maintenance.

Since quitting smoking is a process, and since smokers are at various stages in this process, how might physicians maximize their impact within the time constraints of daily practice? A number of authors proposed specific plans for physicians to follow in helping their patients quit smoking.[8,83,87–89,91–96] There is a great deal of similarity and overlap among these plans. What follows is a plan that most closely approximates the plans of Gritz,[83] Stokes and Rigotti,[8] and the National Cancer Institute publication for physicians.[28]

Specific Physician Interventions

Step 1: Assess Smoking Status/ Initiate Discussion of Smoking

First, and perhaps of primary importance, all patients must be screened for smoking status.[3,97] To do this routinely and systematically, it was proposed that smoking status (current smoker, former smoker, or never smoked) become a new vital sign, along with BP, pulse, temperature, and respiratory rate.[3,93] Considering smoking a vital sign ensures that this topic will be covered at each patient visit.

Even if a patient quit smoking, or never began, it is good practice to confirm nonsmoking status on a regular basis. With patients who do smoke, it is imperative that smoking status be included in every contact with the patient. Chart reminders of those identified as smokers were

---

Table 2

Stop Smoking Checklist

Preparing To Quit

—Make a personal pact with yourself to quit.

—Pick a date for quitting completely (my date is_____).

—Write down, on a card, the three most important reasons for quitting. Carry that card with you from now on. Look at it several times each day.

—Prior to quitting, eliminate smoking completely in two or three of your high risk situations.

—Reduce consumption to one pack per day or less.

—Change to a less desirable brand of cigarettes.

—Discard your lighter; use matches. Carry your cigarettes in a different place.

—Spend a little time each day picturing in your mind stressful events occurring in the future and you not smoking.

Actual Quitting: The First Two Weeks

—Get rid of ALL cigarettes! Put away all smoking related objects such as ashtrays. Ask people you live with not to smoke in your presence for two weeks.

—Spend as much time as possible with non-smoking people.

—Keep busy, especially on evenings and weekends.

—Avoid "high risk" situations (large parties, bars, etc.).

—Spend lots of time in places which prohibit or discourage smoking (e.g. theaters, libraries).

—Drink plenty of fluids.

—Don't substitute food or sugar based products for cigarettes. Use approved substitutions (e.g. ice water, high bulk/low calorie foods, sugarless gum, mouthwash, brushing teeth).

—Begin (or increase) a regular exercise program.

—When experiencing withdrawal effects:

1. Remind yourself of why you are quitting (from your card).

2. Remind yourself that whatever discomfort you are experiencing is only a tiny fraction of the probable discomfort associated with continued smoking (i.e., painful diseases, surgery, chemotherapy).

3. Practice deep breathing or other relaxation techniques.

—Remind yourself that you can free yourself from this unhealthy, expensive, messy habit and become a nonsmoker.

Maintenance of Quitting: After Two Weeks

—Remind yourself that the desire to smoke is linked to a great many situations, people, and emotional states.

—When you do have a desire to smoke, remember that it only lasts a few seconds; distract yourself, and leave the situation if necessary.

—After each desire to smoke has passed, give yourself a "pat on the back"—you have just made progress in breaking your habit forever.

—Save the money you wasted on cigarettes in a "special fund" and buy yourself something nice.

continues

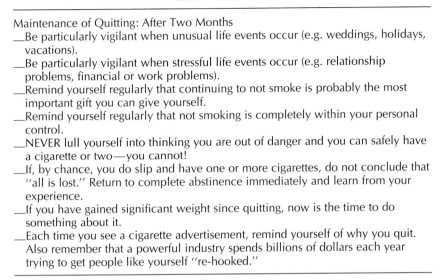

Table 2 Continued

Maintenance of Quitting: After Two Months
__Be particularly vigilant when unusual life events occur (e.g. weddings, holidays, vacations).
__Be particularly vigilant when stressful life events occur (e.g. relationship problems, financial or work problems).
__Remind yourself regularly that continuing to not smoke is probably the most important gift you can give yourself.
__Remind yourself regularly that not smoking is completely within your personal control.
__NEVER lull yourself into thinking you are out of danger and you can safely have a cigarette or two—you cannot!
__If, by chance, you do slip and have one or more cigarettes, do not conclude that ''all is lost.'' Return to complete abstinence immediately and learn from your experience.
__If you have gained significant weight since quitting, now is the time to do something about it.
__Each time you see a cigarette advertisement, remind yourself of why you quit. Also remember that a powerful industry spends billions of dollars each year trying to get people like yourself ''re-hooked.''

Reproduced with permission from Reference 90.

demonstrated to be an effective strategy for helping physicians consistently address the smoking issue at clinical appointments with patients who smoke.[98,99] If the patient is smoking, providing risk-benefit information is important; this information should be personalized as it is relevant to the patient's medical condition.[83] Whereas addressing the patient's smoking status requires only a moment of time, it conveys an important message to the patient—that smoking is an unhealthy behavior that warrants attention. In settings where time available for verbal interventions is severely limited, quality self-help materials should be prominently displayed.[95] However, these should not be considered a substitute for verbal intervention.

Step 2: Assess Patient's Readiness for Smoking Cessation

Smoking patients vary a great deal in their attitudes toward smoking cessation. Some are not even thinking about quitting (precontemplators), some are thinking seriously about quitting but not ready to try (contemplators), and some are ready for action (action stage). The most effective messages from doctors are those that are attuned to the patient's particular stage.[96] If the patient is clearly in the ''precontemplation'' stage—not even thinking of quitting in the next 6 months—they may benefit from information about the risks of smoking and the benefits of quitting. Focus on health effects of smoking may be beneficial, since smokers have significantly more health worries and concerns than nonsmokers.[100] For contemplators who are thinking of quitting but have not yet done so, physicians will need to focus on trying to increase the patient's motivation to quit. Providing the patient with intrinsic motivators (eg, the patient's own desire for health, self-preservation, or self-esteem) is typically more successful in bolstering quitting attempts than the provision of extrinsic motivators (eg, social pressure or monetary reward).[101]

If the patient is in the contemplation stage, less effort may need to be directed toward emphasizing the health issues and more toward underscoring the importance of trying to quit now. Such a patient needs to be encouraged to commit to a specific date for quitting. If the patient is in the action stage—actively attempting to quit—the emphasis needs to be on optimistically conveying the message, "keep at it until you get it right!", at the same time underscoring the need for the patient to learn from their past efforts at quitting.[94]

Patients' confidence that they can quit (ie, self-efficacy) will vary enormously, but virtually all have some doubts. For the patient extremely low in self-efficacy, encouraging patients to keep records of smoking behavior (self-monitoring) and recommending that they disrupt their normal smoking pattern in a variety of ways (eg, not smoking in certain situations, smoking a less-favored brand, or reducing their amount of smoking) can help them develop a partial sense of control leading to enhanced self-efficacy.[102]

Step 3: Advise the Patient to Stop Smoking

Brief but firm advice needs to be given at each and every contact with the patient. It may be framed quite simply: "I want you to stop smoking!"[97] Even for patients in the precontemplation stage who are not ready to take action, hearing this message repeated as often as necessary may eventually induce serious thoughts about quitting. For those patients in the contemplation stage, this recommendation will hopefully be sufficient to propel them into action.

Step 4: Set a Date for Quitting

Setting a specific date for quitting is the most universally agreed upon component of the physician's intervention and the most important for maximizing cessation rates.[83] Encouraging the patient to select and commit to a quitting date within 4 weeks is preferable.[8] The patient may taper down the quantity of smoking before that date but should stop completely when that date arrives. Signing a written contract acknowledging the specific commitment to quit and the date of quitting can be helpful.[83] (Sample contracts are provided as Tables 3 and 4.) The date itself should be during a time when the patient anticipates no unusual stress; however, once selected, the patient should be strongly encouraged to stick with the quitting date regardless of what develops in their life. When possible, involvement of family members or significant others in the patient's life to provide ongoing positive support may facilitate the patient's quitting and maintenance efforts.[82] The physician should keep a written record (or copy) of the patient's commitment as a reminder to follow the patient's progress.

For those remaining in the precontemplation stage, setting a date may not be immediately attainable. These individuals should be encouraged to commit to a date when they will be ready to commit to quitting. Pro-

---

Table 3
Tobacco (Smoking) Cessation Contract

Name: _____   Date: _____

Age: _____   Health Professional: _____

Sex: _____M   _____F

1. Tobacco products (e.g., cigarettes) and rate of current consumption (e.g., one pack per day) _____ .
2. Quit date: "I will totally end my use of tobacco on (specific date within the next month) _____ ."
3. In preparation for my quitting I will eliminate my use of tobacco in the following three situations frequently linked with my tobacco consumption (e.g., talking on the phone, immediately after eating, when bored, etc.):

    1. _____

    2. _____

    3. _____
4. I will call this office the week after quitting and the following week to report on my progress to (health professionals name) _____ . If I experience significant problems during this period I will call (above mentioned person) to obtain advice on how to proceed with quitting.
5. I understand the importance of my ending my tobacco addiction, and know that my motivation and effort are principal components in successfully quitting. I am determined to abide by this contract and will end my tobacco dependence on the quit data I specified above.

    Patient's Signature: _____

Health Professional's Signature: _____

    Date: _____

Table 4
Nonsmoking Contract

I understand that smoking is the single greatest preventable threat to my health. I have been advised by my health professional to end my tobacco addiction and will quit smoking on _____ .
                           (Date)

_____   _____
Patient's Signature   Professional's Signature

                                      _____
                                         Today's Date

---

vision of materials reviewing smoking-related health information and emphasizing the benefits of quitting may be helpful,[88] and these individuals might be encouraged to think about aspects of smoking that they do not like for their next visit. They need to be systematically followed by the physician in the same manner as those who have committed to quitting.

Step 5: Discuss Specific Treatment Strategies

As noted previously, between 85% and 90% of all smokers quit on their own, without the aid of a formal smoking cessation program. For this reason, it makes sense for most smokers to at least try to do it on their own. As discussed earlier, quitting typically involves withstanding some withdrawal symptoms; breaking the associations between smoking and situations, emotions, and persons in the person's life; and gradually coming to realize that the person's psychological meanings of smoking are really myths.

Nicotine replacement may be helpful for the heavily addicted smoker, especially the one who is not able to reduce their smoking to a pack per day or less by the day of quitting. Persons who are prone to depression may also benefit from the use of replacement therapy. When nicotine replacement is recommended, referral to a formal treatment program should be considered, since, as noted previously, pharmacologic aids are most beneficial when they are used as part of a broader smoking cessation program.[24,25]

Individuals who tried repeatedly on their own without successfully quitting or maintaining their quitting might also benefit from referral to a formal smoking cessation program. Multimodal programs that offer a variety of techniques are more likely to be successful than those that rely on a single technique.

Step 6: Arrange Follow-Up

Follow-up visits to the physician or calls from nurses or other appropriate health care personnel can enhance the effectiveness of the physician's advice. Nurse-assisted smoking counseling in medical settings not only appears to be more effective than physician only advice, but it can minimize demands on physicians.[103] Calling the patient on the quit day may be especially helpful.[8] This demonstrates to the patient that the physician is serious about the need for smoking cessation and genuinely supports the patient's attempts to quit. Because many persons have considerable apprehension about quitting, reassurance from the physician or the nurse may be especially welcome at this time. A simple statistic such as "over 46 million smokers quit, I know you can, too," may be quite encouraging.

If the patient is unable to quit or maintain quitting, a nonjudgmental attitude on the part of the physician is in order. The patient should be encouraged to learn from the experience, pick a new quit date, obtain whatever additional assistance may be helpful, and get it right the next time.[94] Notably, personalization of cessation advice and persistence on the part of the physician are the two most important factors associated with eventual success.[74]

Weight Gain

People who work in the field of smoking cessation frequently hear concerns about weight gain. This fear of postcessation weight gain may discourage many smokers from trying to quit and may precipitate relapse among those who already quit.[11] Approximately one-half of both smokers and former smokers agree that smoking helps control weight.[11]

There is ample research evidence to support the notion that smoking helps some people control their weight and that quitting smoking often results in weight gain.[16] A variety of factors may contribute to postcessation weight gain, including increased food consumption, decreased metabolism, and an increased preference for sweet-tasting, high-caloric foods.[16] Smoking cessation may actually raise the body's weight "set point," making some amount of weight gain postcessation difficult to avoid.[104]

However, for most people who quit, the amount of weight gain is considerably less than anticipated. In a recent Surgeon General's Report, which reviewed 15 studies involving a total of 20 000 persons, it was reported that four-fifths of ex-smokers did gain weight, but the average weight gain 1 year later was only 2.3 kg.[11] Less than 4% of those who quit gained more than 9 kg.[11] In terms of health implications, the approximately 2.3-kg average weight gain associated with quitting smoking is minimal, and this small weight gain tends to be accompanied by favorable changes in lipid profiles and in body fat distribution.[11] However, most people are probably more concerned about the cosmetic effects of weight gain than the health effects.

Intensive strategies for combating weight gain during early stages of cessation should be avoided as they may be associated with increased smoking relapse.[105] However, encouragement of healthy lifestyle change, such as exercise and dietary awareness, may help patients to limit post-cessation weight gain. In addition to burning calories, exercise may at least temporarily increase basal metabolic rate, thereby compensating to some degree for the lowered metabolic rate often associated with quitting.[11] Dietary advice would include using appropriate amounts of low-calorie, high-bulk foods in one's diet, and avoiding or eliminating simple sugars and high-fat foods wherever possible.

Perkins[105] provides a recent review of the use of pharmacologic interventions for weight management during smoking cessation. On the basis of his review, he concluded that the nicotine patch does not appear to prevent weight gain. Serotonin-enhancing drugs such as D-fenfluramine and fluoxetine showed some preliminary benefit in prevention of weight gain in the short term, but these do not prevent weight regain after cessation of medication use.[105] Gum chewing may discourage eating by virtue of its incompatibility with eating, but it is not clear that nicotine gum shows an advantage over placebo gum or that gum use yields long-term prevention of weight gain.

Summary and Conclusions

Notwithstanding its highly addictive nature, the money spent to promote it, and the powerful tobacco interests that fight every step of the way to maintain smoking at a high level and thus preserve their profits, smoking is definitely on the decline in the United States. Since 1964, when the first Surgeon General's Report was issued, there was nothing less than a behavioral revolution. Nearly one-half of all living adults who ever smoked quit; between 1964 and 1985 approximately three-quarters of a million smoking-related deaths were postponed or avoided as a result of decisions to quit smoking or not to start.[77] Each of those avoided or postponed deaths represented an average gain in life expectancy of 2 decades.[8] This was preventative health care at its best.

We came a long way in the past 25 years. We have a long way to go. When we eventually succeed in making this a smoke-free society, we will have taken a truly enormous step toward establishing a healthier population. We will have conquered the major preventable source of disability and death. Physicians will then be able to turn their full resources and energies toward treating those whose diseases cannot be prevented.

References

1. US Dept of Health and Human Services. *Reducing the Health Consequences of Smoking: 25 Years of Progress. A Report of the Surgeon General.* Washington, DC: Office on Smoking and Health; 1989. US Dept of Health and Human Services publication CDC 89–8411.
2. Lakier JB. Smoking and cardiovascular disease. *Am J Med* 1992;93(suppl): 8–12.
3. Fiore MC, Pierce JP, Remington PL, et al. Cigarette smoking: the clinician's role in cessation, prevention, and public health. In: *Disease-A-Month.* Chicago, Ill: Year Book Medical Publishers; 1990:4.
4. Cigarette smoking—attributable mortality and years of potential life lost—United States, 1990. *MMWR* 1993;42:645–649.
5. American Heart Association. Active and passive tobacco exposure: a serious pediatric health problem. A statement from the Committee on Atherosclerosis and Hypertension in Children. Council on Cardiovascular Disease in the Young. *Circulation* 1990;90:2581–2590.
6. Cigarette smoking among adults—United States, 1993. *MMWR* 1994;43: 925–930.
7. Medical care expenditures attributable to cigarette smoking—United States. *MMWR* 1994;43:469–473.
8. Stokes J III, Rigotti NA. The health consequences of cigarette smoking and the internist's role in smoking cessation. *Adv Intern Med* 1988;33:431–460.
9. Krupski WC. The peripheral vascular consequences of smoking. *Ann Vasc Surg* 1991;5:291–304.
10. Lassila R, Seyberth HW, Haapanen A, et al. Vasoactive and atherogenic effects of cigarette smoking: a study of monozygotic twins discordant for smoking. *BMJ* 1988;297:955–957.
11. US Dept of Health and Human Services. *The Health Benefits of Smoking Cessation. A Report of the Surgeon General.* Washington, DC: Office on Smoking and Health; 1990. US Dept of Health and Human Services publication CDC 90–8416.
12. Timmreck TC, Randolph JF. Smoking cessation: clinical steps to improve compliance. *Geriatrics* 1993;48:63–70.
13. Rose G, Colwell L. Randomised controlled trial of anti-smoking advice: final (20 year) results. *J Epidemiol Community Health* 1992;46:65–77.
14. Kandel DB, Yamaguchi K. *Developmental Patterns of the Use of Legal, Illegal, and Medically Prescribed Psychotropic Drugs from Adolescense to Young Adulthood.* Washington, DC: US Dept of Health and Human Services; 1986. National Institute of Drug Abuse Research Monograph.
15. Green DE. *Teenage Smoking: Immediate and Long Term Patterns.* Washington, DC: US Dept of Health, Education and Welfare; 1979.
16. US Dept of Health and Human Services. *The Health Consequences of Smoking: Nicotine Addiction. A Report of the Surgeon General.* Washington, DC: Office of Smoking and Health; 1988. US Dept of Health and Human Services publication CDC 88–8406.
17. Silvis GL, Perry CL. Understanding and deterring tobacco use among adolescents. *Pediatr Clin North Am* 1987;34:363–379.
18. Nunn-Thompson CL, Simon PA. Pharmacotherapy for smoking cessation. *Clin Pharm* 1989;8:710–720.
19. Pomerleau OF, Pomerleau CS. Neuroregulators and the reinforcement of smoking: towards a biobehavioral explanation. *Neurosci Behav Rev* 1984; 8:503–513.

20. McKennel AC, Thomas RK. Adults' and adolescents' smoking habits and attitudes. Government Social Survey. London, England: HM Stationery Office.

21. DeNelsky GY, Plesec TL. Smoking and smoking cessation. In: Matzen RN, Lang RS, eds. *Clinical Preventative Medicine.* St. Louis, Mo: Mosby; 1993: 256–283.

22. DiClemente CC, Prochaska JO, Fairhurst SK, et al. The process of smoking cessation: an analysis of precontemplation, contemplation and preparation stages of change. *J Consult Clin Psychol* 1991;59:295–304.

23. Prochaska JO, DiClemente CC. Stages and processes of self-change of smoking: toward an integrative model of change. *J Consult Clin Psychol* 1983; 51:390–395.

24. Schwartz JL. *Review and Evaluation of Smoking Cessation Methods: The United States and Canada, 1978–1985.* Bethesda, Md: US Dept of Health and Human Services; 1987. National Institutes of Health publication 87–2940.

25. Lando HA. A factorial analysis of pregnation, aversion, and maintenance in the elements of smoking. *Addict Behav* 1982;7:143–154.

26. Anglin MD, Brecht ML, Woodard JA. An empirical study of maturing out conditioned factors. *Int J Addict* 1986;21:233–246.

27. Fiore MC, Novothy TE, Pierce JP, et al. Methods used to quit smoking in the United States. *JAMA* 1990;263:2760–2765.

28. Glynn TJ, Manley MW. *How To Help Your Patients Stop Smoking: A National Cancer Institute Manual for Physicians.* Bethesda, Md: National Cancer Institute; 1995. US Dept of Health and Human Services, National Institutes of Health publication 95–3064.

29. Farguhar JW, Maccoby N, Solomon DS. Community applications of behavioral medicine. In: Gentry WD, ed. *Handbook of Behavioral Medicine.* New York, NY: Guilford; 1984.

30. Klesges RC, Somes G, Pascale RW, et al. Knowledge and beliefs regarding the consequences of cigarette smoking and their relationships to smoking status in a biracial sample. *Health Psychol* 1988;7:387–401.

31. Stone S, Perlmutter KJ. Methods for stopping cigarette smoking. Health and Public Policy Committee. American College of Physicians. *Ann Intern Med* 1986;105:281–291.

32. Carmody TP, Brischetto CS, Pierce DK, et al. A prospective five-year follow-up of smokers who quit on their own. *Health Educ Res* 1986;1:101–109.

33. Warner KE. Cigarette advertising and media coverage of smoking on health. *N Engl J Med* 1985;312:384–388.

34. US Department of Health and Human Services. *Vital and health statistics: smoking and other tobacco use.* In: Data from the National Health Survey. Washington, DC: US Dept of Health and Human Services; 1989. Series 10, publication PHS 89–1597.

35. Clarke PBS. Nicotinic receptor blockade therapy and smoking cessation. *Br J Addict* 1991;86:501–505.

36. Hughes JR. Non-nicotine pharmacotherapies for smoking cessation. *J Drug Dev* 1994;6:197–203.

37. Stolerman IP, Goldfarb T, Fink R, et al. Influencing cigarette smoking with nicotine antagonists. *Psychopharmacologia* 1973;28:247–259.

38. Gourlay SG, Benowitz NL. Is clonidine an effective smoking cessation therapy? *Drugs* 1995;50:197–207.

39. Law M, Tang JL. An analysis of the effectiveness of interventions intended to help people stop smoking. *Arch Intern Med* 1995;155:1933–1941.

40. Humfleet G, Hall S, Reus V, et al. The efficacy of nortriptyline as an adjunct to psychological treatment for smokers with and without depressive histories. In: Washington AM, ed. *Problems of Drug Dependence, 1995.* Washington, DC: US Government Printing Office; 1996. National Institute of Drug Abuse Research Monograph Series.

41. Schneider N. Nicotine gum in smoking cessation, efficacy and proper use. *Compr Ther* 1987;13:32–37.

42. Henningfield J, Radzius A, Cooper TM, et al. Drinking coffee and carbonated beverages blocks absorption of nicotine from nicotine polacrilex gum. *JAMA* 1990;264:1560–1564.

43. Silagy C, Mant D, Fowler G, et al. Meta-analysis on efficacy of nicotine replacement therapies in smoking cessation. *Lancet* 1994;343:139–142.

44. Palmer KJ, Faulds D. Transdermal nicotine: a review of its pharmacodynamic and pharmacokinetic properties, and therapeutic use as an aid to smoking cessation. *Drugs* 1992;44:498–529.

45. Hughes JR. Risk/benefit of nicotine replacement in smoking cessation. *Drug Saf* 1993;8:49–56.

46. Fiore MC, Jorenby DE, Baker TB, et al. Tobacco dependence and the nicotine patch: clinical guidelines for effective use. *JAMA* 1994;268:2687–2694.

47. Fortmann ST. Nicotine replacement therapy for patients with coronary artery disease. *Arch Intern Med* 1994;154:989–995.

48. Fiore MC, Smith SS, Jorenby DE, et al. The effectiveness of the nicotine patch for smoking cessation: a meta-analysis. *JAMA* 1994;271:1940–1947.

49. Gourlay SG, McNeil JJ. Antismoking products. *Med J Aust* 1990;153:699–707.

50. Tonnesen P, Norregaard J, Simonsen K, et al. A double-blind trial of a 16-hour transdermal nicotine patch in smoking cessation. *N Engl J Med* 1991; 325:311–315.

51. Wan Po AL. Transdermal nicotine in smoking cessation. *Eur J Pharmacol* 1993;45:519–528.

52. Viswesvaran C, Schmidt FL. A meta-analytic comparison of the effectiveness of smoking cessation methods. *J Appl Psychol* 1992;77:554–561.

53. Levin ED, Westman EC, Stein RM, et al. Nicotine skin patch treatment increases abstinence, decreases withdrawal symptoms, and attenuates rewarding effects of smoking. *J Clin Psychopharmacol* 1994;14:41–49.

54. Transdermal Nicotine Study Group. Transdermal nicotine for smoking cessation. *JAMA* 1991;266:3133–3138.

55. Stapleton JA, Russell MA, Feyerabend C, et al. Dose effects as predictors of outcome in a randomized trial of transdermal nicotine patches in general practice. *Addiction* 1995;90:31–42.

56. Hughes JR. Long-term use of nicotine-replacement therapy. In: Henningfield JE, Stitzer JL, eds. *New Developments in Nicotine-Delivery Systems.* New York, NY: Carlton; 1991.

57. Hajek, P, Jackson P, Belcher M. Long term use of nicotine chewing gum: occurrence, determinants, and effect on weight gain. *JAMA* 1988;260:1593–1596.

58. Cooper TM, Clayton RR. Stop smoking program using nicotine reduction therapy and behavior modification for heavy smokers. *J Am Dent Assoc* 1989;118:47–51.

59. Tonnesen P, Fryd V, Hansen M, et al. Effect of nicotine chewing gum in combination with group counseling on the cessation of smoking. *N Engl J Med* 1988;318:15–18.

60. Basler HD, Brinkmeier U, Buser K, et al. Nicotine gum assisted group therapy in smokers with an increased risk of coronary disease—evaluation in primary care setting format. *Health Educ Res* 1992;7:87–95.

61. Cepeda-Benito A. A meta-analytic review of the efficacy of nicotine chewing gum. *J Consult Clin Psychol* 1993;61:822–830.
62. Lam W, Sze PC, Sacks HS, et al. Meta-analysis of randomised controlled trials of nicotine chewing-gum. *Lancet* 1987;2:27–30.
63. Tang JL, Law M, Wald N. How effective is nicotine replacement therapy in helping people to stop smoking? *BMJ* 1994;308:21–26.
64. Fagerstrom KO. Combined use of nicotine replacement products. *Health Values* 1994;18:15–20.
65. Fagerstrom KO, Schneider NG, Lunell E. Effectiveness of nicotine patch and nicotine gum as individual versus combined treatments for tobacco withdrawal symptoms. *Psychopharmacology* 1993;111:271–277.
66. Kornitzer M, Boutsen M, Dramaix M, et al. Combined use of nicotine patch and gum in smoking cessation: a placebo-controlled clinical trial. *Prev Med* 1995;24:41–47.
67. Hall RG, Sachs DP, Hall SM, et al. Two year efficacy and safety of rapid smoking therapy in patients with cardiac and pulmonary disease. *J Clin Consult Psychol* 1984;52:574–581.
68. McFall RM, Hammen CL. Motivation, structure, and self-monitoring: role of non-specific factors in cigarette smoking. *J Consult Clin Psychol* 1975;37:80–86.
69. Glasgow RE. Smoking. In: Holroyd K, Creer T, eds. *Self-Management of Chronic Disease and Handbook of Clinical Interventions and Research.* Orlando, Fla: Academic Press; 1986:99–126.
70. Carmody TP. Preventing relapse in the treatment of nicotine addiction: current issues and future directions. *J Psychoactive Drugs* 1990;22:211–238.
71. US Dept of Health and Human Services. *The Health Consequences of Smoking: Cardiovascular Disease. A Report of the Surgeon General.* Washington, DC: Office on Smoking and Health; 1983. US Dept of Health and Human Services publication 84–50204.
72. Tiffany ST, Martin EM, Baker TB. Treatments for cigarette smoking: an evaluation of the contributions of aversion and counseling procedures. *Behav Res Ther* 1986;24:437–492.
73. Shiffman S. Relapse following smoking cessation. A situational analysis. *J Consult Clin Psychol* 1982;50:71–86.
74. Kottke TE, Battista RN, DeFriese GH, et al. Attributes of successful smoking cessation interventions in medical practice: a meta-analysis of 39 controlled trials. *JAMA* 1988;259:2883–2889.
75. Epstein LH, et al. Smoking research: basic research, intervention, prevention and new trends. *Health Psychol* 1989;8:705–721.
76. Shiffman S. A cluster-analytic typology of smoking relapse episodes. *Addict Behav* 1986;11:295–307.
77. Shiffman S, Read L, Jarvik ME. Smoking relapse situations: a preliminary typology. *Int J Addict* 1985;20:311–318.
78. Shiffman S. Trans-situational consistency in smoking relapse. *Health Psychol* 1989;8:471–481.
79. Joseph AM, Byrd JC. Smoking cessation in practice. *Prim Care* 1989;16:83–98.
80. Pederson LL, Lefcoe NM. A psychological and behavioral comparison of ex-smokers and smokers. *J Chron Dis* 1976;29:431–434.
81. Cummings KM, Giovino G, Sciandra R, et al. Physician advice to quit smoking: who gets it and who doesn't. *Am J Prev Med* 1987;3:69–75.
82. Frank E, Winkleby MA, Altman DG, et al. Predictors of physicians' smoking cessation advice. *JAMA* 1991;266:3139–3144.

83. Gritz ER. Cigarette smoking: the need for action by health professionals. *Cancer J Clin* 1988;38:194–212.

84. Sachs DP. Smoking cessation strategies: what works, what doesn't. *J Am Dent Assoc* 1990;(suppl):13S–19S.

85. Jelly MJ, Prochazka AV. A survey of physicians' smoking counseling practices. *Am J Med Sci* 1991;301:250–255.

86. Cummings SR, Rubin SM, Oster G. The cost-effectiveness of counseling smokers to quit. *JAMA* 1989;261:75–79.

87. Fiore MC, Baker TM. Smoking cessation treatment and the good doctor club. Editorial. *Am J Public Health* 1995;85:161–163.

88. Goldberg DN, Hoffman AM, Farinha MF, et al. Physician delivery of smoking-cessation advice based on the stage-of-change model. *Am J Prev Med* 1994;10:267–274.

89. Richards JW. Words as therapy: smoking cessation. *J Fam Pract* 1992;24:687–692.

90. DeNelsky GY, Plesec TL. A stop smoking checklist. *Addict Prog Manage* 1990;4:105.

91. Christen AG, Klein JA, Christen JA, et al. How-to-do-it quit-smoking strategies for the dental office team: an eight-step program. *J Am Dent Assoc* 1990;(suppl):20S–27S.

92. DeNelsky GY. Smoking cessation: strategies that work. *Cleve Clin J Med* 1990;57:416–417.

93. Fiore MC. The new vital sign: assessing and documenting smoking status. *JAMA* 1991;266:3183–3184.

94. Marlatt GA, Gordon JR, eds. *Relapse Prevention: Maintenance Strategies in the Treatment of Addictive Behaviors.* New York, NY: Guilford Press; 1985.

95. Mattick RP, Baillie A, Digiusto E, et al. A summary of the recommendations for smoking cessation interventions: the quality assurance in the treatment of drug dependence project. *Drug Alcohol Rev* 13:171–177, 1994.

96. Nett LM. The physician's role in smoking cessation. A present and future agenda. *Chest* 1990;97(suppl):28–32.

97. Hughes TR, Kottle TE. Doctors helping smokers: real world factors. *Minn Med* 1986;69:143–145.

98. Cohen SJ, Christen AG, Katz BP, et al. Counseling medical and dental patients about cigarette smoking: the impact of nicotine gum and chart reminders. *Am J Public Health* 1987;77:313–316.

99. Manley M, Epps RP, Husten C, et al. Clinical interventions in tobacco control. *JAMA* 1991;266:3172–3173.

100. Plesec TL. *Psychological Characteristics of Smokers, Ex-Smokers, and Non-smokers.* Kent, Ohio: Kent State University; 1978. Dissertation

101. Curry S, Wagner EH, Grothaus LC. Intrinsic and extrinsic motivation for smoking cessation. *J Consult Clin Psychol* 1990;58:310–316.

102. Kararck TW, Lichtenstein E. Program adherence and coping strategies as predictors of success in a smoking treatment program. *Health Psychol* 1988;7:557–574.

103. Hollis JF, Lichtenstein E, Mount K, et al. Nurse-assisted smoking cessation in medical settings: minimizing demands on physicians. *Prev Med* 1991;20:497–507.

104. Perkins KA. Weight gain following smoking cessation. *J Consult Clinical Psychol* 1993;61:768–777.

105. Perkins KA. Issues in the prevention of weight gain after smoking cessation. *Ann Behav Med* 1994;16:46–52.

Chapter 13

Antiplatelet and Anticoagulant Therapy in the Prevention of Ischemic Heart Disease

Steven R. Steinhubl, MD
and David J. Moliterno, MD

Introduction

If not for the arterial thrombus, atherosclerosis—the principal cause of mortality in the United States, Europe, and Japan—might be an essentially benign disease. Even though the relation between atherosclerosis and thrombosis was recognized as early as 1852 by von Rokitansky,[1] not until recently was its fundamental role appreciated. A number of investigators have now demonstrated that the disruption of an atherosclerotic plaque with resultant intracoronary thrombus formation is the central pathophysiological process underlying acute myocardial infarction (MI), sudden cardiac death, and unstable angina.[2-5] There is also increasing evidence that asymptomatic plaque fissuring with associated nonocclusive thrombus is the etiology of atherosclerotic plaque progression.[6-9] Fur-

From Robinson K, (ed): *Preventive Cardiology*. Armonk, NY: Futura Publishing Company, Inc. © 1998.

thermore, the plasma levels of several clotting factors are known to be predictors of future cardiac events.[10–12] All of these findings indicate that the prevention of intracoronary thrombosis may be a promising approach to the prevention of coronary artery disease (CAD) and its complications.

The formation of a thrombus on injured arterial endothelium involves a complex interaction between platelets and a cascade of coagulation proteins that result in the production of fibrin. First, the normally thrombosis-resistant endothelium is rendered prothrombotic by atherosclerosis. Disruption of the endothelial monolayer as well as high shear flow that is characteristic of stenosed coronary arteries then induce platelet adhesion and activation, which promotes further platelet aggregation. The platelet plug that rapidly forms following vessel injury is fragile and requires stabilization by the production of a fibrin meshwork. This is accomplished when blood is exposed to subendothelial components and both the intrinsic and extrinsic pathways of coagulation are activated. Both pathways culminate in the formation of the serine protease thrombin, which produces fibrin by the selective cleavage of fibrinogen. Alteration of any one of these components of the thrombotic process would be expected to limit intraarterial thrombosis and its consequences.

A number of antiplatelet and anticoagulant therapies are clinically available. This chapter will present the data available regarding the use of these agents in the prevention of CAD.

Antiplatelet Drugs

Role of Platelets in Thrombosis

The initial platelet binding to the vessel wall (adhesion) is strongly reliant upon specific platelet-membrane glycoprotein binding to adhesive proteins such as von Willebrand factor and collagen.[13] Platelet activation is initiated by several mechanical and chemical stimuli, including thromboxane A_2, thrombin, norepinephrine, collagen, and adenosine diphosphate (ADP). Activation leads to platelet degranulation and the release of serotonin, ADP, and thromboxane A_2, which triggers the recruitment and activation of additional platelets.[14] These platelets ultimately become aggregated into a hemostatic plug by the binding of primarily fibrinogen and von Willebrand factor to glycoprotein IIb/IIIa integrins on adjacent platelets. The membrane surface of the activated platelets also serve to accelerate the conversion of prothrombin to thrombin, thereby promoting the development of an occlusive thrombus containing platelets, thrombin, and fibrin.

There are a number of antiplatelet agents that have been extensively studied in the primary and secondary prevention of the clinical manifestations of CAD. Because each inhibits platelet function by different mechanisms, there is a potential that one may prove more beneficial than another. Aspirin is the antiplatelet agent that was studied the longest and most thoroughly and remains the "gold standard" by which other agents are judged.

Aspirin

The benefits of the use of willow bark as an antipyretic were first reported by Reverend Edmund Stone[15] in 1763. The potential for aspirin to cause a bleeding tendency was recognized as early as 1891,[16] but its inhibitory effect on platelets was not discovered until the late 1960s.[17] Aspirin's first described use in CAD was in 1953,[18] and, even though this nonrandomized observational study of daily aspirin use demonstrated 100% successful prevention of "coronary occlusion" among 1465 asymptomatic male patients, aspirin therapy only recently became a cornerstone of therapy in CAD.

The mechanism by which aspirin induces a functional defect in platelets is through the inhibition of thromboxane A_2 production.[19,20] During platelet activation, the hydrolysis of membrane phospholipids yields arachidonic acid, which is then converted to prostaglandin H_2 (PH_2) by the catalytic activity of the cyclooxygenase enzyme prostaglandin G/H syn-

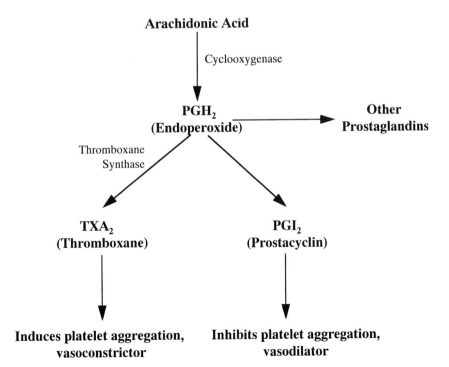

Figure 1. *Arachadonic acid metabolism in platelets and the vascular wall.*

thase[21] (Figure 1). PGH_2 is then converted via thromboxane synthase to thromboxane A_2. By the selective acetylation of a single serine residue within prostaglandin G/H synthase, aspirin causes the permanent inactivation of its cyclooxygenase activity. Because the nonnucleated platelets lack the biosynthetic capabilities necessary to synthesize new protein, the aspirin-induced defect cannot be repaired for the 8- to 10-day life span of the platelet.

The ability of aspirin to inhibit cyclooxygenase activity also accounts for its variety of pharmacologic effects in different tissues. Of particular importance regarding aspirin's use in the prevention of intraarterial thrombosis is its inhibition of endothelial-produced prostacyclin—a vasodilator and inhibitor of platelet aggregation. This potential raises the concern of a possible prothrombotic effect of aspirin therapy. Unlike platelets, because endothelial cells possess the biosynthetic machinery necessary to produce new enzyme, they recover their ability to synthesize prostacyclin within a few hours. Currently there is no evidence to suggest that this effect of aspirin is clinically relevant.

Aspirin for Primary Prevention

The efficacy of aspirin in the prophylaxis of MI in a population of patients without a prior history of a major vascular event (ie, stroke or MI) was evaluated in two large randomized trials involving over 27 000 participants. These trials, the US Physicians' Health Study[22,23] and the British Doctors' Trial[24] enrolled similar cohorts but differed in their design in several ways, including aspirin dose, treatment blinding, end-point definitions, and most importantly, sample size.

In the British Doctors' Trial 5139 male British physicians between ages 50 and 78 participated, beginning in 1978. Two-thirds were randomized to take 500 mg of aspirin daily, and the remaining third were instructed to "avoid" aspirin and products containing aspirin. By the end of the 6-year study there was no significant difference between groups in MI, stroke, the combined end point of adverse vascular events, or total vascular mortality, but the 95% confidence intervals (CIs) were very wide.

On the other hand, the US Physicians Health Study was a double-blind, placebo-controlled trial that utilized a 2×2 factorial design to test simultaneously the effects of aspirin in reducing cardiovascular disease (CVD) and β-carotene in the prevention of cancer. Starting in 1984 a total of 22 071 US male physicians ranging in age from 40 to 84 were randomized to receive 325 mg of aspirin or placebo. The aspirin component of the study was terminated in December 1988 (earlier than the scheduled 1990 completion date) due to a marked reduction in the overall occurrence of an MI [relative risk (RR), 0.56; 95% CI, 0.45–0.70; $P < 0.00001$]. This reduction in risk was apparent only among those over age 50. A trend toward an increased risk of any stroke (RR, 1.22; 95% CI, 0.93–1.60; $P =$

0.15) was observed, influenced primarily by the subgroup with hemorrhagic stroke (RR, 2.14; 95% CI, 0.96–4.77; $P = 0.06$). There was a statistically significant decrease in the rate of fatal MI ($P = 0.004$) in the aspirin group, but this benefit was offset by an apparent increased risk for sudden death ($P = 0.09$), resulting in no reduction in total cardiovascular mortality (44 in both the aspirin and placebo groups). Further analysis demonstrated no impact of aspirin therapy on the clinical characteristics of the nonfatal infarcts[25] nor on the incidence of angina.[26]

An overview was performed to evaluate the data provided by these two trials in combination.[27] Because of the much larger size of the US study, a highly significant 32% reduction in the risk of a nonfatal MI was demonstrated (Table 1). Despite the trend toward an increased risk of stroke in the aspirin arm of both of these studies, the combined data still provided too few end points upon which any firm conclusions could be made. Before generalizing the findings of these trials to the entire male population, it is important to note that the participants in these studies represented a very health-conscious group of individuals. This likely explains the unusually low cardiovascular mortality rate among the participants—approximately 15% of that expected for an age-matched group of white American males. Therefore, given this very low incidence of cardiovascular events, the absolute benefit of aspirin therapy translated to only four important cardiovascular events being prevented for every 1000 patients treated for 5 years.

There are several ongoing studies to further evaluate the role of aspirin in primary prevention. The largest of these is The Women's Health Study, which began in 1992 and randomized approximately 40 000 women in the United States who are >45 years of age to alternate-day 100-mg aspirin or placebo.[28] The additional evidence provided by this trial

Table 1
Aspirin in Primary Prevention of Ischemic Heart Disease

Endpoint	Risk Reduction (% ± standard deviation)		
	U.S. Physicians' Health Study[22]	British Doctors' Trial[24]	Overview of Both Trials[27]
Nonfatal myocardial infarctions	39 ± 9	3 ± 19	32 ± 8
Nonfatal stroke	(19 ± 15)*	(13 ± 24)*	(18 ± 13)*
Total vascular mortality	2 ± 15	7 ± 14	5 ± 10
Important vascular events**	18 ± 7	4 ± 12	13 ± 6

* Not a statistically significant increased risk of nonfatal strokes among aspirin users.
** Nonfatal myocardial infarctions, nonfatal strokes, and vascular deaths combined.

should help to resolve uncertainty regarding the role of aspirin in the primary prevention of CAD. Until these results are available, current data suggest that aspirin therapy should be considered for the primary prevention of ischemic heart disease. However, a substantially greater benefit-to-risk ratio would be expected if such therapy were restricted to patients over age 50 with multiple risk factors for CAD.

Aspirin for Secondary Prevention

Patients with a history of a cardiovascular event are at particular risk for both a subsequent cardiac event as well as a cardiovascular death. A large number of randomized trials were carried out to determine whether aspirin therapy can modify the clinical course of these patients. An overview of 25 of the earliest antiplatelet trials involving approximately 29 000 patients was reported in 1988 by the Antiplatelet Trialists' Collaboration.[30] They concluded that antiplatelet therapy decreased vascular mortality by 15% and nonfatal vascular events (stroke or MI) by 30%. A second overview was reported by this same group in 1994.[31] This updated study included over 145 randomized trials and involved over 100 000 patients. Overall, the results confirmed their earlier findings with a one-third reduction in nonfatal vascular events as well as a one-sixth decrease in vascular deaths in high-risk patients receiving antiplatelet therapy. The larger number of pooled studies and patients allowed the potential benefit in specific subgroups to be discerned.

Stable angina

Three studies prospectively evaluated aspirin therapy in patients with chronic stable angina. A subgroup analysis of the Physician's Health Study[22] evaluated 333 patients who at enrollment had stable angina.[32] Even though aspirin therapy did not influence the frequency or severity of angina episodes over the 4 years of the study, it was associated with a 50% reduction in nonfatal first MIs ($P < 0.019$). All fatal MIs occurred in the placebo group (0 vs 4), whereas, of the 13 strokes that occurred, 11 were among those taking aspirin.

A double-blind, randomized trial by Chesebro et al[33] involved 370 patients with stable CAD and evaluated the impact of combined aspirin and dipyridamole therapy versus placebo over a 5-year period. There was a two-thirds reduction in the incidence of MI ($P = 0.007$) in treated patients as well as a trend for a reduction in new angiographic lesion formation (30% placebo vs 21% treated, $P = 0.06$). The largest trial evaluating aspirin therapy in patients with stable angina was a Swedish trial of 2035 patients.[34] All patients received sotalol, aspirin, or aspirin-placebo and were followed for over 4 years. Patients receiving aspirin demonstrated a 34%

reduction (95% CI, 24% to 49%, $P = 0.003$) in MI and sudden death. In aggregate, these studies suggest that aspirin therapy in 1000 patients with stable angina prevents 51 important cardiovascular events over a 4-year period, a benefit approximately 10 times greater than that seen in primary prevention trials.

Unstable angina and non-Q-wave myocardial infarction

The benefit of aspirin therapy alone or in combination with heparin in the acute treatment of unstable angina was proven in several randomized trials. In the trial by Theroux and colleagues,[35] there was a significant reduction in cardiac death or MI from 11.9% in the placebo group to 3.3% with aspirin alone and 1.6% with the combination of aspirin and heparin ($P = 0.0042$). The Research Group on Instability in Coronary Artery Disease in Southeast Sweden[36] demonstrated a 57% ($P = 0.033$) reduction in MI and death from aspirin compared with placebo, whereas intermittent intravenous heparin showed no significant influence on these end points. One-year follow-up of these patients continued to show an almost 50% reduction ($P < 0.0001$) in death and MI in aspirin-treated patients compared with placebo.[37] The results of these studies and others[38] suggest that aspirin therapy can reduce the occurrence of death and MI by approximately 50% in patients with unstable angina or non-Q-wave MI.

Evolving myocardial infarction and post-myocardial infarction

The ability of aspirin to reduce the risk of recurrent cardiovascular complications in patients who survived an MI was studied in eight trials involving nearly 16 000 patients.[31] When considered collectively, these studies demonstrate a one-third reduction in the risk of nonfatal MI and a one-fourth decrease in the occurrence of MI, stroke, or vascular death. In terms of absolute risk reduction, treatment of 1000 patients with a prior MI for 2 years will prevent 36 major cardiovascular events.

The Second International Study of Infarct Survival (ISIS-2)[39] randomized 17 187 patients to receive streptokinase, aspirin daily for 1 month, neither or both beginning within 24 hours of a suspected MI. Aspirin alone and streptokinase alone decreased 35-day vascular mortality similarly (23% and 25%, respectively), whereas the combination decreased mortality by 42% compared with placebo. Aspirin's role in achieving infarct-artery patency is suggested by a more recent, smaller study suggesting that, when chewed aspirin alone is taken in the hyperacute phase of an MI, stable reperfusion can be achieved in nearly 50% of patients, compared with 25% in controls.[40] These data translate into a reduction of 38 major cardiovascular events per 1000 acute MI patients with 1 month of aspirin therapy.

Congestive heart failure

Patients with left ventricular (LV) dysfunction are an important subgroup of patients with CAD in which aspirin therapy may have a detrimental affect.[41] The Studies of Left Ventricular Dysfunction investigators evaluated the impact of enalapril on mortality and morbidity in a randomized, double-blind trial in over 4200 patients with asympomatic LV dysfunction.[42] Overall, those randomized to enalapril therapy had a 29% reduction in the combined end point of death and development of heart failure. Interestingly, in patients taking concomitant aspirin, there was no improvement in prognosis with enalapril compared with placebo.[43]

A similar interaction was noted between enalapril and aspirin in the Cooperative New Scandinavian Enalapril Survival Study II (CONSENSUS II). This trial of 6090 patients assessed the impact of the early administration of enalapril in acute myocardial infarction.[1] Results of CONSENSUS II demonstrated an overall 10% increase in the relative risk of death with early enalapril administration. When the results were reanalyzed by subgroups defined by the use of aspirin at baseline, a significant negative interaction was found between aspirin and enalapril on survival.[2] In the ~24% of patients not receiving aspirin at baseline, enalapril actually decreased 30-day mortality (Odds ratio 0.86, 95% CI 0.63–1.16, $P = 0.047$).

Although it is possible that these findings could have occurred by chance, there is a physiological basis for postulating that aspirin therapy may negate some of the benefits of angiotensin-converting enzyme inhibition. The production of vasodilating prostaglandins was shown to play an important regulatory role in patients with heart failure,[44] and hemodynamic studies demonstrated that a single dose of aspirin can substantially limit the vasodilator effects of enalapril.[45] The Warfarin Aspirin Study of Heart Failure is a randomized clinical trial being set up that will hopefully provide more conclusive data regarding this concern.[41]

Following revascularization procedures

Approximately one-fifth of saphenous vein coronary artery bypass grafts occlude during the first postoperative year and then a few percent per year thereafter.[46] Fourteen trials involving over 3000 patients evaluated the role of aspirin in preventing bypass graft occlusion.[47] Use of antiplatelet therapy was associated with a reduction of 41% in vascular conduit occlusions ($P < 0.00001$). The majority of these studies began therapy either before or within 24 hours of surgery. Preoperative aspirin therapy is associated with more intraoperative bleeding yet does not appear to add any benefit compared with therapy started early in the postoperative course. Even though the appropriate duration of therapy is unknown, other secondary prevention trials suggest aspirin should be continued indefinitely following revascularization.

Percutaneous transluminal coronary angioplasty (PTCA) is limited by a 4% to 10% acute occlusion rate as well as restenosis within 6 months in 30% to 40%[48,49] of lesions. Because essentially all studies showed a significant decrease in periprocedural Q-wave infarctions with aspirin compared to placebo therapy,[50,51] there is little doubt of the benefit of aspirin therapy at the time of PTCA. On the other hand, the data regarding restenosis is less clear, but the majority of studies support no benefit of aspirin therapy.[52] However, as these patients represent a higher-risk population for further cardiac events, prolonged aspirin therapy is still indicated.

Aspirin Dose and Adverse Effects

Trials of aspirin as preventive therapy in CVD evaluated doses ranging from as little as 30 mg to as much as 1300 mg/day. Despite the study of such a wide range, the optimal dose for initial as well as maintenance therapy is not entirely clear.

As with most medical therapies, but in particular with therapies designed to be preventive in nature, the physician must optimize the benefits while minimizing the risks. Patients who regularly take nonsteroidal anti-inflammatory drugs have an increased risk of gastrointestinal side effects, including bleeding or other events that result in hospitalization or death.[53] The gastrointestinal side effects of aspirin are clearly dose related, with doses even as low as 75 mg/day associated with an increased risk of peptic ulcer disease.[54] A dose-related risk of hemorrhagic stroke was also suggested by several trials evaluating high- and low-dose aspirin.[55,56] Buffered aspirin preparations as well as enteric-coated aspirin are better tolerated and were associated with fewer gastrointestinal side effects than regular aspirin[57,58] but are still associated with peptic ulcers. There is some suggestion that controlled-release preparations currently being evaluated may limit side effects. An interim analysis of the safety results in the first 3667 patients enrolled in the recently completed Thrombosis Prevention Trial demonstrated no excess of gastrointestinal symptoms after an average follow-up of 1.1 years in those treated with 75 mg of enteric-coated, controlled-release aspirin daily compared with placebo.[59] However, no matter which aspirin preparation is utilized, it is clear that to minimize side effects, the lowest effective dose should be used.

Because the cells of the vessel wall, unlike platelets, can synthesize new cyclooxygenase, it was postulated that low-dose, infrequently administered aspirin may preferentially spare vascular prostacyclin production and therefore have greater antithrombotic potential. Contrary to this, studies using quite low aspirin doses (20–40 mg/day) showed inhibition of both thromboxane and prostacyclin.[60–62] The theoretical concern that high-dose therapy may be less antithrombotic because of increased inhibition of prostacyclin synthesis is also not supported by observational studies of rheumatoid arthritis patients consuming large amounts of aspirin.[63,64] A study by Clarke and colleagues[65] showed that through the use of a controlled-release aspirin preparation it is possible to inhibit platelets in the portal circulation but never reach the systemic circulation and impair prostacyclin production. Whether this will translate into improved antithrombotic properties for aspirin is a hypothesis currently being tested in clinical trials.

Unlike the direct relation seen between aspirin dose and side effects, no such relation was shown for clinical efficacy with long-term therapy.[31] The small number of studies that directly compared different doses of aspirin demonstrated no important difference in vascular events. Also, when the protective effects of varying doses of aspirin used in different trials are compared indirectly, the decrease in vascular events of low- (75–150 mg), intermediate- (160–325 mg), and high- (500–1500 mg) dose daily therapy was essentially the same: −26%, 28%, and 21%, respectively. Even though these results suggest that daily therapy of only 75 mg is as effective as higher doses, it is important to note that recent studies demonstrated that individuals vary in their response to different doses of aspirin,[66] and some individuals may develop resistance to previously effective aspirin doses.[67] The clinical implications of these findings have yet to be elucidated.

When starting aspirin therapy, especially in clinical situations such as unstable angina or acute MI when rapid antiplatelet effects are desired, doses of ≥325 mg are recommended. In vitro studies showed that at least 95% inhibition of thromboxane A_2 formation must be achieved to influence thromboxane-dependent platelet activation in vivo[68] and that ≥300 mg is required to accomplish this.[69] To maximize the rapidity of onset, the dose should be chewed. When this is done, even enteric-coated aspirin was shown to inhibit platelet aggregation within 15 minutes.[70]

Finally, for aspirin therapy to be effective it must be prescribed to the patient. Despite the overwhelming evidence supporting its use, as well as its incomparably low cost, recent studies showed that up to one-third of elderly patients do not receive aspirin at the time of an acute MI,[71] and that one-fourth do not receive it chronically following an MI.[72] With over 1 million patients admitted to US hospitals each year with an acute MI, by increasing the use of aspirin to include essentially all patients, nearly 8000 premature deaths each year would be prevented.[73]

Dipyridamole

Dipyridamole is a primidopyrimidine derivative with vasodilator properties that was introduced for the treatment of angina in 1961. Its antithrombotic properties were first reported in 1965.[74] The basis for its antiplatelet and antithrombotic properties is not clear, but may be related to (1) inhibition of platelet phosphodiesterase resulting in an increase in intraplatelet cyclic adenosine monophosphate (cAMP), (2) stimulation of

Table 2

Prospective Randomized Trials Comparing Aspirin Alone with the Combination of Aspirin and Dipyridamole

	Brown et al[127]	Hess et al[128]	Bousser et al[129]	American-Canadian Co-Operative Study Group[130]
Number of patients	147	240	604	890
Patient population	Following coronary bypass grafting	Peripheral vascular disease	Cerebrovascular disease	History of tranient ischemic attacks
Daily aspirin dose (mg)	975	990	1000	1300
Daily dipyridamole dose (mg)	225	225	225	300
End point	1-y angiographic graft patency	2-y arteriographic disease progression	3-year occurrence of cerebrovascular events	CVA or death for up to 5 years follow-up
Results	No benefit of combination therapy	Combination therapy better than aspirin alone	No benefit of combination therapy	No benefit of combination therapy

endogenous prostaglandin release from the endothelium, or (3) inhibition of adenosine uptake with subsequent degradation by the vasculature. Dipyridamole alone is a relatively weak inhibitor of platelet aggregation in vitro.

The potential antithrombotic effect of dipyridamole was assessed in a large number of studies, but typically in combination with aspirin rather than compared directly with a placebo. Doses from 75–400 mg daily in divided doses were investigated. In clinical trials of stroke and CAD in which aspirin alone was compared with the combination of aspirin and dipyridamole, the addition of dipyridamole contributed no benefit, although one study in peripheral vascular disease patients was favorable (Table 2).[75] These results do not support the use of dipyridamole as an antiplatelet agent.

Thienopyridine — Ticlopidine and Clopidogrel

Ticlopidine was first introduced as an antiplatelet agent in the early 1980s. It and its analog, clopidogrel, are thienopyridine derivatives that specifically interfere with ADP-mediated platelet activation and cause an irreversible, noncompetitive inhibition of platelet function. although no clear mechanism of action was determined, current evidence suggests that ticlopidine decreases the ability of ADP to produce the changes in the glycoprotein IIb/IIIa receptor that are responsible for developing a high-affinity ligand binding site.[76] Ticlopidine is usually administered orally in doses of 250 mg twice daily. Inhibition of platelet aggregation is both dose and time related, with onset of activity 24–48 hours following oral administration and maximal activity at 3–5 days. Because thienopyridines are inactive in vitro, and minimally active when administered intravenously, their effects may be due to an unstable metabolite that is produced after oral ingestion.[77]

Ticlopidine was studied in a number of controlled trials for the secondary prevention of stroke, MI, peripheral arterial occlusive disease, and primary treatment of unstable angina.[78–83] All of these studies demonstrated a benefit with ticlopidine compared with placebo. The results of the Ticlopidine Aspirin Stroke Study[78] demonstrated significantly fewer primary end points (new cerebral ischemic event, stroke, or death) at 5-year follow-up for patients taking ticlopidine compared with those on aspirin, suggesting that ticlopidine may be superior to aspirin in stroke prevention. The role of thienopyridines in secondary prevention has recently been evaluated in the Clopidogrel versus Aspirin in Patients at Risk for further Ischemic Events (CAPRIE) trial.[3] This was a prospective, randomized, blinded study involving over 19,000 patients with atherosclerotic vascular disease. Patients with a recent ischemic stroke or myocardial infarction or with symptomatic peripheral vascular disease were randomly assigned to either daily aspirin or clopidogrel therapy. After a mean follow-up of ~2 years those receiving clopidogrel had an annual risk of ischemic stroke, myocardial infarction, or vascular death of 5.3% compared with 5.8% for those receiving aspirin ($P = 0.043$). These results suggest that for every 1000 patients with manifestations of atherosclerotic vascular disease receiving antiplatelet therapy for secondary prevention, clopidogrel would be expected to prevent five more major clinical events per year than aspirin with a decreased incidence of side effects.

Recently, ticlopidine therapy became a major component of antiplatelet therapy following intracoronary stent placement for the prevention of stent thrombosis. Although its combined use with aspirin was initially emperic, recent studies demonstrated a decrease in both cardiac events and hemorrhagic complications when this combination was compared with combined anticoagulant and aspirin therapy.[84,85]

Ticlopidine has several noteworthy adverse effects, the most frequent (~20% of patients) being diarrhea. The most serious adverse effect is neutropenia, which reportedly occurs in 2.4% of patients and is severe in 0.85% of patients. This typically occurs within the first 3 months of treatment and appears to be reversible when the drug is discontinued.[86] Close monitoring of the white blood cell count is therefore necessary during the first 3 months of therapy. Interestingly, clopidogrel does not appear to share ticlopidine's side-effects profile. The CAPRIE study demonstrated an incidence of rash and diarrhea of only 0.26% and 0.23%, respectively, and neutropenia occurred less frequently than in the aspirin group, 0.10% versus 0.17%.

Despite the disadvantage of increased cost relative to aspirin, its limited usefulness in the acute setting, and the potential for severe neutropenia, in the aspirin-intolerant patient, ticlopidine and clopidogrel provide an effective antiplatelet alternative.

Sulfinpyrazone

Sulfinpyrazone was discovered in 1957 as a metabolite of the antiinflammatory phenylbutazone and first used for the treatment of gout. Its effect on platelets was first reported in 1965[87] when it was noted that it normalized the shortened platelet survival associated with gout. Further investigation determined that sulfinpyrazone or its metabolite is a weak inhibitor of platelet cyclooxygenase.[88] Two randomized, placebo-controlled trials carried out in the mid-1970s evaluated the impact of sulfinpyrazone therapy in survivors of acute MI.[89,90] Even though both trials demonstrated an improvement in outcome compared with placebo, inconsistent findings between the studies leave the results in doubt. At best, sulfinpyrazone provides no greater benefit than aspirin, and it is not recommended for routine antiplatelet therapy.

Inhibitors of Thromboxane Formation and/or Binding

Because of the theoretical disadvantage of aspirin inhibiting endothelial cyclooxygenase and therefore the production of platelet-inhibitory prostacyclin, specific inhibitors of thromboxane A_2 synthase were postulated to potentially induce greater platelet inhibition than aspirin. When thromboxane A_2 synthase is inhibited, arachidonic acid metabolism in the stimulated platelet leads to the buildup of prostaglandin endoperoxides, which are then shunted to endothelial prostacyclin production. In fact, it is this enhanced generation of the platelet-inhibitory prostacyclins and not the blockade of thromboxane A_2 production that appears to determine the antiplatelet effects of thromboxane A_2 synthase inhibitors.[91] However, because accumulating prostaglandin endoperoxides can also produce platelet activation directly by acting on the thromboxane A_2 receptor,[92] combined-mode agents that both inhibit thromboxane synthase as well as block thromboxane receptors would likely offer the greatest antiplatelet potential.

Clinical trials were carried out evaluating the thromboxane synthase inhibitor, sulotroban,[93] the thromboxane receptor antagonist, vapiprost,[94] and the combined-mode agent, ridogrel.[95] The first two trials demonstrated no benefit of these agents on restenosis following PTCA. The third study compared ridogrel with aspirin in acute MI patients treated with streptokinase. Although ridogrel was not superior to aspirin in terms of its impact on fibrinolytic efficacy, a post hoc analysis demonstrated a significantly lower incidence of new ischemic events (reinfarction, recurrent angina, or ischemic stroke) in the ridogrel group. Based on these results, the authors concluded that ridogrel could be considered an acceptable alternative to aspirin for patients intolerant of aspirin with an acute MI.

Platelet Glycoprotein IIb/IIIa Receptor Inhibitors

The newest and one of the most promising family of antiplatelet agents currently being evaluated are the glycoprotein IIb/IIIa receptor inhibitors. As already noted, platelet aggregation can be initiated by a number of pathways. However, the final common pathway of aggregation—irrespective of how it is initiated—involves the binding of the IIb/IIIa receptors of adjacent platelets. By blocking these receptors, platelet aggregation can be effectively prevented. Several trials in coronary angioplasty and acute coronary syndromes are currently under way or were recently completely and yielded very encouraging results.[96–100] In the setting of coronary angioplasty, these agents (abciximab, integrilin, tirofiban) have reduced ischemic events an additional ~35% beyond that with aspirin therapy alone. Over 30 agents in this family are in development, many of which are expected to reach clinical trials in the next several years. Their role in primary and secondary prevention appears promising and awaits further clinical testing as oral agents are further developed.

Anticoagulant Agents

The formation of intracoronary thrombi requires not only platelet aggregation but also the integral involvement of the coagulation cascade. The culmination of the multiple enzymatic reactions of this cascade is the conversion of prothrombin to thrombin. Thrombin not only causes additional platelet activation, but it also converts fibrinogen to fibrin, which is ultimately responsible for platelet plug stabilization. The presence of thrombin also causes the further amplification of the coagulation cascade by activating factors V and VIII. Consequently, agents that either prevent the formation or inhibit the action of thrombin would be anticipated to be effective in the prevention of coronary thrombosis and its complications.

The two most commonly used anticoagulant drugs in clinical practice today are the coumarin derivatives and heparin. Heparin's anticoagulant action is due to the binding of heparin to antithrombin III; the heparin-antithrombin III complex inhibits free thrombin and other coagulant proteins. Coumarin derivatives (primarily warfarin in the United States) are vitamin K antagonists. By inhibiting the vitamin-K-dependent post-translational modification of clotting factors II, VII, IX, and X, their activation is prevented, which leads to a substantial reduction in thrombin generation.

Heparin

Because heparin is only available parenterally, there are understandably little data available regarding its prolonged use in a preventative role. Only one large randomized study compared long-term heparin therapy after an MI with a control group.[101] A total of 728 patients were entered at a mean of 11 months after MI and randomly assigned to 12,500 IU of daily unfractionated heparin subcutaneously or no heparin for an average of 23 months. Heparin treatment reduced the cumulative mortality by a nonsignificant 34% on an intention-to-treat basis but by 48% on an "on-treatment" basis ($P < 0.05$). The reinfarction rate was also significantly reduced by 61% ($P = 0.05$) in the heparin group.

The benefit of heparin in combination with aspirin as short-term treatment in unstable angina has recently been clarified by Oler and co-workers[4] through a meta-analysis of 6 trials involving 1353 patients. Compared with patients only receiving aspirin, those receiving heparin and aspirin had a reduced risk of myocardial infarction or death (odds ratio 0.67; 95% CI, 0.44–1.02; $P = 0.06$). This translates into an absolute risk reduction for death or myocardial infarction of ~3% with the addition of heparin to aspirin in the treatment of patients with unstable angina.

Compared with unfractionated heparin, low molecular weight (LMW) heparin offers the advantages of greater bioavailibility and more predictable anticoagulant response. In the treatment of deep vein thrombosis it has been shown to be more effective and safer than dose-adjusted unfractionated heparin.[5] In patients with unstable angina, several studies have recently shown LMW heparin to be more efficacious than unfractionated heparin in preventing myocardial infarction or death.[6,7] Unfortunately, parenteral dosing still remains an issue regarding long-term compliance.

Warfarin

In the 1920s, cattle in North Dakota and Alberta, Canada, were discovered to be dying because of fatal bleeding.[102] The cause was traced to improperly cured hay made from common varieties of sweet clover and was therefore referred to as "hemorrhagic sweet clover disease." In 1939 bishydroxycoumarin (dicumarol) was isolated and shown to be the responsible agent. Interestingly, early studies incorrectly suggested that its "hypoprothrombinemic" effects were due to its metabolism to salicylic acid.[103] By 1942, animal experiments demonstrated the ability of dicumarol to decrease experimentally induced thrombosis, and use in humans quickly followed. Warfarin—derivative number 42 of dicumarol that was initially promoted for rodent control— became the anticoagulant of choice in North America following the reported case in 1951 of an army inductee who ingested 567 mg of the compound and was successfully treated with vitamin K.[104]

Warfarin in Primary Prevention

Because of the direct association between the level of factor VII coagulant activity and the risk of subsequent ischemic heart disease demonstrated in the Northwick Park Heart Study[11] as well as other trials, long-term low-dose anticoagulant therapy was postulated to be potentially effective in the primary prevention of ischemic heart disease. A randomized, double-blind pilot study by Meade et al[105] involving 441 high-risk men was begun in 1984 to evaluate the feasibility and safety of such a trial. In patients randomized to warfarin, an average daily dose of 4.6 mg was used to achieve an international normalized ratio (INR) of about 1.5 and to lower factor VII activity to approximately 70%. No difference was noted in the number of patients reporting bleeding episodes between the warfarin and placebo groups. Based on these results, the TPT was initiated to evaluate primary prevention with either low-dose aspirin (75 mg daily), low-dose warfarin (INR target of 1.5), combination of these, or placebo in

45- to 69-year-old men at "greater than average risk" for ischemic heart disease.[29] Recruitment was completed in 1994 with the entry of 5499 men. Results after a median follow-up of 6.8 years demonstrated that all three treatment groups demonstrated a significant decrease in ischemic cardiac events (coronary death or non-fatal MI) compared with placebo (placebo 13.3%, warfarin 10.3%, aspirin 10.2%, warfarin and aspirin 8.7%).[8] The combination arm of aspirin and warfarin had the greatest reduction, but this was not significant compared with aspirin alone and was associated with a nonsignificant increase in strokes. Major bleeding complications were similar in all groups, but intermediate bleeding epsidoes were significantly increased in both the warfarin only and combination arms compared with placebo, but not compared with aspirin. Minor bleeding episodes were increased in all three treatment groups. The results of this study confirm that long-term treatment with warfarin—alone or in combination with aspirin—for primary prevention can prevent three to five ischemic cardiac events among 1000 patients treated for 1 year.

Warfarin in Secondary Prevention

Encouraging reports of the use of dicumarol in patients with CAD in 1946[106] and 1947[107] led to the endorsement of anticoagulant use in acute MI by the American Heart Association in 1948.[108] Over the two decades that followed, it would have been considered unethical not to use anticoagulants in patients with an MI. However, beginning in the late 1960s, anticoagulant use started becoming much more controversial with the publication of major methodological criticisms of earlier trials[109] as well as a trial by the British Medical Research Council,[110] which showed no improvement in mortality compared with controls. Based on these findings, along with their risk of bleeding complications, anticoagulant use post-MI was abandoned in many countries.

A gradual resurgence of interest in the use of warfarin as secondary prevention therapy following MI began in 1980 with the publication of the Sixty Plus Reinfarction Study.[111] This study equally randomized 878 patients who were on anticoagulant therapy for at least 6 months (mean 6 years) since an MI to placebo or to continued anticoagulant therapy. After 2 years of follow-up these investigators reported a 43% lower total mortality (7.6% vs 13.4%, $P = 0.017$) and a 64% reduction in recurrent MI (5.7% vs 15.9%, $P = 0.0001$) for those continued on anticoagulants compared with placebo.

The Warfarin Re-infarction Study (WARIS)[112] and Anticoagulants in the Secondary Prevention of Events in Coronary Thrombosis (ASPECT) trial[113] were prospective, randomized, double-blind, placebo-controlled trials carried out to evaluate the impact of long-term anticoagulant therapy on mortality and reinfarction in patients after an MI. Combined, these studies evaluated over 4600 patients with a target INR range of 2.4–4.8. Both trials reported their results after a mean follow-up of 37 months. The smaller WARIS trial demonstrated a 24% reduction (95% CI, 4% to 44%, $P < 0.03$) in total mortality with oral anticoagulants compared with placebo, whereas the ASPECT trial showed a nonsignificant 10% reduction (95% CI, −11% to 27%). However, both trials did demonstrate a significant decrease in reinfarctions with anticoagulant therapy—a 34% reduction in the WARIS trial and 53% in the ASPECT study.

Very few patients in the WARIS study and only one-fourth of the ASPECT trial patients received thrombolytic therapy due to the early years of recruitment. Whether previous thrombolytic therapy might influence the clinical benefits of anticoagulant treatment was addressed in the Antithrombotics in the Prevention of Reocclusion in Coronary Thrombolysis Study (APRICOT).[114] In this trial 300 patients who had a recent MI were randomized to either aspirin, placebo, or coumadin. At 3-month follow-up reinfarction occurred in 3% of patients on aspirin, 8% for those on coumadin, and 11% on placebo (aspirin vs placebo, $P < 0.025$; other comparisons, $P =$ not significant). An event-free clinical course was seen in 93% of aspirin patients, 82% with coumadin, and 76% with placebo (aspirin vs placebo, $P < 0.001$; aspirin vs coumadin, $P < 0.05$). An important problem with this study was the low dose of heparin initially administered and the fact that five of the seven reinfarctions in the coumadin group occurred during the heparin infusion. Nonetheless, the results do raise the possibility that acute thrombolytic treatment could influence the benefit of post-MI anticoagulant therapy.

Only two other previous long-term trials attempted to directly compare aspirin and oral anticoagulation therapy after an MI.[115,116] Although both of these trials showed no significant difference in mortality between the aspirin and oral anticoagulant groups, the impact of these results is limited by their open design, small size, suboptimal quality of anticoagulation, and prethrombolytic era study dates.

Warfarin Dose and Adverse Effects

Treatment with oral anticoagulant agents requires a delicate balance between minimizing the risk of bleeding and maximizing antithrombotic effect. Bleeding complications were shown to be directly related to the level of anticoagulation achieved, with one study demonstrating a 42% increase in the risk of major bleeding for every 1.0 rise in the INR.[117] Increasing age was also thought to increase the risk of bleeding complications, but recent data do not support this.[118] On the other hand, the risk of thromboembolic events is inversely related to the level of anticoagulation maintained. Data from the ASPECT trial were evaluated to assess the optimal intensity of oral anticoagulant therapy for secondary prevention that best balances the risks and benefits.[119] By giving equal weight to

hemorrhagic and thromboembolic events, Azar and colleagues[119] identified that the best risk/benefit ratio for long-term treatment following an
MI was achieved with an INR between 2.0 and 4.0, with a trend toward
3.0 to 4.0 being optimal.

Combination Antiplatelet and Anticoagulant Therapy

Because both platelets and the coagulation cascade are integral in the
pathophysiology of intracoronary thrombosis, therapy using a combination of antiplatelet and anticoagulant agents may offer a substantial synergistic benefit. This hypothesis is supported by studies among patients
with prosthetic heart valves that demonstrated a decreased risk of thromboembolic complications in patients receiving combination therapy.[120]

The Antithrombotic Therapy in Acute Coronary Syndromes (ATACS)
Research Group studied the combination of aspirin and anticoagulant
therapy (heparin followed by warfarin) versus aspirin alone in 214 nonprior aspirin users with either unstable angina or non-Q-wave MI.[121]
Those randomized to receive warfarin had a target INR of 2 to 3, and
active treatment was maintained for 12 weeks. although combination therapy significantly reduced the incidence of primary ischemic events within
the first 14 days (27% aspirin alone, 10% combination therapy, $P = 0.004$),
by 12 weeks there was only a trend favoring combination therapy (28%
aspirin alone, 19% combination therapy, $P = 0.09$). These results are consistent with the benefit demonstrated by other studies[35] of the acute treatment of unstable angina with a combination of aspirin and heparin, but
they do not offer strong support for prolonged oral anticoagulant therapy
for these patients.

The role of low-dose anticoagulation along with aspirin therapy for
the prevention of the progression of saphenous vein graft disease was
recently evaluated by The Post Coronary Artery Bypass Graft Trial Investigators.[9] In this study, 1351 patients who had undergone bypass surgery 1–11 years prior were randomized using a two-by-two factorial design to either aggressive or moderate cholesterol lowering therapy, and
either warfarin or placebo. All patients were "encouraged" to take 81 mg
of aspirin daily. The warfarin dose was regulated to maintain the INR <2.
After a mean duration of follow-up of 4.3 years, with 88% angiographic
follow-up and 98% clinical follow-up, randomly assigned to warfarin
showed no significant difference in angiographic outcomes compared
with placebo. Although these results cannot exclude a benefit of more
aggressive long-term anticoagulation, they do not support low-dose combination therapy over aspirin alone.

There are currently five trials, involving over 25 000 patients, designed to evaluate the combination of aspirin and anticoagulant therapies
in post-MI patients[122] (Table 3). One study, the Coumadin Aspirin Rein-

Table 3

Current Trials of Combined Antiplatelet and Anticoagulant Therapy

Trial	CARS	CHAMP	WARIS-2	ASPECT-2	APRICOT-2
Number of patients	8803	4000	6000	9000	300
Aspirin-alone dose (mg daily)	160	160	75	80	80
Combination therapies	80	80	75	80	80
Aspirin Dose (mg daily)					
Oral anticoagulant dose	1 or 3 mg daily	Titrated to INR 1.5–2.5	Titrated to INR 2.0–2.5 or 2.8–4.2	Titrated to INR 2.0–2.5 or 2.8–4.8	Titrated to INR 2.0–2.5
Follow-up	4 y	4 y	2 y	3 y	3 mo

INR = international normalized ratio.

farction Study (CARS) was recently prematurely terminated because of a lack of efficacy in the combination arms versus aspirin alone.[10] Importantly, compared with the other studies, the combination arms of this study used rather low, set doses (1 or 3 mg) of warfarin (median INR for 3-mg group only 1.19), which may have limited its efficacy. Further analysis of the other ongoing investigations should aid considerably in determining the optimal antithrombotic regimen for secondary prevention.

Conclusion

Antiplatelet and anticoagulant agents offer valuable therapeutic options in the prevention of ischemic heart disease. However, the 20% reduction in recurrent MIs made possible with long-term antithrombotic agents must be weighed against the associated bleeding complications as well as the benefits achievable through the modification of other risk factors such as cholesterol reduction,[123] antihypertensive therapy,[124] and smoking cessation.[125,126]

Antithrombotic therapy, as it is currently used, prevents heart attacks and saves lives. For every 1000 individuals free of diagnosed atherosclerotic disease treated with aspirin over a 5-year period, four important cardiac events will be prevented. More importantly, by targeting preventative therapy to those at higher risk, a 10-times greater benefit can be achieved. In fact, when aspirin is used in patients following MI or with unstable angina, an almost one-fourth reduction in mortality can be realized. Even though aspirin is extremely inexpensive, generally well tolerated, and at least as effective as all other currently studied antithrombotic preventative regimens, there are those individuals in whom it is not a viable therapeutic option. Chronic warfarin therapy can provide a benefit similar to aspirin's as secondary prevention in those patients with other indications for prolonged anticoagulant therapy, and ticlopidine is an effective antiplatelet alternative for those who are aspirin intolerant. Undoubtedly, the results of numerous current trials should help better define the optimal preventative antithrombotic therapy in a number of patient groups. Just as the last 50 years of antithrombotic therapy in CAD allowed for some dramatic changes in treatment philosophy, as our understanding of the pathophysiology of all aspects of CAD continues to grow, further innovations in antithrombotic therapy will lead to even more dramatic results in the prevention of ischemic heart disease.

References

1. Swedberg K, Held P, Kjekshus J, et al. Effects of early administration of enalapril on mortality in patients in acute myocardial infarction: results of the Cooperative New Scandinavian Enalapril Survival Study II (CONSENSUS II). *N Engl J Med* 1992;327:678–684.

2. Nguyen KN, Aursnes I, Kjekshus J. Interaction between enalapril and aspirin on mortality after acute myocardial infarction: Subgroup analysis of the Co-operative New Scandinavian Enalapril Survival Study II (CONSENSUS II). *Am J Cardiol* 1997;79:115–119.

3. CAPRIE Steering Committee. A randomised, blinded trial of clopidogrel versus aspirin in patients at risk of ischemic events (CAPRIE). *Lancet* 1996; 348:1329–1339.

4. Oler A, Whooley MA, Oler J, et al. Adding heparin to aspirin reduces the incidence of myocardial infarction and death in patients with unstable angina. *JAMA* 1996;276:811–815.

5. Lensing AWA, Prins MH, Davidson BL, et al. Treatment of deep venous thrombosis with low-molecular-weight heparins: a meta-anlysis. *Arch Intern Med* 1995;155:601–607.

6. Cohen M, Demers C, Gurfinkel EP, et al. A comparison of low-molecular-weight heparin with unfractionated heparin for unstable coronary artery disease. Efficacy and Safety of Subcutaneous Enoxaparin in Non-Q-Wave Coronary Events Study Group. *N Eng J Med* 1997;337(7):447–452.

7. FRISC Study Group. Low-molecular-weight heparin during instability in coronary artery disease. *Lancet* 1996;347:561–568.

8. The Medical Research Council's General Practice Research Framework. Thrombosis prevention trial: randomises trial of low-intensity oral anti-coagulation with warfarin and low-dose aspirin in the primary prevention of ischemic heart disease in men at increased risk. *Lancet* 1998;351:233–241.

9. The Post Coronary Artery Bypass Graft Trial Investigators. The effect of aggressive lowering of low-density lipoprotein cholesterol levels and low-dose anticoagulation on obstructive changes in saphenous vein coronary artery bypass grafts. *N Engl J Med* 1997;336:153–162.

10. Coumadin Aspirin Reinfarction Study (CARS) Investigators. Randomised double-blind trial of fixed low-dose warfarin with aspirin after myocardial infarction. *Lancet* 1997;350:389–396.

11. Meade TW, Ruddock V, Stirling Y, et al. Fibrinolytic activity, clotting factors, and long term incidence of ischaemic heart diasease in the Northwick Park Heart Study. *Lancet* 1993;342:1076–1079.

12. Ernst E, Resch KL. Fibrinogen as a cardiovascular risk factor: a meta-analysis and review of the literature. *Ann Intern Med* 1993;118:956–963.

13. Kaplan AV, Leung LL-K, Leng W-H, et al. Roles of thrombin and platelet membrane glycoprotein IIb/IIIa in platelet-subendothelial deposition after angioplasty in an ex vivo whole artery model. *Circulation* 1991;84:1279–1288.

14. Holmsen H, Weiss HJ. Secretable storage pools in platelets. *Annu Rev Med* 1979;30:119–134.

15. Stone E. An account of the success of the bark of the willow in the cure of agues. *Philos Trans R Soc Lond Biol Sci* 1763;53:195–200.

16. Binz C. *Vorlesungen Ueber Pharmakologie.* 2nd ed. Berlin, Germany: 1891.

17. Weiss HJ, Aledort LM. Impaired platelet-connective-tissue reaction in man after aspirin ingestion. *Lancet* 1967;2:495–497.

18. Craven LL. Experiences with aspirin (acetylsalicylic acid) in the nonspecific prophylaxis of coronary thrombosis. *Mississippi Valley Med J* 1953;75:38–44.

19. Vane JR. Inhibition of prostaglandin synthesis as a mechanism of action for aspirin-like drugs. *Nature* 1971;231:231–235.

20. Smith JB, Willis AL. Aspirin selectively inhibits prostaglandin production in human platelets. *Nature* 1971;231:235–237.

21. Patrono C. Aspirin as an antiplatelet drug. *N Engl J Med* 1994;330:1287–1294.

22. Steering Committee of the Physicians' Health Study Research Group. Final report on the aspirin component of the ongoing Physicians' Health Study. *N Engl J Med* 1989;321:129–135.
23. Steering Committee of the Physicians' Health Study Research Group. Preliminary report: findings from the aspirin component of the ongoing Physicians' Health Study. *N Engl J Med* 1988;318:262–264.
24. Peto R, Gray R, Collins R, et al. Randomised trial of prophylactic aspirin in British male doctors. *BMJ* 1988;296:313–316.
25. Ridker PM, Manson JE, Buring JE, et al. Clinical characteristics of nonfatal myocardial infarction among individuals on prophylactic low-dose aspirin therapy. *Circulation* 1991;84:708–711.
26. Manson JE, Grobbee DE, Stampfer MJ. Aspirin in the primary prevention of angina pectoris in a randomized trial of United States physicians. *Am J Med* 1990;89:772–776.
27. Hennekens CH, Peto R, Hutchison GB, et al. An overview of the British and American aspirin studies. *N Engl J Med* 1988;318:923–924.
28. Buring JE, Hennekens CH. The Women's Health Study: summary of the study design. *J Myocardial Ischemia* 1992;4:27–29.
29. Meade TW, Miller GJ. Combined use of aspirin and warfarin in primary prevention of ischemic heart disease in men at high risk. *Am J Cardiol* 1995;75:23B–26B.
30. Antiplatelet Trialists' Collaboration. Secondary prevention of vascular disease by prolonged antiplatelet therapy. *BMJ* 1988;296:320–331.
31. Antiplatelet Trialists' Collaboration. Collaborative overview of randomised trials of antiplatelet therapy. I. Prevention of death, myocardial infarction, and stroke by prolonged antiplatelet therapy in various categories of patients. *BMJ* 1994;308:81–106.
32. Ridker PM, Manson JE, Gaziano JM, et al. Low-dose aspirin therapy for chronic stable angina. A randomised, placebo-controlled clinical trial. *Ann Intern Med* 1991;114:835–839.
33. Chesebro JH, Webster MWI, Zoldhelyi P, et al. Antithrombotic therapy and progression of coronary artery disease. Antiplatelet versus antithrombins. *Circulation* 1992;86:III-100–III-111.
34. Juul-Moller S, Edvardsson N, Johnmatz B, et al. Double-blind trial of aspirin in primary prevention of myocardial infarction in patients with stable chronic angina pectoris. *Lancet* 1992;340:1421–1425.
35. Theroux P, Ouimet H, McCans J, et al. Aspirin, heparin or both to treat acute unstable angina. *N Engl J Med* 1988;319:1105–1111.
36. The RISC Group. Risk of myocardial infarction and death during treatment with low dose aspirin and intravenous heparin in men with unstable coronary artery disease. *Lancet* 1990;336:827–830.
37. Wallentin LC. Aspirin (75 mg/day) after an episode of unstable coronary artery disease: long-term effects on the risk of myocardial infarction, occurrence of severe angina and the need for revascularization. *J Am Coll Cardiol* 1991;18:1587–1593.
38. Lewis HD Jr, Davis JW, Archibald DG, et al. Protective effects of aspirin against acute myocardial infarction and death in men with unstable angina: results of a Veterans Administration Cooperative Study. *N Eng J Med* 1983;309:396–403.
39. ISIS-2 Collaborative Group. Randomised trial of intravenous streptokinase, oral aspirin, both, or neither among 17 187 cases of suspected acute myocardial infarction: ISIS-2. *Lancet* 1988;2:349–360.
40. Freifeld A, Rabinowitz B, Kaplinsky E, et al. Aspirin-induced reperfusion in acute myocardial infarction. Abstract. *J Am Coll Cardiol* 1995:310.

41. Cleland JGF, Bulpitt CJ, Falk RH, et al. Is aspirin safe for patients with heart failure? *Br Heart J* 1995;74:215–219.
42. The SOLVD Investigators. Effect of enalapril on mortality and the development of heart failure in asymptomatic patients with reduced left ventricular ejection fractions. *N Engl J Med* 1992;327:685–691.
43. Pitt B. Use of converting enzyme inhibitors in patients with asymptomatic left ventricular dysfunction. *J Am Coll Cardiol* 1993;22:158A–161A.
44. Dzau VJ, Packer M, Lilly LS, et al. Prostaglandins in severe congestive heart failure. Relation to activation of the renin-angiotensin system and hyponatremia. *N Engl J Med* 1984;310:347–352.
45. Hall D, Zeitler H, Rudolph W. Counteraction of the vasodilator effects of enalapril by aspirin in severe heart failure. *J Am Coll Cardiol* 1992;20:1549–1555.
46. Fuster V, Chesebro JH. Role of platelets and platelet inhibitors in aortocoronary vein graft disease. *Circulation* 1986;73:227–232.
47. Antiplatelet Trialists' Collaboration. Collaborative overview of randomised trials of antiplatelet therapy. II. Maintenance of vascular graft or arterial patency by antiplatelet therapy. *BMJ* 1994;308:159–168.
48. Holmes DR Jr, Vlietstra RE, Smith HC, et al. Restenosis after percutaneous transluminal angioplasty (PTCA): a report from the PTCA registry of the National Heart, Lung, and Blood Institute. *Am J Cardiol* 1984;53:77C–81C.
49. Detre K, Holubkov R, Kelsey S, et al. Percutaneous Transluminal Coronary Angioplasty Registry: percutaneous transluminal angioplasty in 1985–1986 and 1977–1981: the National Heart, Lung, and Blood Institute Registry. *N Engl J Med* 1988;318:265–270.
50. Barnathan ES, Schwartz JS, Taylor L, et al. Aspirin and dipyridamole in the prevention of acutecoronary thrombosis complicating coronary angioplasty. *Circulation* 1987;76:125–134.
51. Schwartz L, Bourassa MG, Lesperance J, et al. Aspirin and dipyridamole in the prevention of restenosis after coronary angioplasty. *N Engl J Med* 1988;318:1714–1719.
52. Meier B. Prevention of restenosis after coronary angioplasty: a pharmacological approach. *Eur Heart J* 1989;10:64–68.
53. Gabriel SE, Jaakkimainen L, Bombardier C. Risk of serious gastrointestinal complications related to nonsteroidal anti-inflammatory drugs: a meta-analysis. *Ann Intern Med* 1991;115:787–796.
54. Weil J, Colin-Jones D, Langman M, et al. Prophylactic aspirin and risk of peptic ulcer bleeding. *BMJ* 1995;310:827–830.
55. The Dutch TIA Study Group. A comparison of two doses of aspirin (30 mg vs 283 mg a day) in patients after transient ischemic attack or minor ischemic stroke. *N Engl J Med* 1991;325:1261–1266.
56. Farrell B, Godwin J, Richards S, et al. The United Kingdom transient ischemic attack (UK-TIA) aspirin trial: final results. *J Neurol Neurosurg Psychiatry* 1991;54:1044–1054.
57. Hofteizer JW, Silvoso GR, Burks M, et al. Comparison of the effects of regular and enteric coated aspirin on gastroduodenal mucosa of man. *Lancet* 1980;2:609–612.
58. Leonards JR, Levy G. Effect of pharmaceutical formulation on gastrointestinal bleeding from aspirin tablets. *Arch Intern Med* 1972;129:457.
59. Meade TW, Roderick PJ, Brennan PJ, et al. Extracranial bleeding and other symptoms due to low dose aspirin and low intensity oral anticoagulation. *Thromb Haemost* 1992;68:1–6.
60. Kyrle PA, Eichler HG, Jager U, et al. Inhibition of prostacyclin and thromboxane A_2 generation by low-dose aspirin at the site of plug formation in man in vivo. *Circulation* 1987;75:1025–1029.

61. Preston FE, Whipps S, Jackson CA, et al. Inhibition of prostacyclin and platelet thromboxane A$_2$ after low dose aspirin. *N Engl J Med* 1981;304:76–79.
62. Weksler BB, Tack-Goldman K, Subramanian VA, et al. Cumulative inhibitory effect of low-dose aspirin on vascular prostacyclin and platelet thromboxane production in patients with atherosclerosis. *Circulation* 1985;71:332–340.
63. Wood L. Aspirin and myocardial infarction. *Lancet* 1972;2:1021–1022.
64. Linos A, Worthington JW, O'Fallon W, et al. Effect of aspirin on prevention of coronary and cerebrovascular disease in patients with rheumatoid arthritis. A long-term follow-up study. *Mayo Clin Proc* 1978;53:581–586.
65. Clarke RJ, Mayo G, Price P, et al. Suppression of thromboxane A$_2$ but not systemic prostacyclin by controlled-release aspirin. *N Engl J Med* 1991; 325:1137–1141.
66. Buchanan MR, Brister SJ. Individual variation in the effects of ASA on platelet function: implications for the use of ASA clinically. *Can J Cardiol* 1995; 11:221–227.
67. Helgason CM, Bolin KM, Hoff JA, et al. Development of aspirin resistance in persons with previous ischemic stroke. *Stroke* 1994;25:2331–2336.
68. Reilly IAG, FitzGerald GA. Inhibition of thromboxane formation in vivo and ex vivo: implications for therapy with platelet inhibitory drugs. *Blood* 1987;69:180–186.
69. Buerke M, Pittroff W, Meyer J, et al. Aspirin therapy: optimized platelet inhibition with different loading and maintenance doses. *Am Heart J* 1995; 130:465–472.
70. Jimenez AH, Stubbs ME, Tofler GH, et al. Rapidity and duration of platelet suppression by enteric-coated aspirin in healthy young men. *Am J Cardiol* 1992;69:258–262.
71. Krumholz HM, Radford MJ, Ellerbeck EF, et al. Aspirin in the treatment of acute myocardial in elderly medicare beneficiaries. Patterns of use and outcomes. *Circulation* 1995;92:2841–2847.
72. Krumholz HM, Radford MJ, Ellerbeck EF, et al. Aspirin for secondary prevention after acute myocardial infarction in the elderly: prescribed use and outcomes. *Ann Intern Med* 1996;124:292–298.
73. Hennekens CH, Jonas MA, Buring JE. The benefits of aspirin in acute myocardial infarction: still a well kept secret in the US *Arch Intern Med* 1994;154:37–39.
74. Emmons PR, Harrison MJG, Honour AJ, et al. Effect of dipyridamole on human platelet behaviour. *Lancet* 1965;2:603–606.
75. FitzGerald GA. Dipyridamole. *N Engl J Med* 1987;316:1247–1257.
76. Hardisty RM, Powling MJ, Nokes TJC. The action of ticlopidine on human platelets: studies on aggregation, secretion, calcium mobilization and membrane glycoproteins. *Thromb Haemost* 1990;64:150.
77. Defreyn G, Bernat A, Delebasse D, et al. Pharmacology of ticlopidine: a review. *Semin Thromb Hemost* 1989;15:159.
78. Hass WK, Easton JD, Adams HP Jr, et al. A randomized trial comparing ticlopidine hydrochloride with aspirin for the prevention of stroke in high risk patients. *N Engl J Med* 1989;321:501–507.
79. Knudsen JB, Kjoller E, Skagen K, et al. The efect of ticlopidine on platelet functions in acute myocardial infarction. A double blind controlled trial. *Thromb Haemost* 1985;53:332–336.
80. Balsano F, Rizzon P, Violi F, et al. Antiplatelet treatment with ticlopidine in unstable angina. A controlled multicenter clinical trial. *Circulation* 1990; 82:17–26.
81. Sadowski Z, Luczak D, Dyduszynski A, et al. Comparison of ticlopidine and aspirin in unstable angina. Abstract. *Eur Heart J* 1995;16:259.

82. Janzon L, Bergqvist D, Boberg J, et al. Prevention of myocardial infarction and stroke in patients with intermittent claudication; Effects of ticlopidine. Results from STIMS, the Swedish Ticlopidine Multicentre Study. *J Intern Med* 1990;227:301–308.

83. Gent M, Blakely JA, Easton JD, et al. The Canadian American Ticlopidine Study (CATS) in thromboembolic stroke. *Lancet* 1989;1:1216–1220.

84. Colombo A, Hall P, Nakamura S, et al. Intracoronary stenting without anticoagulation accomplished with intravascular ultrasound guidance. *Circulation* 1995;91:1676–1688.

85. Schomig A, Neumann F, Kastrati A, et al. A randomized comparison of antiplatelet and anticoagulant therapy after placement of coronary-artery stents. *N Engl J Med* 1996;334:1084–1089.

86. Haynes RB, Sandler RS, Larson EB, et al. A critical appraisal of ticlopidine, a new antiplatelet agent. *Arch Intern Med* 1992;152:1149–1156.

87. Smythe HA, Orgryzlo MA, Murphy EA, et al. The effect of sulfinpyrazone (Anturane) on platelet economy and blood coagulation in man. *Can Med Assoc J* 1965;92:818.

88. Ali M, McDonald JWD. Effects of sulfinpyrazone on platelet prostoglandin synthesis and platelet release of serotonin. *J Lab Clin Med* 1977;89:868.

89. Anturane Reinfarction Italian Study. Sulphinpyrazone in post-myocardial infarction. *Lancet* 1982;1:237.

90. Anturane Reinfarction Trial Group. Sulfinpyrazone in the prevention of sudden death after myocardial infarction. *N Engl J Med* 1980;302:250.

91. Sills T, Heptinstall S. Effects of a thromboxane synthase inhibitor and a cAMP phosphodiesterase inhibitor, singly and in combination, on platelet behaviour. *Thromb Haemost* 1986;55:305–308.

92. Mayeux PR, Morton HE, Gillard J, et al. The affinities of prostaglandin H_2 and thromboxane A_2 for their receptors are similar in washed human platelets. *Biochem Biophys Res Commun* 1988;157:733–739.

93. Savage MP, Goldberg S, Bove AA, et al. Effect of thromboxane A_2 blockade on clinical outcome and restenosis after successful coronary angioplasty. Multi-Hospital Eastern Atlantic Restenosis Trial (M-HEART II). *Circulation* 1995;92:3194–3200.

94. Serruys PW, Rutsch W, Heyndrickx GR, et al. Prevention of restenosis after percutaneous transluminal coronary angioplasty with thromboxane A_2 receptor blockade: a randomized, double-blind placebo-controlled trial. *Circulation* 1991;84:1568–1580.

95. The RAPT Investigators. Randomized trial of ridogrel, a combined thromboxane A_2 synthase inhibitor and thromboxane A_2/prostaglandin endoperoxide receptor antagonist, versus aspirin as adjunct to thrombolysis in patients with acute myocardial infarction. The Ridogrel Versus Aspirin Patency Trial (RAPT). *Circulation* 1994;89:588–595.

96. Coller BS. Blockade of platelet GPIIb/IIIa receptors as an antithrombotic strategy. *Circulation* 1995;92:2373–2380.

97. Lefkovits J, Plow EF, Topol EJ. Platelet glycoprotein IIb/IIIa receptors in cardiovascular medicine. *N Engl J Med* 1995;332:1553–1559.

98. Lefkovits J, Topol EJ. The clinical role of platelet glycoprotein IIb/IIIa receptor inhibitors in ischemic heart disease. *Cleve Clin J Med* 1996;63:181–189.

99. The EPIC Investigators. Use of a monoclonal antibody directed against the glycoprotein IIb/IIIa receptor in high-risk coronary angioplasty. *N Engl J Med* 1994;330:956–961.

100. Topol EJ, Califf RM, Weisman HF, et al. Randomised trial of coronary intervention with antibody against platelet IIb/IIIa integrin for reduction of clinical restenosis: results at six months. *Lancet* 1994;343:881–886.

101. Neri Serneri GG, Rovelli F, Gensini GF, et al. Effectiveness of low-dose heparin in prevention of myocardial infarction. *Lancet* 1987;1:937–942.

102. Link KP. The discovery of dicumarol and its sequels. *Circulation* 1959;19:97.

103. Link KP, Overman RS, Sullivan WR, et al. Studies on the hemorrhagic sweet clover diesease. XI. Hypoprothrombinemia in the rat induced by salicylic acid. *J Biol Chem* 1943;147:463–474.

104. Fiore L, Deykin D. Anticoagulant therapy. In: Beutler E, Lichtman MA, Coller BS, et al, eds. *Williams Hematology.* New York, NY: McGraw-Hill; 1994: 1562–1584.

105. Meade TW, Wilkes HC, Stirling Y, et al. Randomized controlled trial of low dose warfarin in the primary prevention of ischemic heart disease in men at high risk: design and pilot study. *Eur Heart J* 1988;9:836–843.

106. Wright IS. Experiences with dicumarol [3,3'-methylene-bis-(4-hydroxycoumarin)] in the treatment of coronary thrombosis with myocardial infarction. *Am Heart J* 1946;32:20.

107. Nichol ES, Fassett DW. An attempt to forestall acute coronary thrombosis. Preliminary note on the continuous use of dicumarol. *South Med J* 1947;40:631–637.

108. Wright IS, Marple CD, Beck DF. Report of the committee for the evaluation of anticoagulants in the treatment of coronary thrombosis with myocardial infarction: (a progress report on the statistical analysis of the first 800 cases studied by this committee). *Am Heart J* 1948;36:801–815.

109. Gifford RH, Feinstein AR. A critique of methodology in studies of anticoagulant therapy for acute myocardial infarction. *N Engl J Med* 1969;280:351–357.

110. Working Party on Anticoagulant Therapy in Coronary Thrombosis. Assessment of short-term anticoagulant administration after cardiac infarction. *BMJ* 1969;1:335–342.

111. The Sixty Plus Reinfarction Study Group. A double-blind trial to assess long-term oral anticoagulant therapy in elderly patients after myocardial infarction. *Lancet* 1980;2:989–994.

112. Smith P, Arnesen H, Holme I. The effect of warfarin on mortality and reinfarction after myocardial infarction. *N Engl J Med* 1990;323:147–152.

113. Anticoagulants in the Secondary Prevention of Events in Coronary Thrombosis (ASPECT) Research Group. Effect of long-term oral anticoagulant treatment on mortality and cardiovascular morbidity after myocardial infarction. *Lancet* 1994;343:499–503.

114. Meijer A, Verheugt FWA, Werter CJPJ, et al. Aspirin versus coumadin in the prevention of reocclusion and recurrent ischemia after successful thrombolysis: a prospective placebo-controlled angiographic study. *Circulation* 1993;87:1524–1530.

115. EPSIM Research Group. A controlled comparison of aspirin and oral anticoagulants in prevention of death after myocardial infarction. *N Engl J Med* 1982;307:701–708.

116. Breddin K, Loew D, Lechner K, et al. Secondary prevention of myocardial infarction. A comparison of acetylsalicylic acid, placebo and phenprocoumon. *Haemostasis* 1980;9:325–344.

117. van der Meer FJM, Rosendaal FR, Vandenbroucke JP, et al. Bleeding complications in oral anticoagulant therapy: an analysis of risk factors. *Arch Intern Med* 1993;153:1557–1562.

118. Fihn SD, Callahan CM, Martin DC, et al. The risk for and severity of bleeding complications in elderly patients treated with warfarin. *Ann Intern Med* 1996;124:970–979.

119. Azar AJ, Cannegieter SC, Deckers JW, et al. Optimal intensity of oral anti-coagulant therapy after myocardial infarction. *J Am Coll Cardiol* 1996; 27:1349–1355.
120. Chesebro JH, Fuster V, McGoon DC, et al. Trial of combined warfarin and dipyridamole or aspirin therapy in prosthetic heart valve replacement: danger of aspirin compared with dipyridamole. *Am J Cardiol* 1983;51:1537–1541.
121. Cohen M, Adams PC, Parry G, et al. Combination antithrombotic therapy in unstable rest angina and non-Q-wave infarction in nonprior aspirin useers. Primary end points analysis from the ATACS trial. *Circulation* 1994;89:81–88.
122. Altman R, Rouvier J, Gurfinkel E. Oral anticoagulant treatment with and without aspirin. *Thromb Haemost* 1995;74:506–510.
123. Lipid Research Clinics Program. The Lipid Research Clinics Coronary Primary Prevention Trial results. I. Reduction in incidence of coronary heart disease. *JAMA* 1984;251:351–364.
124. Yusuf S, Lessem J, Jha P, et al. Primary and secondary prevention of myocardial infarction and strokes: an update of randomly allocated, controlled trials. *J Hypertens* 1993;11(suppl):61–73.
125. Rosenberg L, Kaufman DW, Helmrich SP, et al. The risk of myocardial infarction after quitting smoking in men under 55 years of age. *N Engl J Med* 1985;313:1511–1514.
126. Rosenberg L, Palmer JR, Shapiro S. Decline in the risk of myocardial infarction in women who stop smoking. *N Engl J Med* 1990;322:213–217.
127. Brown BG, Cukingnan RA, DeRouen T, et al. Improved graft patency in patients treated with platelet-inhibiting therapy after coronary bypass surgery. *Circulation* 1985;72:138–146.
128. Hess H, Mietaschk A, Deichsel G. Drug-induced inhibition of platelet function delays progression of peripheral occlusive arterial disease. A prospective double-blind arteriographically controlled trials. *Lancet* 1985;1:415–419.
129. Bousser MG, Eschwege E, Haguenau M, et al. "AICLA" controlled trial of aspirin and dipyridamole in the secondary prevention of athero-thrombotic cerebral ischemia. *Stroke* 1983;14:5–14.
130. The American-Canadian Co-Operative Study Group. Persantine aspirin trial in cerebral ischemia. II. Endpoint results. *Stroke* 1985;16:406–415.

Chapter 14

Organizational Design and Operations of a Preventive Cardiology Clinic

Dennis L. Sprecher, MD
JoAnne Micale Foody, MD
and Robert Hunter, MA

Introduction

Recent changes in the delivery of health care in the United States and new scientific evidence strongly supporting the role of preventive interventions in the maintenance of health focused much-needed attention and efforts on cardiovascular prevention programs. The field of cardiology is making a gradual transition from a technology driven, intervention-oriented perspective to a preventive perspective. As new evidence is becoming available that preventive measures affect a considerable decrease in the incidence of both primary and secondary cardiac events and mortality, there is widespread acknowledgment that health care providers must initiate preventive strategies in the management of their patients. Additionally, as physicians and health care providers are faced with an increasingly limited health care dollar, they must focus attention on strategies to reduce health care costs through the reduction of hospitalizations, procedures, and clinical events. There are new financial incentives and

From Robinson K, (ed): *Preventive Cardiology*. Armonk, NY: Futura Publishing Company, Inc. © 1998.

fiscal imperatives to keep people disease-free. These factors provide new motivation for an organization to implement preventive interventions that manage the patient with or without coronary heart disease (CHD) in a cost-effective manner.

In 1995, our organization began a preventive cardiology program, the goals of which are to provide a multidisciplinary approach to the management of risk factors in the patient with CHD. As envisioned, our program is interdepartmental, nurse and physician-assistant based, algorithm driven, cost centered, and outcome evaluated. In this chapter we will discuss the mission and strategy of our program as well as review the major studies and scientific evidence upon which our strategies are based. Recent developments in the delivery of health care had a dramatic effect on the conceptualization and implementation of this program. We will address these issues as well as programmatic issues in the actual implementation of the program. Finally, we will discuss potential future directions for the field of preventive cardiology and the possible impact of coordinated clinical programs such as our own.

Background

In the United States alone, CHD claims the lives of 500 000 men and women each year. The prevalence of CHD and congestive heart failure increased during the last decade. During the same time period, technical advances in the field of cardiology vastly improved. These technical advances, with improvements in care, came at a significant cost. Annual cardiovascular health care expenditures in the United States currently exceed $100 billion, largely resulting from hospitalizations and revascularization procedures.[1] Increasing costs in medical care led to cost shifting and a reevaluation of clinical outcomes, cost-effectiveness, and health care delivery systems. Highlighting this paradigm shift in health care delivery is the contrast between current health care dollars spent for cardiovascular intervention procedures and preventive or lifestyle interventions. For every dollar spent on cardiovascular disease (CVD) in this country, only 6 cents is spent on out-of-hospital medical therapy and on reinforcing healthy lifestyles.[1]

History

Preventive cardiology has only come into its own in the last several years in response to new evidence that medical interventions do in fact alter the course of CVD and new imperatives in health care resource allocation. The preventive cardiology field was fragmented. It was traditionally driven by cardiac rehabilitation and was exercise and diet based. Rehabilitation programs, specifically targeting those CHD patients following coronary artery bypass grafting (CABG), percutaneous transluminal coronary angioplasty (PTCA), or myocardial infarction (MI) were focused on exercise and only recently expanded to include diet, cholesterol reduction, and the management of obesity. Interventions were outlined by the American Association of Cardiovascular and Pulmonary Rehabilitation and the American College of Sports Medicine. These organization were traditionally separate from the American Heart Association (AHA) and American College of Cardiology (ACC). Lipids and lipoproteins were traditionally in the realm of internal medicine and endocrinology and to a lesser extent cardiology, whereas hypertension was traditionally the realm of nephrology and internal medicine, with again cardiology to a lesser extent. Thrombosis and extracoronary atherosclerotic processes were governed by vascular medicine. As mounting evidence suggests that cardiovascular illness is the result of multiple disease processes acting unfavorably on the process of atherosclerosis, cardiologists must become well versed in all aspects of this process. A collaborative effort to reduce cardiovascular risk would be more clinically and cost-effective.

Clinical Studies

Until recently, the literature did not support protecting patients through cholesterol reduction.[2] Early primary prevention trials tested the hypothesis that a decrease in total cholesterol leads to a decrease in cardiovascular events. Three early studies—the Oslo, the World Health Organization Primary Prevention Tria, and the Upjohn trial—all demonstrated a decrease in total cholesterol and a decrease in the CHD events (Figure 1).

In the early 1980s, two additional large-scale primary trials were conducted: the Lipid Research Clinics-Coronary Primary Prevention Trial (LRC-CPPT)[3] and the Helsinki Heart Study (HHS).[4] The LRC-CPPT was a randomized, double-blind placebo-controlled trial of diet plus cholestyramine versus diet and placebo. This landmark study conclusively showed that reducing cholesterol by diet and a pharmacological regimen reduced the risk of CHD in men with hypercholesterolemia. Specifically, a 10% to 15% reduction in serum cholesterol may result in a 20% to 30% reduction in risk for CHD. The HHS was a double-blind, placebo-controlled primary prevention trial than randomized men without CHD to receive either placebo or gemfibrozil. Overall, a 34% reduction in the incidence of CHD was observed. Importantly, the HHS identified a subgroup of patients with high risk for cardiac events. This group was characterized by a low-density lipoprotein cholesterol (LDL-C):high-density lipoprotein cholesterol (HDL-C) ratio >5 and triglyceride >200 mg/dL and experienced a 71% reduction in CHD event rate with treatment. These studies demonstrated significant reductions in lipids and an associated

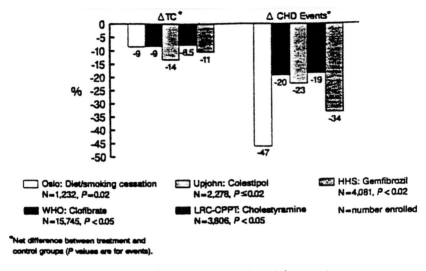

Figure 1. *Early primary prevention trials: overview.*

decrease in CHD events. They provide clear evidence of the clinical benefits associated with the primary prevention of CHD.

Over the last two decades, several large, randomized controlled trials assessed the effect of cholesterol reduction in the prevention of primary coronary events and in the prevention of subsequent CHD events among CHD patients. With the development of 3-hydroxy-3-methylglutaryl coenzyme A reductase inhibitors, greater LDL-C reductions were attainable than with other agents. Three large-scale trails were conducted to evaluate the effect of LDL-C lowering on clinical events. The West of Scotland Coronary Prevention Study (WOSCOPS)[5] was a primary prevention trial; both the Scandinavian Simvastatin Survival Study (4S)[6] and the the Cholesterol and Recurrent Events (CARE)[7] Study were secondary prevention trials. CARE was designed to examine the effects of LDL-C lowering in CHD patients with only minimal elevations in LDL-C. All three of these lipid-lowering trials achieved a significant reduction in clinical events. Between 24% and 42% in nonfatal and fatal CHD events were observed in patients being treated with statins (Figures 2, 3, and 4).

Early trials of lipid-lowering therapy demonstrated cardiovascular benefit but were not of sufficient power to show a reduction in total mortality. The 4S, a secondary prevention study, decisively resolved this issue. It showed a significant 30% reduction in total mortality and a 42% reduction in coronary mortality in 4444 CHD patients randomized to lipid-lowering therapy or placebo for an average of 5.4 years. Especially important was a 37% reduction in revascularization procedures and a 34%

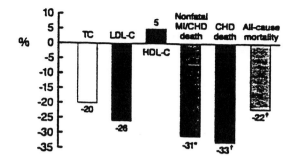

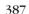

*P < 0.0005
†P < 0.05
‡P = 0.051

Figure 2. *WOSCOPS: effect of lipid lowering on coronary events in primary prevention trial in men.*

reduction in hospital days (Figure 5). Importantly, these improvements began early, only 1 to 2 years after the initiation of therapy.

Furthermore, a cost analysis of the 4S trial data was conducted to determine the economic impact of lipid-lowering therapy. Fewer hospitalization (1403 vs 1905) and shorter hospital stays occurred in those patients receiving simvastatin, resulting in a 34% decrease in hospital days ($P < 0.0001$). There was also a 32% reduction in hospitalization for acute CHD events. The reduction in hospitalization costs during the study would correspond to a reduction of $3872 per patient. When these savings are applied to the cost of simvastatin for the 5-year study period, the

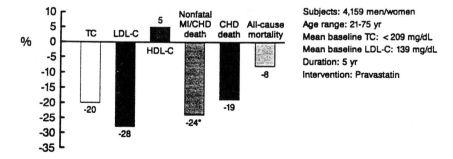

*P < 0.002

Figure 3. *Cholesterol and recurrent events: effect of lipid lowering on coronary events in secondary prevention trial in men and women.*

Reductions observed in:	%	P
Fatal CHD or nonfatal MI*	24	0.003
Confirmed nonfatal MI	23	0.02
MI, fatal and nonfatal	25	0.006
CABG	26	0.005
PTCA	23	0.01
Total CHD events	18	0.0001

Figure 4. *Cholesterol and recurrent events: event rates.*

effective cost was reduced to $0.28/day; it increases to $0.41/day over 5 years when the costs of routine lipid measurements are included (Figure 6). The significant findings from the 4S trial pointed to an impressive relation between clinical and economic considerations. In general it appears that reductions in LDL-C are positively associated with reductions in CHD events, hospitalization rates, and health care costs.[8]

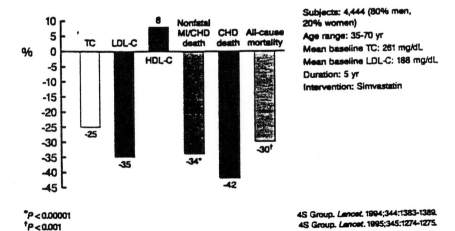

Figure 5. *4S: effect of low-density lipoprotein cholesterol lowering on coronary events in secondary prevention trial in men and women.*

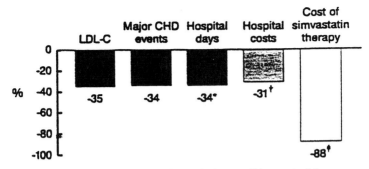

Figure 6. *4S: clinical and economic benefits of treatment over 5-year period.*

Recent advances in vascular biology and molecular biology suggested that medical interventions to arrest the atherosclerotic process must address not only obstruction but, perhaps more importantly, plaque stabilization. Interestingly, therapy that lowers cholesterol by 20% results in a significant decrease in cardiovascular event within 1–2 years. However, the angiographic change in stenoses associated with these impressive clinical event reductions is remarkably insignificant, on the order of 1% to 2% (eg, 0.2 mm).[9,10] Stabilization of high-risk plaques appears to account for the impressive reduction in cardiovascular events,[11,12] and aggressive modification of risk alters endothelial dysfunction, an early change in the course of atherosclerosis. Lowering LDL, estrogen replacement therapy, and smoking cessation all act to improve endothelial function. The major effects of lipid-lowering therapy appear related to stabilization of high-risk plaques and improvement in abnormal endothelial function.

There are other risk-reduction strategies with similar ability to improve the outlook for patients with CHD. Angiotensin-converting enzyme inhibitor therapy after MI in patients with symptomatic and asymptomatic left ventricular failure, β-blockers in the post-myocardial patient, aspirin therapy, and antihypertensive treatment all show reductions in mortality and morbidity in the CHD patient.

Unfortunately, most patients in the health care system do not receive comprehensive risk-reduction therapies. Despite all the research in vascular and molecular biology, the well-designed clinical trials showing a decrease in cardiovascular events, and the consensus panels and statements emphasizing the importance of preventive strategies, most patients do not receive the risk-reduction therapies proven to prolong life and reduce morbidity.

Risk Factor Management

The concept of risk as it applies to medicine is firmly entrenched in clinical medicine and public perception. Based upon data from numerous epidemiological studies and clinical trials, the 27th Bethesda Conference in 1996 summarized 21 risk factors of CVD. It is beyond the scope of this chapter to review the literature on risk factor for CVD. However, it is important for clinicians in the field of preventive cardiology to develop a framework from which to evaluate and apply new data on clinical interventions. We propose that the clinician be guided by three factors: the strength of the scientific data, the ability of the clinician or therapies to modify the risk factor, and finally the cost-effectiveness of intervention. To illustrate, we will review two specific modifiable risk factors and their cost-effectiveness.

Cholesterol Reduction

Both diet and drug therapy are successful in the reduction of LDL-C, and both result in reduction in cardiac events.[13] Diet was viewed as notoriously difficult to implement and monitor. Despite the challenges presented by diet modification, it appears that the overall reduction in cardiac events over the last 20 years was in large part the result of reductions in per capita fat intake (from ~40% of total calories to ~33% of daily calories). These reductions were brought about by continued campaigns waged by the health care establishment. The mean reduction of cholesterol achieved through diet by a patient after initial consultation with a physician is approximately 5%. Careful scrutiny of the data suggests that only a small percentage (<10% of the population) achieves >10% reduction in cholesterol. The vast majority realizes only 5% to 10% reductions in cholesterol, whereas another 10% realizes virtually no long-term improvement in cholesterol levels. This is the result of both genetic heterogeneity in the responsiveness of cholesterol to diet as well as large variations in compliance. New genetic testing [eg, apolipoprotein (apo) AIV and apo E isoforms][14] may aid in the identification of those best served by dietary instruction and modification. Data instruments to assess behavior and preferences may also be helpful in discerning which patients have the greatest chance of maintaining a diet lower in calories or overall fat content.[15]

Drug therapy was previously discussed, and all evidence suggests that reduction of LDL-C to the target levels recommended by the National Cholesterol Education Program Adult Treatment Panel (NCEP-ATP) is easily accomplished by the physician, resultsin a significant reduction in cardiac events, and is cost-effective.

Cigarette Smoking

The data concerning the deleterious effects of cigarette smoking are overwhelming. According to the Coronary Artery Surgery Study,[16] cigarette smokers with coronary artery disease (CAD) realized a 50% reduction in the risk for recurrent cardiac events with discontinuation of the habit. Today, about 25% of the adults in this country smoke cigarettes, whereas approximately 40% with CAD smoke cigarettes. Sixty percent of those subjects with CAD who smoke (24% of the total population of smokers) discontinue the habit after an MI with only a comment from their physician. Only another 10% to 15% terminate their habit with general cigarette cessation programs (4% to 6% of the total population).[17] Given these statistics and the low rate of success of smoking interventions in the general population, are these interventions an economically reasonable use of health care resources?

Two analyses addressed the cost-effectiveness of smoking interventions.[18,19] Cummings and colleagues[18] assessed the cost-effectiveness of counseling smokers to quit. Based on the assumption that counseling would increase the cessation rate by 2.7%, 10% of patients who quit would relapse and that counseling would cost $10 in physician time and $2 in printed materials, the cost-effectiveness ratio of physicians counseling was found to be $705–$988 per year of life saved for men and $1204–$2058 per year of life saved for women, depending upon the patient's age at intervention. The incremental cost of a $30 follow-up visit was $421–$5051 per year of life saved for men and $772–$9259 per year of life saved for women.

Oster and colleagues[19] analyzed the cost-effectiveness of nicotine gum as an adjunct to physician counseling against smoking. Their analysis calculated that the incremental cost of nicotine gum therapy per year of life saved was $4113–$6465 for men and $6880–$9473 for women, depending upon age at intervention. Despite the difficulties of implementation of a smoking cessation program and poor results in the general population, smoking remains a highly cost-effective medical intervention.

The question of which patients are most appropriate for medical intervention and which will have the largest benefit of therapy is in large part based on cost-effectiveness of the interventions. The decision tree for prevention will additionally be based upon the prevention program in place. Our approach is to consider all patients with CAD at particularly high risk and to enroll them in a program in which various other risk factors are identified and an overall risk is estimated.

The cost strategy, assuming a capitated environment, hinges on the estimated yearly rate of cardiac events (MI, CABG, PTCA, etc.) in the population treated. For a general population of males between ages 45 and 65, the general incidence of MI is 0.6% as identified by the Framingham Study. However, in the presence of CAD, this incidence rate increases tenfold to >6%. In an otherwise-healthy subject with four or more risk factors for CAD, the incidence of MI is approximately 4% per year. A simplistic approach to cost analysis would be to consider a continuum of risk in a patient population ranging from <1% to 6% per year for the development of cardiac events. The larger the burden of risk in a given population, the larger and more cost-effective would be a series of interventions.

Of particular note in the development of our prevention program is the value of a computer-based database used at various critical points in patient management, patient, nurse and physician feedback, and cost-effectiveness and outcomes analysis. The cost of a computer system and the development of a database to serve both clinical and research needs of the prevention program may make the cost of a program prohibitive; however, we should emphasize the value of a database as a mandatory part of the program. Only with a robust database can we adequately manage large volumes of patients in a cost-effective manner, provide valuable feedback to health care providers, and measure quality and outcomes of the program.

Cost-effectiveness analysis improves clinical practice and aids in the development of clinical guidelines and health policy on a larger level and in the development of individual prevention programs by providing information about the value of alternative health interventions in specific high-risk populations. It should not be considered the sole basis for resource allocation but serve as a guide.

Various forms of cues or reminders were used to identify patients in need of preventive services. We designed our clinical database to assist in issues of patient compliance as well as physician and nurse-follow-up. It was demonstrated that cholesterol values identified as abnormal by the laboratory computer were more likely to lead to follow-up treatment than those values not described as abnormal.[20] In general, cue and reminder systems appear to improve the implementation of preventive services by assisting both the nurse and physician in utilizing preventive strategies.[21-25]

More sophisticated computer-based clinical decision-making and clinical support systems had more equivocal results. Johnston et al[26] concluded that the success of a computer-based clinical support system was variable but did improve physician performance in four of six studies designed to enhance the quality of preventive care.

Our computer-monitoring systems provide data for individual and organizational feedback and reinforcement and improve the potential for

Table 1

Key Measures for Quality of Preventive Care

1. Smoking status should be documented in all patients with coronary heart disease (CHD), cerebrovascular disease (CVD), or peripheral vascular disease (PVD)
2. Organizations should have a smoking cessation program available for patients and their families
3. All eligible patients should have documentation of a physician offer of advice and self-help materials to stop smoking
4. All patients with CHD, CVD, or PVD should have a fasting lipoprotein profile documented within the first 3 months after onset of disease if the patient is deemed appropriate for pharmacologic intervention
5. All patients with CHD, CVD, or PVD should be offered nutritional evaluation and counseling at the time of diagnosis
6. All patients with CHD, CVD, or PVD who have an LDL-C level >130 mg/dL after nutritional therapy should be prescribed lipid-lowering medication if appropriate
7. All patients with CHD, CVD, or PVD should be assessed and provided with exercise counseling or prescription at the time of diagnosis if appropriate
8. Aspirin therapy should be offered to all eligible patients. If aspiration is not indicated, the contraindication should be documented in the medical record
9. All patients with CHD, CVD, or PVD should have two blood pressure (BP) measurements recorded at every visit
10. If an average of three BP measurements is ≥140 mm Hg *systolic* or 90 mm Hg *diastolic,* lifestyle and pharmacologic therapy treatment plans should be offered and documented at the time of diagnosis

success. Computerized records in a preventive setting facilitate quality assurance and management efforts to provide performance data and to reinforce organizational and provider behavior.

Quality-assurance programs are readily applicable to primary and secondary prevention programs, and the assessment of quality is more accurately performed with a database that monitors key measures of quality. As proposed by Pearson et al[27] in Task Force 8 of the Bethesda Conference, quality should be measured by ten key indicators (Table 1).

Program Concepts

We attempted to design a program based on sound clinical practice guided by current scientific evidence that reduces risk in a clinically as well as cost-effective manner. Our program design and its ongoing development are based upon nine key concepts (Table 2). These concepts were conceptualized based on available scientific data, effectiveness of interventions, and economic considerations.

Table 2
Key Concepts in the Design of a
Preventive Cardiology Clinic

Dedicated prevention unit
Multidisciplinary physician management
Physician-extender staffing
Risk factor modification
Algorithm-driven treatment
Behavior modification
Outcome-based analysis
Cost-effectiveness
Active research program

Dedicated Prevention Unit

The reason for referral to a dedicated preventive unit rather than having the primary local contact provide such services is severalfold. First, the prevention nursing staff can allocate the time necessary to treat behaviorally related factors. This relatively large time commitment redirected to the unit can free up the physician to spend more time with diagnostic issues. Second, the nurse practitioner can initially evaluate the patient, revisit as often as necessary, and use the phone to remind patients about compliance. Thus the prevention unit becomes focused on outcomes and can be more effective than typically observed in the more traditional setting. Furthermore, by cultivating a team under the direction of specialists with up-to-date expertise in the various risk factor areas, the clinic can promote and deliver cutting edge treatment.

The arguments against a dedicated unit includes the patient's perception of fragmented care and the inconvenience of a referral to a separate geographic area. This is time consuming and less appealing for the medical care consumer. If specialty diagnostics and treatment can be brought immediately into the primary physician's office, this may be a feasible and appropriate compromise where the needs of both the physician and the patient are advanced.

The challenge for the primary care physician is to provide preventive interventions to an appropriate subset of patients. Preventive cardiology is only one area of prevention. Continued scrutiny of the high cost of medical care has limited preventive measures to those identified as being at high risk. This was emphasized by the American College of Physicians, which suggests that cholesterol measurement and treatment be strictly reserved for those with current vascular disease or who are at very high risk for its development.[28]

For this and other reasons, our group decided to treat all CAD patients with one or more risk factors as well as those without CAD who have at least two or three risk factors or over 2% annual risk in a dedicated prevention unit. We propose that a specialized unit can provide these service very economically and should produce well above an average 20% risk reduction.

Multidisciplinary Physician Involvement

Patient care is provided by physicians. Members of the physician staff are assigned to a particular clinic.

Each physician is assigned two nurse practitioners or physician extenders. The current staff is composed of three cardiologists, one endocrinologist/diabetologist, one vascular medicine specialist, one hypertension/nephrologist, and a general internist. Physician staffing can be determined based on the particular population being treated as well as institutional resources.

In addition to patient care, the staff physicians are integrally involved in the management of the program. These generalists and specialists reached a consensus on the goals of the program, baseline algorithms, and identified data elements to be collected. Their backgrounds include extensive experience in clinical practice, teaching, and research. Physician diversity and broad experience of physician staff provide a strong base for program development.

Physician Extender-Based Staffing

Staffing of a prevention unit is similar to most general internal medicine or cardiology clinics. Patients are seen by both a nurse/physician extender as well as a physician. Current reimbursement guidelines do not allow for a solely nurse/physician-extender-based visit. Ultimately, we envision that an effective, clinically sound preventive program would principally utilize physician extenders as the main health care provider. A preventive clinic provides an ideal environment for physician extenders. Physician extenders were shown to be more consistent and more accurate in providing routine care. Physician extenders are less expensive than general internists. Given a limited budget for the performance of multiple tasks and interventions, costs savings achieved through the use of physician-extender staffing can be translated into additional interventions.

Risk Factor Modification

Controversy surrounds the effectiveness and value of reducing a single risk factor versus intervening on multiple risks. Meta-analyses of the treatment of hypertension indicate that a 17% reduction in CAD end points occurs when blood pressure (BP) is controlled in hypertensive subjects. The Framingham data showed greater benefits when older hypertensive patients (over age 50) were examined 10 years after prescribed treatment. The risk of death from CVD was 60% lower in treated versus nontreated subjects. However, it was suggested that the concomitant presence of hyperlipidemia[29,30] is perhaps central to the overall impact of hypertension. Once lipids are corrected, BP control may not be as critical in terms of incremental reduction in risk.

When programs focused efforts on multiple risk factor targets rather than a single predominant risk factor target, the benefit achieved only minimally exceeded those achieved through modification of a single risk factor. Combined programs targeting cigarettes, lipids, and exercise reveal no more than a 40% benefit.[10] Most participants indeed have only one risk factor, however, those with multiple risk factors do not appear to experience risk reduction beyond that of a single risk factor.

Given the large risk reduction achieved by cholesterol reduction, we chose to focus predominantly on cholesterol and use adjunctive therapies secondarily for the modification of other risk factors in our patients with CAD. This is not to say that other risk factors are less important in the assessment of risk, however, cholesterol reduction provides a medically feasible cost-effective intervention.

In addition to aggressive modification of lipids, the clinic focuses on a strategy to identify additional risk factors in the patient with CAD. A short summary of dietary goals as well as dietary information is provided to patients. Each patient compiles a food-frequency questionnaire in the interval between visits. The overall fat/saturated fat percentage of total daily calories is assessed at each visit through the completion and analysis of the Gladys Block questionnaire utilizing data provided by the patient.

Supervised nutritional counseling was documented to lower cholesterol levels by 5%. Dietary manipulation in conjunction with drug therapy produces a reduction in cholesterol beyond that of drugs alone.[31] We believe that efforts targeting dietary modification remain valuable.

Algorithm-Driven Treatment

CVD prevention in some respects is an ideal application for algorithm treatment plans. When treating CVD, prevention is complex and involves multiple body systems and diseases such as hypertension, diabetes, coronary artery, and both cerebrovascular as well as peripheral vascular disease. Baseline algorithms for the diagnosis and management of hypertension, hyperlipidemia, diabetes, and vascular disease were developed based on standard clinical practice guidelines provided by the NCEP, Fifth Joint National Committee on Detection, Evaluation, ACC, and AHA.

Defined pathways for elevated cholesterol and BP values[32] are available to permit algorithmic-driven, nurse-run programs.[33-36] Similar pathways for diabetes and postmenopausal hormone replacement therapy were developed. These algorithms add to the clinical efficiency of a preventive program.

Behavior Modification

Treatments that require chronic behavioral modifications are extremely difficult to maintain unless there is chronic behavioral intervention.[37] Questionnaires can be filled out on all major compliance items including medication use, diet, weight control, cigarette cessation, and exercise. Behaviorists and/or psychologists are useful adjuncts to the clinic operation. Counseling becomes a crucial intervention in a population at risk. The effectiveness of behavior modification is difficult to assess. Outcomes analysis will focus on quantitative markers for behavior modification initially and then move toward psychosocial profiles and health status scores ultimately. For example, cotinine is a marker for cigarette use,[38] and red blood cell membranes can be assessed for fatty acid composition.[39] Metabolic assessments can be made for exercise activity.[40]

Focus on Outcomes

The positive effects of cholesterol reduction were clearly established. However, the transferability of these results to a clinical setting remains a critical question. If third-party payers are going to reimburse organizations, if primary care physicians are going to refer patients, or if organizations are going to fund these programs in a capped environment, we must answer that question.

By collecting data on all patients who come through the program as well as monitoring their progress, an extensive database will be developed that leads to outcome measures and, as a consequence, refinement of the process. Whenever possible, the data are being collected using scientific methods and using quality-control and uniform data collection techniques. Parts of the program that do not have clear benefit will be discontinued. The program's algorithms will be validated or adjusted based upon actual patient data collected and analyzed in a real-life practice setting.

Cost-Effectiveness

It is essential that programs such as this operate in a cost-effective manner. The program can operate efficiently and at a low cost due to its reliance on computers for repetitive tasks, use of nurse practitioners, and careful view on outcomes to define those clinical measures and interventions that are most effective. Many of these components in an overall health care system overlap the traditional domains of primary care and specialty care. However, the narrow focus on issues that are treatable and relevant toward CVD make such a program valuable for both the generalist as well as the specialist. The cost-effective nature of this clinical approach, however, rests on the characteristics of the target population.

Active Research Program

Preventive cardiology is a dynamic field. As such, a prevention unit, in our estimation, must provide the framework and the ability to conduct significant clinical research in the area of clinical efficacy, health care outcomes, and management strategies. By designing a program that collects data on its population and compiles a robust clinical data set that is easily accessible to the clinician, clinical research can proceed in an efficient manner. The research component of a prevention clinic is likely to incur significant cost; however, these costs, at least initially, are necessary for self-assessment and ultimately for the advancement of the field of prevention.

Programmatic Issues

The programmatic issues can be broken down into five general areas: patient flow through the program, clinical database, resources required, patient recruitment, and financial considerations. This section will focus on the general rather than the specific and will serve to provide a framework on which to establish a program in preventive cardiology.

Patient Flow

Referral patterns at most institutions are similar for the cardiac patient. In general, patients are referred to a preventive cardiology unit from one of four general referral sources. First, patients can be referred from a partner within the organization from several different departments including internal medicine, endocrinology, cardiology, and hypertension and nephrology. Second, the patient can be referred after an acute episode or a recent cardiac procedure, ie, CABG, angioplasty, transplantation, or vascular surgery. The third source would be general internists or other physicians outside the institution. The fourth source of patients is through self-referral.

Our major source of referrals are in-house cardiologists who identified the patient as one who would benefit from risk-factor modification. Referring cardiologists determine the lipid profile, BP, cigarette use, postmenopausal estrogen use, and body mass index prior to referring the patient to the prevention program. Currently, a critical pathway for the management of lipids and modification of risk in cardiac patients does not exist, but it is envisioned that one will ultimately exist. In general, patients referred to the clinic have at least three risk factors: LDL >160 mg/dL, HDL <35 mg/dL, male age >45 years, female age >55 years, diabetes mellitus, BP > 140/90, and or cigarette use. The Framingham database[41] is useful in establishing a risk-stratification schema.

Prior to the patient's appointment, a letter describing the program and reviewing instructions for laboratory measurements is sent to all new patients. Relevant data-abstraction tools including an 11-page medical/family history questionnaire and a seven-page nutritional assessment form (Gladys Block) are included in the mailing.

At the initial visit, all forms are reviewed for completeness and data are scanned into the patient database. Patients then complete a nurse or physician-extender visit and a care plan based on data obtained from the patient-completed questionnaire, and the medical history and examination are presented to the staff physician. In general, these care plans are developed based on the application of the series of algorithms developed for clinic use. The algorithms have a series of different phenotypes (eg, increase LDL or increased BP) with specific treatment (both pharmacologic and otherwise), a series of goals (potentially targeted toward the initial visit and follow-up visit), and laboratory assays for day of visit and for follow-up visits.

The patient flow is similar for our follow-up visits: information on compliance with medication (ie, pills for each risk factor category missed per week), dietary and exercise compliance, and cigarette use and/or date of discontinuation. We use these follow-up visits to motivate and educate. A return visit date is decided and recorded on the data form.

Resource Requirements—Facilities, Space, and Personnel

Individual and group processing of patients should be feasible within the space of the clinic. In general, the following space requirements aid in the efficient flow of patients through the clinic.

1. A phlebotomy room (ie, approximately 36 m²). This should include a desktop centrifuge, phlebotomy chair, 4°C refrigerator, −20°C freezer, and general supplies including tubes and syringes for blood draw.
2. Reception desk supported with computer for appointment scheduling, laboratory retrieval, and database entry.
3. Two dietitians' conference rooms or offices for patient counseling.
4. Four clinical examination rooms.
5. One waiting room to accommodate 10–15 people.

Each examination room has an examination table, wall ophthalmoscope, BP monitor with three different-sized cuffs, and a laptop computer. Nurse practitioners perform an initial evaluation of the patients. The staff physician reviews the recommended treatment approach determined by the nurse practitioner.

This entire process on a new patient should not take more than 2 hours. For former patients it should take <45 minutes. Other valuable additions to the clinical operation include an electrocardiogram machine and office space for the physicians and nurse practitioners, X-ray viewing box, and medical record viewing area. The total space requirement for such a clinic is approximately 225 m². This allows for some storage and a filing area. The addition of exercise space for rehabilitation, educational areas, or other rooms dedicated to alternate critical pathways would invariably increase the space needs. Personnel needs include

One physician who will oversee the nurse practitioners

Two or three nurse practitioners or physician assistants

One data coordinator

Two dietitians

One phlebotomist

One receptionist/secretary/scheduler

Clinical/Research Database

The database is an integral part of the program. The organization's central appointment system populates the clinic database with patient demographics. A patient-specific questionnaire is created via the database and mailed to the patient. The night prior to the appointment, the computer generates a patient-specific data entry form. On the day of the visit findings from the visit are entered and a patient summary note is produced to assist the physician and nurse in treating the patient. In addition, a clinical note of the visit is generated for inclusion in the patient's chart. The visit results, dietary assessment, laboratory results, and medications are recorded in the same database. Finally, the computer system generates approximately 90% of a comprehensive letter to the referring physician, a patient letter, as well as a detailed monograph on the patient's cardiovascular risk factors.

Significantly, the database used by the program was designed by physicians, nurses, administrators, front desk personnel, biostatisticians, and support personnel. It was expressly designed to meet the research mission of the program as well as meet the clinic needs of the program. It provides a robust source of clinical information from which to monitor program success, aids in the identification of subsets patients at clinically significant increased risk, and finally provides a base from which to perform clinical research trials.

Patient Recruitment and Marketing

A successful recruitment and marketing strategy hinges on the ability to assess the community needs and to formulate a plan with specific objectives. In a tertiary-care facility such as ours, four sources of patients referred to the program were identified. Each major referral population requires a specific marketing strategy tailored to its specific needs and objectives. With the assistance of the organization's marketing department, a comprehensive marketing plan was developed and implemented.

Financial Considerations

There are two major financial aspects of the program, traditional budgeting and cost analysis. Budgeting for the program follows traditional budget practices and is the same method used by all programs at this institution. Revenues were estimated, based upon patient volume projections, personnel and other expenses were allocated, and a contribution margin was calculated. Figure 7 shows patient recruitment during the first 48 weeks of the program along with our initial volume goal.

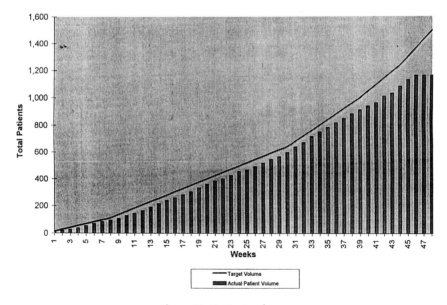

Figure 7. *Patient volume.*

We show volume to illustrate two points. Prevention programs at this time initially do not make a return on investment. Physician expenses are higher than general internal medicine clinics, and these programs require more ancillary support than specialty clinics (nurses, secretarial, data management, and supervisory support). The second financial aspect of the program concerns cost-effectiveness. Cost-effectiveness analysis is a widely used method of determining the value of a health intervention.[42] Using well-established methods, both screening and treatment programs can be evaluated in terms of the cost-effectiveness of the intervention.[7,27]

Definitive cost analyses in the field of preventive cardiology were done by Goldman et al.[42] Task Force 6 of the 27th Bethesda Conference, chaired by Goldman, discusses the fundamentals of cost-analysis as it applies to preventive cardiology. The Task Force concluded that screening programs for hypertension and treatment programs for smoking cessation, hypertension, aspirin, and cholesterol lowering were cost-effective. As was mentioned above, from a financial perspective, these programs are at best a break-even endeavor. For these programs to be effective, they must demonstrate they are cost-effective for the organization. Using the principals and methods of cost-effectiveness, program directors will be able to provide their organizations with a method of analyzing the program not from the microdepartmental or program level but from the macro- or overall organizational perspective. Using a hypothetical intervention costing $2000/year and producing a 50% reduction in the risk of MI, CABG, and other events in 10 000 patients over 5 years, their example calculated an approximate cost per year of life saved of $11 500. If instead the cost per year per patient were reduced to $600, the same method could show a cost savings of $500 per life saved.

Like many of the aspects of preventive cardiology, cost-effectiveness analysis has enormous possibilities for study and application. It is reasonable to conclude that cost-effectiveness is a legitimate method of definitively establishing the financial viability of preventive cardiology programs.

Conclusion

Recent changes in resource allocation and new evidence demonstrating the unequivocal efficacy of medical intervention in the prevention of cardiac events focused attention on the growing field of preventive cardiology. We provided a brief overview of the establishment, implementation, and programmatic issues that faced us as we developed preventive cardiology at the Cleveland Clinic Foundation.

References

1. American Heart Association. *Heart and Stroke Facts: 1994 Statistical Supplement.* Dallas, Tex: American Heart Association; 1994.

2. Oliver M. Doubts about preventing coronary heart disease. Multiple interventions in middle aged men may do more harm than good. *BMJ* 1992;304:393–394.
3. Lipid Research Clinics Program. The Lipid Research Clinics Coronary Primary Prevention Trial results. II. The relationship of reduction in incidence of coronary heart disease to cholesterol lowering. *JAMA* 1984;251:365–374.
4. Frick MH, Elo O, Haapa K, et al. Helsinki Heart Study. Primary-prevention trial with gemfibrozil in middle-age men with dyslipidemia. *N Engl J Med* 1987;317:1235–1245.
5. Shepherd J, Cobbe SM, Ford I, et al. Prevention of coronary heart disease with pravastatin in men with hypercholesterolemia. *N Engl J Med* 1995;333:1301–1307.
6. Scandinavian Simvastatin Survival Study Group. Randomised trial of cholesterol lowering in 4444 patients with coronary heart disease: the Scandinavian Simvastatin Survival Study (4S). *Lancet* 1994;344:1383–1389.
7. Pfeffer M, Sacks F, Lemuel A, et al. Cholesterol and recurrent events: a secondary prevention trial for normolipidemic patients. *Am J Cardiol* 1995;98C–106C.
8. Pederson T, Kjekshus J, Berg K, et al. Cholesterol lowering and the use of healthcare resources. Results of the Scandinavian Simvastatin Survival Study. *Circulation* 1996;93:1796–1802.
9. Watts G, Lewis B, Brunt J, et al. Effects on coronary artery disease of lipid-lowering diet, or diet plus cholestyramine, in the St. Thomas Atherosclerosis Regression Study (STARS). *Lancet* 1992;339:563–569.
10. Haskell W, Alderman E, Fair J, et al. Effects of intensive multiple risk factor reduction on coronary atherosclerosis and clinical cardiac events in men and women with coronary artery disease. The Stanford Coronary Risk Intervention Project (SCRIP). *Circulation* 1994;89:975–990.
11. Levine G, Keaney JJ, Vita J. Cholesterol reduction in cardiovascular disease: clinical benefits and possible mechanisms. *N Engl J Med* 1995;332:512–521.
12. Philbin E, Pearson T. How does lipid lowering therapy rapidly reduce ischemic events? *J Myocardial Ischemia* 1994;6:13–18.
13. Law M, Wald N. An ecological study of serum cholesterol and ischaemic heart disease between 1950 and 1990. *Eur J Clin Nutr* 1994;48:305–325.
14. McCombs R, Marcadis D, Ellis J, Weinberg R. Attenuated hypercholesterolemic response to a high-cholesterol diet in subjects heterozygous for the apolipoprotein A-IV$_2$ allele. *N Engl J Med* 1994;331:706–710.
15. Rosenthal SL, Knauer-Black S, Stahl MP, et al. The National Cholesterol Education Program pediatric guidelines: behavioral considerations. *J Dev Behav Pediatr* 1992;13:288–289.
16. Cavender J, Rogers W, Fisher L, et al. Effects of smoking on survival and morbidity in patients randomized to medical or surgical therapy in the Coronary Artery Surgery Study (CASS): 10-year follow-up. CASS Investigators. *J Am Coll Cardiol* 1992;20:287–294.
17. Stafford R, Becker C. Cigarette smoking and atherosclerosis. In: Fuster V, Ross R, Topol E, eds. *Atherosclerosis and Coronary Artery Disease.* Philadelphia, Pa: Lippincott-Raven; 1996:303–321.
18. Cummings S, Rubin S, Oster G. The cost-effectiveness of counseling smokers to quit. *JAMA* 1989;261:75–79.
19. Oster G, Huse D, Delea T, Colditz G. Cost-effectiveness of nicotine gum as an adjunct to physician's advice against cigarette smoking. *JAMA* 1986;256:1315–1318.

20. Reed R, Jenkins P, Ta P. Laboratory's manner of reporting serum cholesterol affects clinical care. *Clin Chem* 1994;40:847–848.
21. Davidson R, Fletcher S, Retchin S, Duh S. A nurse-initiated reminder system for the periodic health examination. Implementation and evaluation. *Arch Intern Med* 1984;144:2167–2170.
22. Cheney C, Ramsdell J. Effect of medical records' checklist on implementation of periodic health measures. *Am J Med* 1987;83:129–136.
23. Harris R, O'Malley M, Fletcher S, et al. Prompting physicians for preventive procedures: a five-year study of manual and computer reminders. *Am J Prev Med* 1990;6:145–152.
24. McDonald C. Protocol-based computer reminders, the quality of care and the non-perfectibility of man. *N Engl J Med* 1976;295:1351–1355.
25. Williams B. Efficacy of a checklist to promote preventive medicine approach. *J Tenn Med Assoc* 1981;74:489–491.
26. Johnston M, Langton K, Haynes R, et al. Effects of computer-based clinical decision support systems on clinician performance and patient outcome. A critical appraisal of research. *Ann Intern Med* 1994;120:135–142.
27. Pearson T, McBride P, Miller N, et al. Task Force 8. Organization of preventive cardiology services. *J Am Coll Cardiol* 1996;27:1039–1047.
28. Physicians ACo. Guidelines for using serum cholesterol, high density lipoprotein cholesterol, and triglyceride levels as screening tests for preventing coronary heart disease in adults. *Ann Intern Med* 1996;124:515–517.
29. Sytkowski P, D'Agostino R, Belanger A, et al. Secular trends in long-term sustained hypertension, long-term treatment, and cardiovascular mortality. The Framingham Heart Study 1950–1990. *Circulation* 1996;93:697–703.
30. Chobanian A. Adaptive and maladaptive responses of the arterial wall to hypertension: the 1989 Corcoran Lecture. *Hypertension* 1990;15:666–674.
31. Grundy S. Lipids, nutrition, and coronary heart disease. In: Fuster V, Ross R, Topol E, eds. *Atherosclerosis and Coronary Artery Disease.* Philadelphia, Pa: Lippincott-Raven; 1996:45–68.
32. National Cholesterol Education Program. *Report of the Expert Panel on Blood Cholesterol Levels in Children and Adolescents.* Bethesda, Md: US Dept of Health and Human Services; 1991.
33. Reichgott M, Pearson S, Hill M. The nurse practitioner's role in complex patient management: hypertension. *J Natl Med Assoc* 1983;75.
34. Blair T, Bryant F, Bocuzzi S. Treatment of hypercholesterolemia by a clinical nurse using a stepped-care protocol in a nonvolunteer population. *Arch Intern Med* 1988;148:1046–1048.
35. Weinberger M, Kirkman M, Samsa G, et al. A nurse-coordinated intervention for primary care patients with non-insulin-dependent diabetes mellitus: impact on glycemic control and health-related quality of life. *J Gen Intern Med* 1995;10:59–66.
36. Taylor C, Houston-Miller N, Killen J, et al. Smoking cessation after acute myocardial infarction: effects of a nurse-managed intervention. *Ann Intern Med* 1990;113:118–123.
37. van Elderen-van Kemenade T, Maes S, van den Broek Y. Effects of a health education programme with telephone follow-up during cardiac rehabilitation. *Br J Clin Psychol* 1994;33:367–378.
38. Pre J. Markers for smoking. *Pathol Biol* 1992;40:1015–1021.
39. Theret N, Bard J, Nuttens M, et al. The relationship between the phospholipid fatty acid composition of red blood cells, plasma lipids, and apolipoproteins. *Metabolism* 1993;42:562–568.

40. Young J. Exercise prescription for individuals with metabolic disorders. Practical considerations. *Sports Med* 1995;19:43–45.
41. Anderson K, Wilson P, Odell P, et al. An updated coronary risk profile: a statement for health professionals. *Circulation* 1991;83:356–362.
42. Goldman L, Weinstein M, Goldman P, et al. Cost-effectiveness of HMG-CoA reductase inhibition for primary and secondary prevention of coronary heart disease. *JAMA* 1991;265:1145–1151.

Index